KU-825-973

Gynaecological Cytology

E05439

Gynaecological Cytology

A Textbook and Atlas

Mathilde E Boon and
Mette Lise Tabbers-Boumeester

© Mathilde E. Boon and Mette Lise Tabbers-Boumeester 1980

All rights reserved. No part of this publication may be reproduced or transmitted, in any form or by any means, without permission

First published 1980 by
THE MACMILLAN PRESS LTD
London and Basingstoke
Associated companies in Delhi Dublin
Hong Kong Johannesburg Lagos Melbourne
New York Singapore and Tokyo

Typeset in 10/12pt Press Roman by
STYLESET LIMITED
Salisbury, Wilts
and Printed in Hong Kong

British Library Cataloguing in Publication Data

Boon, Mathilde E
   Gynaecological cytology.
   1. Generative organs, Female — Diseases — Diagnosis
   2. Diagnosis, Cytologic
   I. Title   II. Tabbers-Boumeester, Mette Lise
   618.1'07'582   RG107.5.C/

   ISBN 0–333–26117–8
   ISBN 0–333–26118–6 Pbk

EAST GLAMORGAN GENERAL HOSPITAL
CHURCH VILLAGE, near PONTYPRIDD

This book is sold subject to the standard conditions of
the Net Book Agreement

The paperback edition of this book is sold subject to the condition that
it shall not, by way of trade or otherwise, be lent, resold, hired out, or
otherwise circulated without the publisher's prior consent in any form of
binding or cover other than that in which it is published and without a similar
condition including this condition being imposed on the subsequent purchaser

Preface

The basis for this book was laid in 1969, when the first course in diagnostic cytology was given in Leiden. In subsequent years the lectures were under constant revision to incorporate the endless stream of questions, comments and criticism from trainee analysts and pathologists as well. To illustrate the modern concepts of cytopathology we included also examples of more advanced approaches such as transmission electron microscopy, scanning electron microscopy, DNA measurements, morphometry and immunopathology.

We believe that the time has come to publish these lectures and thus to offer our experiences in the field of education and our insights into diagnostic cytology to a wider public. The lectures are coordinated with the photographs in the Atlas section, in which a great variety of relevant examples of cytology, histology, colposcopy (Dr J. M. van Meir, Rotterdam), scanning electron microscopy (Dr C. A. Rubio, Stockholm) and transmission electron microscopy (Dr D. Ruiter, Leiden and Dr C. R. Laverty, Sydney) are presented. At the end of each chapter is a list of references which is based purely on the personal preferences of the authors.

Many have helped to complete the text of this book: H. Craane assisted in writing the chapter on cell biology; G. P. J. Beyer and Dr J. Wildschut provided the groundwork for the chapters 'The Development of the Female Genital Tract' and 'Sex Differentiation'; J. G. Moggré-Kastelein and Dr S. J. C. Dunlop cooperated on the section on microbiological flora in chapter 7; Dr C. Cornelisse contributed to chapter 9. Professor J. Janssens kindly assisted in writing the 'Clinical Aspects of Cervical Carcinoma'; P. W. Arentz assisted in the completion of the technical section. The morphometric measurements were performed by M. van der Voorn-den Hollander and the DNA measurements by H. R. de Koning. The drawings in this book were made by Dr M. E. Boon, H. Craane and E. Vysma. The graphs and charts were prepared by W. C. van Kleef and J. J. Magdelijns. The English text was prepared by Mrs C. F. Bieger-Smith. This book came into being through the combined efforts of all our associates in the Department of Cytopathology at Leiden University, the Leiden Cytological Laboratory and the S.S.D.Z. in Delft. Finally, the indefatigable optimism and energy of M. de Rooy, B. Flaton and Th. H. A. Witte ensured that the numerous new versions were re-typed quickly. Special thanks are due to Professor A. Schaberg, Dr B. N. Naylor and C. H. Fox for their support of our work and their constructive criticism.

We hope that this book will provide an insight into the problems of diagnosis in gynaecological cytology and will stimulate further activity in this field. We realise that the last word on diagnostic cytology has not yet been written, that is why we will be grateful to receive comments from our readers.

Leiden University, 1979

M. E. Boon
M. L. Tabbers-Boumeester

Foreword

More than half a century has passed since Papanicolaou presented his first paper on the cytological diagnosis of uterine cancer. Yet it was not until the 1940s that this preliminary work kindled the idea that the cytological approach to the diagnosis of uterine cancer might have an important practical application. Much has taken place since then to confirm this idea. The development and application of clinical cytology is now regarded as one of the most significant advances in the morphological diagnosis of cancer of this century. Not only does it enable us to diagnose symptomatic cancers of various organs quickly and efficiently, but it also makes it possible to diagnose uterine cervical cancer in its presymptomatic and curable stage.

This monograph is written for those who wish to continue this success story, that is, for those who wish to familiarise themselves with the principles and methods of cytological diagnosis as they are applied to the female genital tract. Drs Boon and Tabbers-Boumeester are widely experienced in the practical realities and demands of cytopathology. Not only are they capable diagnosticians but they are also experienced teachers who have imparted their knowledge and their skills to numerous cytotechnologists, pathology residents and pathologists in the Netherlands and elsewhere.

Their interest in clinical cytology of the female genital tract is expansive as evidenced by the scope of this monograph which includes discussion of the anatomy, physiology, pathology, epidemiology, and cyto-pathology of a variety of gynaecological diseases.

The authors have expressed themselves lucidly and their text is well supplied with excellent illustrations coupled with generous and appropriate references. For those who are about to embark on the demanding discipline of gynaecological cytopathology, this book will serve as a most useful guide and reference.

Bernard Naylor,
Professor of Pathology,
The University of Michigan,
Ann Arbor, Michigan, USA

Contents

Contents

Preface

Part One

Part One

1

Cell Biology

1.1 Introduction

1.1.1 The Discovery of the Cell

In the seventeenth century Robert Hooke reported to the Royal Society that a thin slice of cork consists of microscopically tiny 'rooms' which he called 'cellulae' (cellula – little cavity, tiny room). In the same century others carried out similar studies of plants and found that *living* cells are not hollow spaces but are filled with sap, called protoplasm. Otherwise there was little real progress in cellular morphology until the nineteenth century when Brown described a structure in the cell which today we know as the *nucleus*. Other structures were discovered in the cell, such as Golgi's reticular apparatus.

In 1861 Max Schultze defined a cell as a 'lump of protoplasm containing a nucleus'. At that time it was known that unicellular organisms also exist in addition to the plants and animals which are made up of aggregates of cells arranged according to certain laws. In an important publication in 1885, Virchow defended the theory of Schwann and Schleiden and proposed that 'every cell originates from another cell' ('omnis cellula e cellula'). In 1890 Waldeyer proved that the principle of most cell divisions is the formation of 'nuclear filaments' or *chromosomes*. Germ cells were discovered, as well as the principle of fertilisation in plants and animals. Ultimately this led to the theory that the nucleus of the cell is the carrier of the hereditary factors.

1.1.2 Light Microscopy

The growing awareness that organisms consist of cells was clearly related to the discovery and development of the microscope. In the seventeenth century van Leeuwenhoek worked with a simple microscope (magnifying glass), whereas today we use a compound microscope with two or more lenses. Before cells and tissues can be studied under the light microscope, various procedures are sometimes necessary, such as fixation and staining. Although these procedures bring about changes in the living material (artefacts), it is often possible to use the light microscope to gain insight into the structure of the original living tissue.

Fixation is necessary to preserve the tissue or the cells. The tissue is then dehydrated and embedded in paraffin or in plastics. Instruments, called microtomes, have been developed to cut thin slices of tissue (thin sections). Staining is usually used to see specific structures in the cell. With other types of microscopes it is possible to study *living cells*, for instance, cells in division or cells in motion.

1.1.3 Electron Microscope

As a result of the development of the electron microscope (1932–52) detailed knowledge of cellular morphology below the limits of resolution of the light microscope became available. With the light microscope it is only possible to discriminate between two particles if they are separated by at least 0.25 μm, whereas under the electron microscope particles that are separated by at least 3 Å (1Å = $10^{-4}\mu$m) can be resolved. This apparatus made it possible to see many new cell constituents. Together with developments in the field of biochemistry the electron microscope has contributed enormously to our knowledge of the mechanisms which play a role in the form and function of the cell.

The electron microscope uses beams of electrons, which are refracted by electromagnets comparable to the refraction of light beams by glass lenses. The introduction of the electron microscope led to new technical problems because the preparation of the tissue or the cells (see transmission electron micrographs) now had to satisfy new and stricter requirements. It became necessary to develop special fixatives, microtomes and staining methods. For fixation osmium tetroxide and glutaraldehyde are often used. A *true* dye is not applied. Instead, treatment with heavy metal compounds (such as lead citrate) produces certain constrasts which absorb electrons. For this reason one refers to 'electron-dense' structures.

The use of *transmission* electron microscopy has been supplemented by the use of *scanning* electron microscopy. With the transmission electron microscope one looks through a thin slice of cells or tissue whereas the scanning electron microscope is specifically designed to show surface detail. It gives a three-dimensional effect (see SEM micrographs in the atlas section). With transmission electron microscopy ultrastructural changes in the cell surfaces are evident only along the cell margins (see transmission electron micrographs in the Atlas section).

1.2 General Architecture of the Cell

1.2.1 Introduction

The definition of a cell as used here is 'the smallest unit of living material which can survive independently in favourable surroundings that contains enough genetic information for its reproduction'. This implies interactions with the environment around the cell. Many cells consist of a nucleus and cytoplasm. The cell is enclosed by a membrane. The *nucleus* is essential for the survival of the cell and for cell division; in the *cytoplasm* processes, such as the formation of cell constituents (for instance, tonofilaments in squamous cells, see section 2.3.1.3), the production of energy and the exchange of gases, take place. These processes involve *organelles*, which are organised cytoplasmic components such as mitochondria, endoplasmic reticulum, etc. The cytoplasm also contains inclusions such as reserve food and metabolic products (Bloom and Fawcett, 1975).

The nucleus and other organelles as well as the entire cell are enclosed in membranes which, when seen in the electron microscope, appear to be constructed according to the same principle, that of the so-called 'unit membrane'. These membranes react with osmium tetroxide (*osmiophilic*). Most of the membranes consist of three layers: two osmiophilic layers separated by a nonosmiophilic layer. Biochemically these three layers appear to correspond to two layers of regularly arranged fat molecules enclosed within two layers of protein (figure 1.1). The fat molecules have polar and nonpolar ends: the nonpolar (hydrophobic) ends are directed towards each other and the polar (hydrophilic) ends are directed towards the protein layers. The heavy metal compounds appear to be deposited on the outer layers in particular, so that the electron microscope reveals the characteristic pattern of the 'unit membrane': two black lines

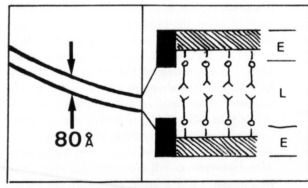

figure 1.1   Schematic representation of a unit membrane. Left, as seen with the electron microscope. Right, the biochemical structure. (E = protein layer; L = lipid component)

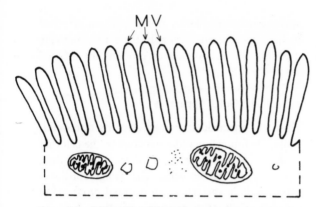

MV

figure 1.2   Microvilli (MV). Bulges in the cell membrane which serve to increase the surface. There are also several mitochondria

with the light microscope. What is observed with this microscope is a condensation of the cytoplasm along the cell membrane. For this reason it is better to refer to cell *margins* or *borders*. The true cell membrane can only be seen directly with the electron microscope; it is constructed like a standard type membrane. In some places on the surface we find thin finger-like *microvilli* (figure 1.2) which increase the surface of the cell. Several sorts of specific structures (desmosomes, close contacts, etc.) are seen under the electron microscope where the cells are attached to each other; for further details consult the textbooks listed in the references.

1.2.3 Cell Organelles

1.2.3.1 Mitochondria

Mitochondria supply much of the cell's energy. With the light microscope their structure can barely be observed (see LM figure 1.3). As seen with the electron microscope, mitochondria consist of a double membrane system of the standard type. They measure about 0.5–4 μm across. The inner membrane has many bulges or *cristae* (figure 1.3). The number of mitochondria as well as the number of cristae depends on the energy requirements of the cell and can therefore vary markedly from cell to cell (Novikoff and Holtzman, 1970).

enclosing a space of varying width. The composition of these membranes is not identical in every cell, which is why the term *'standard type'* membrane should be used instead of unit membrane. Imbedded in the lipid bilayer are many types of enzymes and other macromolecules so that many membranes are a 'mosaic' of molecular types.

1.2.2 Cell Membrane

The cell membrane separates the cell from its surroundings and plays a role in the release and absorption of various substances. The cell requires raw materials not only for self-maintenance but also for processing into secretory products. The absorption of these raw materials is partly passive (for example, by diffusion) and partly active, so that energy is required to take up or give off metabolites. In addition the absorption of solid particles (*phagocytosis*) or droplets (*pinocytosis*) also occurs. These processes are also called *endocytosis* while the term *exocytosis* is used for the opposite process, the release of particles or products by the cell. In phagocytosis the particle to be absorbed is surrounded by bulges in the membrane which then merge so that the particle becomes intracellular (see also under 'lysosomes', section 1.2.3.6).

The cell membrane is too thin (80 Å) to be seen

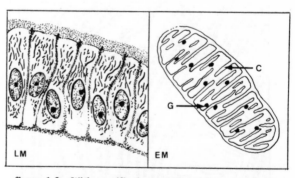

figure 1.3   With specific dyes mitchondria appear under the light microscope (LM) in the cytoplasm as tubes and rods. The electron microscope (EM) reveals cristae (C) and granules (G)

1.2.3.2 The Endoplasmic Reticulum

The endoplasmic reticulum is particularly prominent in cells which produce proteins, for instance, secretory cells. A distinction can be made between the *granular endoplasmic reticulum* (or *ergastoplasm* in early terms) and the *agranular or smooth endoplasmic reticulum.*

(1) *Granular endoplasmic reticulum.* The electron microscope reveals that the ergastoplasm consists of a compact system of flat parallel spaces (*cisternae*) enclosed by standard type membranes. Attached to the outer surface of these membranes are round bodies about 150 Å in diameter (figure 1.4). These are the *ribosomes.*

(2) *Agranular endoplasmic reticulum.* The agranular endoplasmic reticulum possibly functions as a channelling system regulating diffusion and transport within the cell.

1.2.3.3 Ribosomes

Ribosomes play a role in protein synthesis. It is here that protein is assembled from various amino-acids. From the nucleus the ribosomes receive information that orders the sequence of the amino acids in a protein. Ribosomes cannot be observed with the light microscope because they are only 150 Å across. However, it is possible to see where they are by making use of their chemical properties; they are made up of *ribonucleic acid* (RNA) on a protein core. Ribosomes

also occur independently in the cell, not attached to the ergastoplasm. Probably these ribosomes are used for the production of proteins for internal use in the cell.

1.2.3.4 The Golgi Apparatus

This cell organelle is named after its discoverer, Golgi. He found a net-like structure in the cell that could be seen by means of silver impregnation, especially in active cells. The Golgi apparatus plays a role in the release of material produced in the cell. Cells that produce secretions have an extensive Golgi apparatus when they are active. With the light microscope the Golgi apparatus is seen as an optically empty area, referred to as a *negative Golgi area.* A plasma cell, for example, often has a clearly visible negative Golgi area (figure 1.5).

The electron microscope reveals that the Golgi apparatus consists of a system of flat regular membranes (cisternae) which lie close together. At one or both ends the membranes dilate to form wide cavities. In some places these cavities seem to have become detached, forming sacs or bubbles (*vesicles*). Microvesicles are also seen (figure 1.6).

There is a functional relationship between the Golgi apparatus, the endoplasmic reticulum and ribosomes. The proteins which are formed on the ribosomes migrate via the cisternae of the endoplasmic reticulum to the Golgi apparatus. Here a change takes place, a 'concentration' occurs, and the protein is 'packed' in a detached membrane of

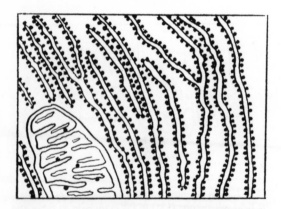

figure 1.4   The endoplasmic reticulum consists of a double membrane covered with granules (ribosomes)

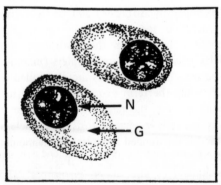

figure 1.5   Two plasma cells. The lighter area near the nucleus (N) is the site of the Golgi apparatus (G)

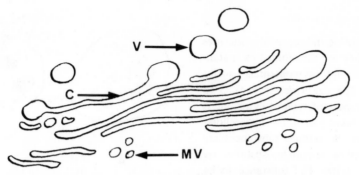

figure 1.6   Schematic representation of the Golgi apparatus as seen with an electron microscope. It consists of cisternae (C), large sacs or vesicles (V) and small vesicles (MV)

the Golgi apparatus (a *concentration vacuole*). By means of exocytosis this product can be delivered to the surrounding cellular environment (figure 1.7).

1.2.3.5 Centrosome

The centrosome can be seen under the light microscope under some circumstances as two tiny granules (*centrioles*). The centrosome lies fairly close to the nucleus (figure 1.8) and plays a part in cell division. Under the electron microscope the centrosome has a characteristic structure, consisting of two perpendicular cylinders, the centrioles, which are 1500 Å in diameter and on average 4000 Å long. The cylinders are closed at one end. Each centriole is in fact a group of conected tubes lying in a highly regular arrangement (figure 1.9).

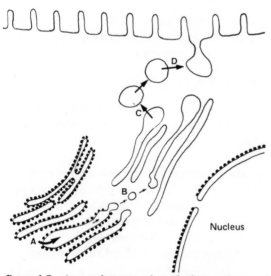

figure 1.7   A protein passes through the membrane of the endoplasmic reticulum (A) and migrates via the cisternae in the direction of the Golgi apparatus. A vesicle separates from the cisternae (B) and passes on to the Golgi apparatus. From the Golgi apparatus vesicles detach themselves (C) forming the so-called *concentration vacuoles*. By means of fusion with the cell membrane (D) the product can be released

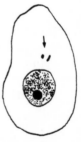

figure 1.8   The position of the centrosome (arrow)

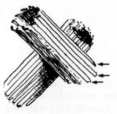

figure 1.9   The centrosome consists of two perpendicular cylinders (centrioles) each consisting of small tubes arranged in groups (arrows)

1.2.3.6 Lysosomes

In the cytoplasm are round or oval structures called *cytosomes*. They are surrounded by a standard type membrane and the content is usually highly osmiophilic. The size varies from 0.25 to 0.5 μm. The most important type of cytosome is the *lysosome* which takes part in the intracellular breakdown processes. Sometimes substances are digested which the cell membrane has absorbed via phagocytosis (figure 1.10). The substance to be absorbed is surrounded by the bulging cell membrane until it is intracellular; it is subsequently enclosed by a detached segment of cell membrane. Such a particle is called a *phagosome*.

Lysosomes attach themselves to a phagosome by a process in which the membranes of the phagosome and the lysosome merge together. Then, within the membrane of the lysosome, the breakdown process can begin. We can distinguish between *primary lysosomes*, in which a breakdown process has not yet occurred, and *secondary lysosomes*, after such a process has taken place (figure

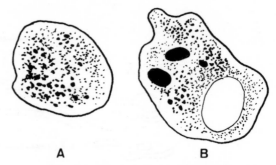

figure 1.11   A primary lysosome (A) and a secondary lysosome (B) with remnants of undigested material

1.11). Undigested remnants remain behind in the lysosome (*residual bodies*) while the materials useful to the cell are released into the cytoplasm. When the membranes of the lysosomes are damaged, the cytoplasm will be destroyed by the contents of the lysosome (*autolysis*).

1.2.4 Cell Inclusions

1.2.4.1 Pigments

Cells may contain many different kinds of coloured materials such as the pigment haemoglobin in red blood cells (*erythrocytes*).

1.2.4.2 Cell Products

Secretory cells are able to produce substances that leave the cell. These secretions might consist mainly of protein — ergastoplasm is then plentiful in the cell — or mainly of carbohydrates, as in mucus-producing cells. Such cells have an extensive Golgi apparatus. The secretory products can often be seen under the microscope, such as the immunoglobulins often found in plasma cells.

1.2.4.3 Substances Involved in Cell Metabolism

Glycogen and fats are examples of reserve food. They can be demonstrated with specific stains. Fat often appears in the cytoplasm as small droplets. When the droplets merge to form one large fat vacuole, the nucleus and the cytoplasm will be pushed aside forming a narrow rim around the fat globule.

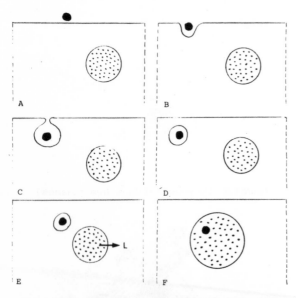

figure 1.10   Schematic representation of phagocytosis. The cell membrane surrounds the substance to be absorbed (B and C); subsequently the continuity of the cell membrane is restored (D). The phagosome (D and E) is surrounded by a detached part of the cell membrane. After fusion of the membranes of the phagosome and the lysosome (F) the breakdown process can begin

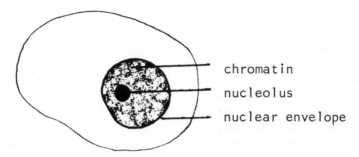

figure 1.12 Cell with nucleus as seen by light microscope

1.3 The Nucleus

The nucleus regulates cell division and the processes which take place in the cytoplasm. The nucleus is easily distinguished from the cytoplasm under the light microscope. Within the nuclear membrane there is a deeply staining granular mass, the *chromatin*, and in active cells the *nucleoli* can often be seen; in between is the *karyolymph* (figure 1.12). Multinucleate cells also occur (figure 1.13).

The architecture of a nucleus as described here refers to a *nondividing nucleus* or an *interphase nucleus*. When the nucleus divides, chromosomes form and an entirely different pattern is seen (see section 1.4.2) (Fawcett, 1966).

1.3.1 Architecture of the Nucleus

1.3.1.1 Nuclear Membrane

The outline of the nuclear membrane is much easier to see with the light microscope than is the cell membrane. However, what is seen is not the nuclear membrane itself but a condensation of the

chromatin along the membrane. In the light microscopical descriptions we will use the term 'nuclear membrane' (see also section 9.5.1.3). The electron microscope shows that the nuclear membrane or envelope consists of two membranes of the standard type. The space between them probably communicates with the cisternae of the endoplasmic reticulum (figure 1.14). In the nuclear membrane there are pores, whose structure is complicated; there seems to be a thin diaphragm which often closes off the pore. There is often a nucleolus near the pores.

1.3.1.2 Chromatin

The light microscope shows that the nucleus contains a fine granular mass, the chromatin, which in some places has condensed to form

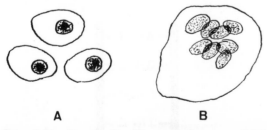

figure 1.13 Several cells with one nucleus per cell (A) and one cell with several nuclei (B)

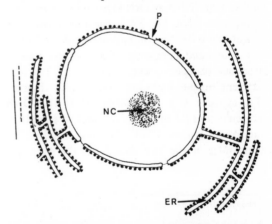

figure 1.14 Illustration of a nucleus with a nucleolus (NC) as seen with an electron microscope. It appears that there are pores (P) in the nuclear membrane and also that the nuclear membrane communicates with the endoplasmic reticulum (ER)

chromocentres (see also section 9.5.1.1). Chromatin consists of a chain of nucleic acids (DNA, the so-called *deoxyribonucleic acid*, which are bound to protein. Basic dyes stain chromatin intensely. With the electron microscope thread-shaped structures with local condensations are seen. The structure of chromatin at the molecular level is only now becoming clear and many interesting books and specialised reviews may be found on the subject.

1.3.1.3 Nucleolus

A nucleus may contain one or more nucleoli which appear under the light microscope as small, round, dense structures. The size of a nucleolus can vary markedly and depends on the degree of synthetic activity of the cell. The nucleolus can also be stained with basic dyes due to the presence of other nucleic acids (RNA, *ribonucleic acid*) bound to protein. Under the electron microscope the nucleolus appears as a skein-like structure – the *nucleolonema*. It consists mainly of grains which are ±150 Å across and closely resemble ribosomes.

1.3.2 Chemistry of the Nucleus

1.3.2.1 DNA

Chromatin and the nucleolus are made up of nucleic acids (DNA and RNA) bound to complexes of proteins. DNA, like RNA, has a high molecular weight and is built up of *nucleotides*. A nucleotide is a compound consisting of an organic base, a sugar and phosphoric acid (figure 1.15). The four different organic bases are adenine (A), thymine (T), cytosine (C) and guanine (G). The DNA molecule consists of a double spiral of strands of nucleotides (figure 1.16): the *double helix*. The nucleotides in the two strands of the spiral are

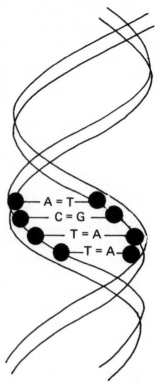

figure 1.16　The double helix

arranged in a specific sequence. The bases are always directed towards each other, whereby adenine always lies opposite thymine, guanine always lies opposite cytosine and the pairs are joined by hydrogen bonds (figure 1.17). Thus one strand is a reflection of the other and they are called *complementary strands*. In this manner DNA can store a wealth of information in code,

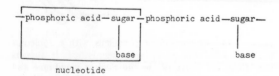

figure 1.15　Composition of nucleotides

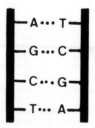

figure 1.17　Complementary strands

based on the sequence of the nucleotides. Since there are four different bases there are numerous possibilities.

The DNA contains all data required by the cell in order to continue to exist and to function. In the event of cell division, this information is transferred with the DNA. A beautiful and fascinating presentation of the entire function of the nucleus and its contents can be found in Watson (1975).

1.3.2.2 RNA

RNA is constructed in the same manner as DNA. In contrast to DNA, most RNA consists of a *single* strand of nucleotides. As far as the bases are concerned, uracil (U) is found instead of thymine which, like thymine, is located opposite adenine. The sugar, a deoxyribose (pentose) in DNA, is a ribose in RNA (figure 1.18). RNA is found both in the nucleus (mainly in the nucleolus) and in the cytoplasm (on the ribosomes).

1.3.2.3 Protein Synthesis

The architecture and function of a cell is determined by the nature of the proteins produced in the cytoplasm. This includes functional proteins (enzymes necessary for cell functioning) and specific secretory products. In protein synthesis the cell nucleus, the mitochondria and the ergastoplasm with its ribosomes work closely together. The mitochondria ensure the necessary energy. Protein synthesis consists of the combining of amino acids in a specific sequence.

The data present in the DNA molecule are transmitted to the RNA system by means of a copying system or a *transcription* involving enzymes. The sequence of the nucleotides in the RNA is determined by the sequence of the nucleotides in the DNA. The transcription occurs in the nucleus. The RNA transmits the code message, stored in the sequence of the nucleotides, to the cytoplasm; this RNA is called the messenger RNA (mRNA). All protein production based on this information occurs on the ribosomes. Some of the ribosomes consist of *ribosomal RNA (rRNA)*, which is also formed in the nucleus – probably in the nucleolus. In addition to rRNA there is also *transport RNA (tRNA)*. The tRNA transports the amino acids which must be incorporated in a protein. Each tRNA, molecule transports on amino acid. At the ribosome the amino acid is bound to the amino acid chain already present. Upon release from the tRNA, a protein has been formed. This process is shown schematically in figure 1.19. The complex story of protein synthesis has been interestingly described by Lehninger (1976).

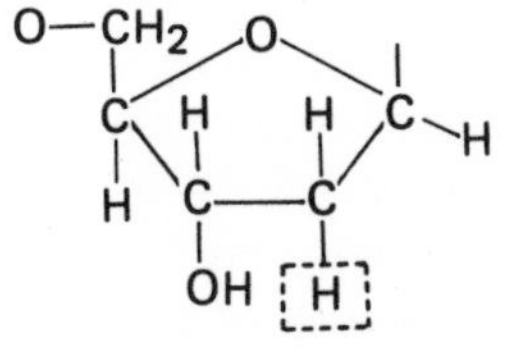

1.4 Cell Division

Cells are in general capable of increasing in number by means of division. One of the reasons why this is necessary is that cells are destined genetically to die after completing their biological function (differentiation). The lifetime of the different cells can vary from several days (epithelial cells in the intestine) to several months (cells from, for instance, the liver). There are also several types of cell which no longer divide, such as nerve cells, but most living creatures are rebuilt several times before they die.

deoxyribose

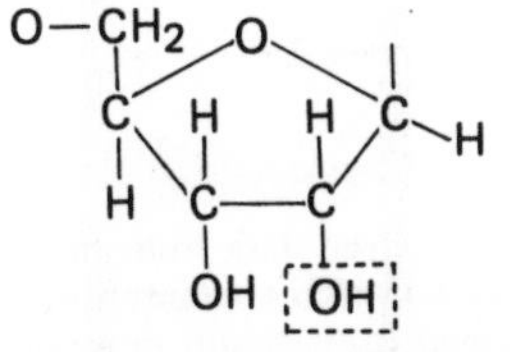

ribose

figure 1.18   Sugar in DNA and RNA

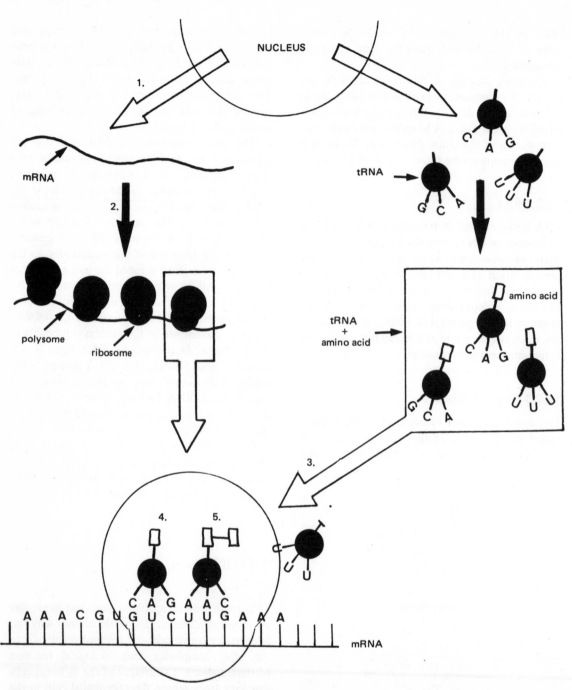

figure 1.19   Schematic representation of protein synthesis. 1. The mRNA has received data from that part of the DNA which is specific for a certain protein, and moves to the cytoplasm. 2. Ribosomes with rRNA (transcription probably in the nucleolus) attach themselves to the long-chain mRNA; thus polysomes are formed (usually not more than about 30 ribosomes). 3. Specific tRNA, which is bound to a specific amino acid, moves toward the mRNA. The tRNA contains a specific group of three nucleotides in sequence which is the code for the amino acid. 4. This group of three nucleotides seeks the complementary group on the mRNA. 5. The various amino acids, each still joined to a tRNA molecule, are released and bound together by means of enzymes so that a protein is formed

1.4.1 Cell Cycle

At any given time most cells are in *interphase*, which is the phase between two mitotic divisions. During this phase the cell may appear to be inactive morphologically, but preceding mitosis the nucleus must double its content of DNA and the events of this 'cell cycle' are divided into four different phases (figure 1.20).

(1) The *G1 phase* (G = gap). Most cells are usually in this phase since many of the cell populations do not reproduce actively.

(2) The *S phase* (S = synthesis). During this phase which lasts 6–9 hours, the DNA molecules duplicate. This is necessary in order to provide the daughter cells with enough nuclear material.

(3) The *G2 phase*. The cell prepares itself for division. In this period the cell has twice its normal amount of DNA (duration: 0.5–2 hours).

(4) *Mitosis*, whereby two cells originate from one cell, each having the same amount of DNA as the original cell. Mitosis lasts about 0.5–2 hours.

For the many variations of the cell cycle see Prescott (1976).

1.4.2 Mitosis

In the light microscope as mitosis begins the chromatin is seen to condense to form *chromo-* somes. These chromosomes divide during mitosis into two equal halves, the *chromatids*, which are drawn to the two poles of the cell. New nuclei develop around the chromatids so that ultimately two identical daughter cells are formed. During division a number of phases can be distinguished in stained or living cells (figure 1.21).

(1) *Prophase*. The granular chromatin yields thread-like structures, the chromosomes. The nuclear membrane disappears. Outside the nucleus, the centrioles have already duplicated and now move to opposite sides of the cell, where they become the anchoring points of a spindle.

(2) *Prometaphase*. From the disorganised skein easily recognised chromosomes finally emerge and subsequently migrate to the 'equatorial plate'. Between the centrioles a spindle configuration develops consisting of hollow fibres about 150 Å thick. In the prometaphase the nucleolus disappears.

(3) *Metaphase*. The chromosomes, now situated in the equatorial plate, lie in a radial pattern.

(4) *Anaphase*. The two halves of each chromosome (the chromatids) migrate away from each other to the two poles of the cell. The spindle disappears.

(5) *Telophase*. The cell becomes constricted in the equatorial plate. Two daughter cells are formed with chromosomal material. This material changes later into nuclei with recognisable nucleoli. The daughter cells are in interphase.

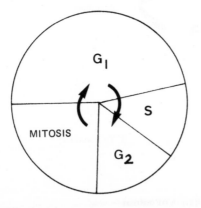

figure 1.20 **Schematic representation of the cell cycle. During the S phase DNA is duplicated**

1.4.3 Meiosis

The fusion of a spermatozoon and an ovum produces a cell with the normal number (46) of chromosomes (a *diploid* cell). To achieve this it is necessary that beforehand the number of chromosomes in the ova and spermatozoa is divided in two by means of a process called meiosis. It results in '*haploid*' cells that contain only half the usual diploid amount of genetic material. For the intricate details of meiosis and its many variants see De Robertis *et al.*, 1975.

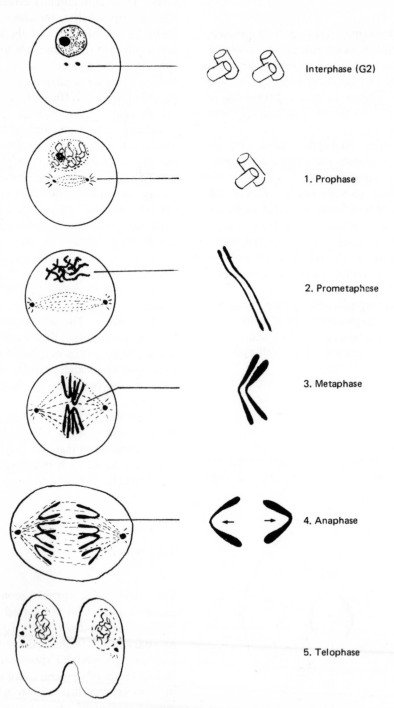

Interphase (G2)

1. Prophase

2. Prometaphase

3. Metaphase

4. Anaphase

5. Telophase

figure 1.21   Schematic representation of mitosis

References

Bloom, W. and Fawcett, D. W. (1975). *A textbook of Histology*, Saunders, Philadelphia and London

Fawcett, D. W. (1966). *The Cell*, Saunders, Philadelphia and London

Lehninger, W. (1976). *Biochemistry*, Worth Publishers, New York

Novikoff, A. B. and Holtzman, E. (1970). *Cells and Organelles*, Holt, Rinehart and Winston, New York

Prescott, D. (1976). *Reproduction of Eukaryotic Cells*, Academic Press, London

De Robertis, E. D. P., Nowinski, W. W. and Saez, F. A. (1975). *General Cytology*, Saunders, Philadelphia and London

Watson, J. D. (1975). *Molecular Biology*, Benjamin Inc., New York

2

Anatomy, Histology and Cytology of the Female Genital Tract

2.1 Introduction

In gynaecological cytodiagnosis cervical cellular samples are usually prepared by scraping the uterine cervix and smearing the cells thus obtained on to glass slides. With these smears it is possible to study the constitution of the cervical epithelium.

Because the superficial layers of the epithelium shed continuously, the smear will contain not only cells scraped off with the spatula but also cells that have been spontaneously *exfoliated* (literally 'the falling of leaves'). Many surface epithelia of women are influenced by the concentration of circulating hormones; consequently they undergo cyclic changes during a woman's menstrual years. Cytopathology demands a knowledge of the macroscopic and microscopic anatomy and the dynamics of the female genital tract.

2.2 Macroscopic and Microscopic Anatomy

The female genital tract consists of *external genitalia* and *internal genitalia*. The former are visible on external examination, whereas the latter cannot be seen this way. The external genitalia are also referred to as the *vulva*. The internal genitalia consist of the vagina, uterus, fallopian tubes and ovaries (figure 2.1).

2.2.1 Vulva

The vulva may be divided into the mons veneris, labia majora, labia minora, clitoris and vestibule (figure 2.2). The labia majora and labia minora are folds of skin covered with *keratinising squamous epithelium*. The inner sides of the labia minora are lined with *stratified squamous epithelium* without a stratum corneum. The vagina and the urethra open into the vestibule, and on either side of the vaginal orifice are Bartholin's glands embedded in the subdermal tissues.

2.2.2 Vagina

The vagina is a fibromuscular tube about 10 cm long which extends from the vestibule to the uterus. On the anterior and posterior sides of the uterus, the vagina terminates in the anterior fornix and the posterior fornix. Secretions and exfoliated cells will collect in the deep posterior fornix. On the anterior side, the vagina lies adjacent to the urinary bladder; on the posterior side it is next to the rectum (figure 2.1). The lymphatics of the lower third of the vagina drain into the inguinal lymph nodes; the lymphatics of the upper two-thirds, like those of the cervix, drain into the lymph nodes of the pelvis minor. The wall of the vagina consists of three layers: a layer of connective tissue, a muscular layer and a mucous membrane

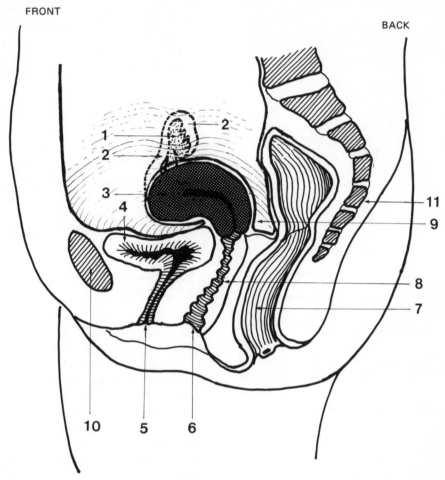

FRONT

BACK

figure 2.1 Diagram of the female genital tract; sagittal section. 1. Ovary; 2. fimbriae and fallopian tube; 3. uterus; 4. bladder; 5. urethral orifice; 6. vaginal orifice; 7. rectum; 8. vagina; 9. pouch of Douglas (Cul de sac); 10. pubic bone; 11. coccyx

of *stratified squamous epithelium* which lines the vagina.

The vagina normally contains no glands. The epithelium of the vagina is subject to cyclic changes under the influence of the sex hormones.

2.2.3 Uterus

The uterus (womb) is a pear-shaped hollow muscular organ about 8 cm long which is held in position in the pelvis minor by various ligaments consisting of bands of connective tissue. The folds of con-

nective tissue on each side of the uterus are called the *parametrium*. The uterus consists of the cervix and the corpus (body).

2.2.3.1 Cervix

The cervix opens into the vagina through the *external os* (figure 2.3). It can be divided into the *ectocervix* (portio), which is the part of the çervix that is continuous with the vagina, and the *endocervix*, which contains the *endocervical canal* with its mucus-producing glands or crypts. The endocervical canal is narrow, being only a few mm wide, and can be obstructed by a plug of mucus.

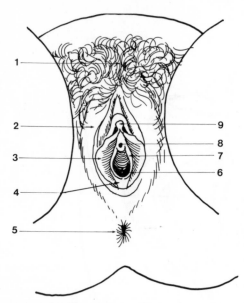

figure 2.2   Diagram of the vulva. 1. Mons veneris; 2. labia majora; 3. labia minora; 4. Bartholin's glands; 5. anus; 6. vestibule with the orifices of 7 and 8; 7. vaginal orifice; 8. urethral orifice; 9. clitoris

The endocervical canal extends upwards to the *uterine cavity*; the *internal os* marks the transition between the two (figure 2.3). The cervix lies in close anatomical relationship to the bladder and

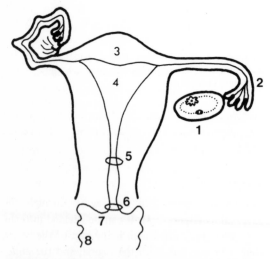

figure 2.3   Schematic diagram of the uterus and adnexa in coronal section. 1. Ovary; 2. fallopian tube; 3. uterine cavity; 4 fundus; 5. internal os of the endocervix; 6. external os of the endocervix: between 5 and 6 is the endocervical canal; 7. ectocervix; 8. vagina

the ureters. Lymphatic drainage from the cervix and uterine body is similar, that is via the pelvic lymphnodes.

Examination with a speculum (see section 15.3.1) allows the clinician to see the ectocervix with its external os and the entrance of the endocervical canal.

The ectocervix is covered mainly with stratified squamous epithelium, whereas the endocervix is lined with columnar epithelium which changes only slightly during the menstrual cycle. The junction of squamous epithelium and columnar epithelium takes place at the *squamocolumnar junction* (figure 2.4), which is also the boundary of the endocervical glands ('original' squamocolumnar junction).

2.2.3.2 Transformation Zone and Squamocolumnar Junction

The location of the squamocolumnar junction varies in different women. It can be situated within the endocervical canal, at the external os, or on one or both sides of the ectocervix (figure 2.5A and B), even extending on to the vaginal walls. In pregnancy, for example, the cervix increases its dimensions with subsequent eversion of the columnar epithelium (Coppleson *et al.*, 1976). In these women, therefore, part of the ectocervix will be covered with the much thinner *columnar epithelium* imparting eroded appearance (ectopy). The most distal part of the columnar epithelium may be replaced by squamous epithelium. This process of replacing another kind of epithelium by stratified squamous epithelium is extremely common and is called *squamous metaplasia* (see

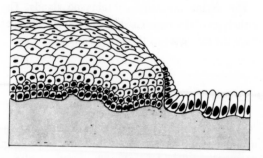

figure 2.4   Histological pattern of the squamocolumnar junction

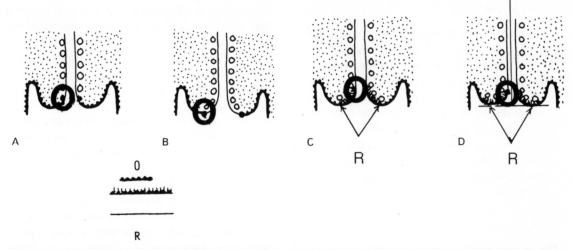

figure 2.5   The site of the squamocolumnar junction and the various 'points of reference'. The transition from squamous epithelium to endocervical columnar epithelium is indicated by a circle. A. Squamocolumnar junction within cervical canal. B. Squamocolumnar junction on the ectocervix. C. Reference point (arrows) used by Johnson *et al*. (1964) and Burghardt (1970), namely, the location of the last glandular duct. D. Point of reference (arrows) used by Reagan and Patten (1962). At C and D part of the columnar epithelium has been replaced by squamous metaplastic epithelium

section 7.4.2). Underneath this metaplastic epithelium the glandular ducts remain with their lining of columnar epithelium. The original squamocolumnar junction is situated at the position of the last glandular duct and can usually be identified with the colposcope (Coppleson *et al.*, 1976). The area of metaplastic epithelium, located proximal to the original squamocolumnar junction, is referred to as the *transformation zone*. This zone 'precisely defines the field of neoplastic potential' (Coppleson *et al.*, 1976).

In the literature the transition between the endocervix and the ectocervix is described in various ways. Burghardt (1970) and Johnson *et al.* (1964) used the location of the last endocervical glandular duct, that is, the original squamocolumnar junction (figure 2.5C). In some women (figure 2.5A, B) this point coincides with the transition from squamous to columnar epithelium. In others the original squamocolumnar junction has changed into a squamosquamous junction, separating native squamous epithelium from metaplastic epithelium (figure 2.5C). Assuming the endocervical canal is lying horizontally, Reagan and Patten (1962) used another reference point: the intersection of a horizontal line in the axis of the cervical canal and a perpendicular line that touches the lowest part of the ectocervix (figure 2.5D).

2.2.3.3 Corpus

The corpus (or body) consists of the fundus above and the uterine cavity. One fallopian tube opens into each side of the uterine cavity (see figure 2.3), which becomes continuous with the endocervical canal below. The wall of the corpus consists of three layers: a layer of connective tissue (the perimetrium), a muscular layer (the myometrium) and a mucosal layer (the endometrium) which lines the uterine cavity and is continuous with the endocervical mucous membrane. The upper part of the corpus is covered externally by the serosa, a layer of connective tissue containing the blood vessels and nerve supply to the uterus. This in turn is covered by the peritoneum, which becomes reflected posteriorly to form the *pouch of Douglas* (see figure 2.1). The endometrium is subject to cyclic changes. For lymphatic drainage see cervix.

2.2.4 Adnexa

The adnexa include the fallopian tubes and ovaries.

2.2.4.1 Fallopian Tubes

One fallopian tube is situated on each side of the fundus of the uterus. The proximal ends enter the uterine cavity and the distal ends consist of fimbriae which open directly into the abdominal cavity; thus there is a direct communication between the vagina and the abdominal cavity. The walls of the tubes consist of three layers: a mucosal lining, a muscular layer (the muscularis and the adventitia) and a serosal coat. The mucosal layer is composed of high columnar epithelium containing both ciliated and basal cells.

2.2.4.2 Ovaries

The ovaries are almond-shaped organs about 3 cm long, which lie in the vicinity of the fimbriae of the fallopian tubes. Like the tubes, the ovaries are held in place by folds of peritoneum. The lymphatics of the tubes and the ovaries drain into the lymph nodes in the pelvis minor and along the aorta. The ovaries consist of a cortex where the primitive ova are situated (oogonia) and the medulla. The medulla contains blood vessels and nerve fibres as well as follicles in various stages of maturity, the corpora lutea and the corpora albicantia.

The ovaries of sexually immature girls contain many thousands of primordial follicles consisting of an oocyte (egg cell) enclosed in a layer of flat follicle cells. During the period of sexual maturity a small number (400–500) of these primordial follicles can develop into mature follicles at intervals of about one month; the rest atrophy. After the menopause (see section 4.3.5) the ovaries are devoid of ova.

The ripening process of a primordial follicle, which is accompanied by a marked increase in size, is as follows.
(1) *Primary follicle.*   This is an oogonium which is surrounded by a single layer of cuboidal epithelium.
(2) *Secondary follicle.*   Between the ovum and the cuboidal epithelium is a thick transparent zone, the *zona pellucida*.
(3) *Tertiary follicle.*   The cuboidal epithelial cells (granulosa cells) produce a fluid which accumulates to one side in the follicle. The eccentric egg ends up in a 'mound' of granulosa cells (cumulus oophorus). The fluid-filled cavity is still lined with cuboidal epithelium. Around the follicle, the connective tissue forms a double layer, the *theca interna* and the *theca externa*.
(4) *Graafian follicle.*   The fluid-filled cavity distends, enlarging the follicle until it becomes a body about 5 mm across with an envelope of granulosa cells, the theca interna and the theca externa.
(5) *Ovulation.*   The graafian follicle ruptures; the egg, caught in a cloud of granulosa cells, is released and adheres to the fimbriae of the tubes. The remaining cells of the follicle form a gland with internal secretion, the *corpus luteum*. At the end of the cycle hormone secretion is discontinued in the corpus luteum which, via involution, then becomes the *corpus albicans*.

Under normal conditions only one egg cell is released during ovulation; the remaining follicles gradually degenerate.

2.3 Histology and Cytology of the Epithelia of the Female Genital Tract

As far as the uterus and the vagina are concerned, different epithelia can be distinguished: *stratified squamous epithelium* that covers part of the ectocervix, the vagina and the inner sides of the labia minor; *columnar epithelium* which lines the endocervix, the glandular ducts and eventually part of the portio; and finally the *endometrial epithelium* which lines the uterine cavity. These epithelia, especially the stratified squamous epithelium and the endometrial epithelium, are markedly influenced by hormones. Their histological and cytological patterns vary considerably during the different phases of life.

2.3.1 Stratified Squamous Epithelium

2.3.1.1 Histology

In a sexually mature female stratified squamous epithelium consists more or less of three layers:

the deepest layer from which regeneration of the epithelium takes place, a middle layer which determines the thickness of the epithelium and a superficial layer (figure 2.6). The stratified squamous epithelium provides a barrier against external injuries and stores nutrients (glycogen). Only under abnormal conditions will this epithelium produce a cornified layer. Squamous epithelium can mature in about 4 days under the influence of oestrogen.

The *germinal* (deepest) layer which adheres to the basement membrane is composed of a thin layer of small narrow cells which show signs of active growth: in the nuclei there are nucleoli and chromocentres, and mitotic figures may be seen. During maturation the amount of cytoplasm in proportion to the area of the nucleus increases. When the epithelium is mature, it is possible to distinguish a layer of *(para)basal cells* and a layer of *intermediate cells*. The cells in these layers are bound by intercellular bridges. The *superficial layer* consists of cells which do not mature any further. Intercellular bridges are not highly developed so that the cell bonds are weaker. The superficial cells are dead or dying and will exfoliate spontaneously. Interposed between the intermediate and the superficial cell layer a granular cell layer may be present (Patten, 1978). These cells may display dark blue granules in their cytoplasm (H and E stain).

Underneath the squamous epithelium is the *stroma*, which is separated from the epithelium by a *basement membrane*. The squamous epithelium may form an even epithelial layer on the basement membrane or may bulge into the stroma (Rubio *et al.*, 1976). The term 'rete pegs' is used to describe these sawtoothed irregularities.

The thickness of the epithelium depends on the hormonal status. In young girls and elderly women the epithelium is not usually stimulated and is only several cell layers thick (*atrophic epithelium*). During the sexually mature period, as a result of the hormone progesterone, the intermediate cell layer will increase markedly in thickness and may become rich in glycogen; the superficial layer will also develop under the influence of oestrogen. The *vulva* is covered by *keratinising stratified squamous epithelium* covered with a horny layer, the *stratum corneum*.

2.3.1.1.1 Keratinisation

Keratin and keratinisation are terms that may cause some confusion. Keratin is a chemical substance: a fibrous protein that occurs in epidermal tissues such as hair and nails. Keratin proteins were used by Corey and Pauling (1955) to establish the first three-dimensional model of a biochemical substance (it forms an alpha helix). Keratin in cells forms long bundles of fibres that are related in origin to keratohyaline bodies in the cytoplasm. Synthesis of keratin fibres probably begins when cells are still in the basal layers (Fitzpatrick *et al.*, 1971). As epithelial cells differentiate and proceed to migrate to the upper layers of an epithelial surface, increasing amounts of keratin may be synthesised. The amounts of keratin in a cell may be related to how rapidly the cell differentiates and the type of epithelium in which it occurs. Cells of mucous membranes such as in the mouth usually show little keratinisation whereas cells of intensely cornified epidermis may consist entirely of keratin fibres (Fawcett, 1966). There is recent evidence that most epithelial cells have some potential for synthesis of keratin or its precursors (Franke *et al.*, 1979; Osborn *et al.*, 1977) and that keratin is an important factor in the formation of the epithelial cytoskeletal fibres.

On the other hand, pathologists refer to keratin and keratinisation as a morphological process in which cells synthesise large amounts of cyto-

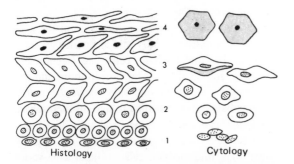

figure 2.6   Schematic drawing of nonkeratinising stratified squamous epithelium. 1. reserve cells; 2. parabasal cells; 3. intermediate cells; 4. superficial cells

plasmic keratin while the nucleus of the cell becomes pyknotic, dies, and disappears, leaving the anucleate husk of the cell behind (anucleate squames). We shall retain the pathological description of keratinisation, but with the understanding that the difference is probably quantitative and that many epithelial cells contain keratin in some form.

2.3.1.2 Cytology

The various types of cells corresponding to the various layers described above (figure 2.6) will now be discussed. For cytological examination, the Papanicolaou* stain is most often used, so the description of the various cell types given below is based on the use of this stain.

(1) *Primitive or reserve cells.*   We have chosen to use the term 'reserve cells' to indicate those cells in the epithelium that are analogous to stem cells in the haemopoetic system. They originate in the basal layers and are the parent cells of those cells that will subsequently be 'exported' to the surface, die and exfoliate. Contrary to the superficial cells, reserve cells might also be called 'primitive cells', 'keratinoblasts' or 'non differentiating prokeratinocytes'. The nuclear area varies from 25 to 55 μm^2; the ratio of nuclear to cytoplasmic area (N/C ratio) is high (figure 2.7 and 2.11). The cytoplasm is very sparse and ill-defined without visible signs of maturation (Langley and Crompton, 1973) or is altogether absent. The absence of cytoplasm is not due to a degenerative change but to mechanical damage of the fragile cytoplasm during smear preparation (see section 2.3.1.3). The nuclei are fairly narrow and oval usually, but sometimes they have a curved side and a straight side.

The chromatin pattern of the nuclei is fine; several chromocentres may be present. The pattern of exfoliation of these cells is highly characteristic: the nuclei often lie in rows or pairs so that nuclei partly overlap (like shingles). One nucleus may seem to be indented by other nuclei; the so-called *moulding effect*.

These cells are found in less than 0.5 per cent

* George N. Papanicolaou, 1883–1962, an American of Greek birth who was the father of cytopathology.

(see section 10.3.1, Table 10.3) of the smears from sexually mature females often at the time of ovulation. We use the term *immature cells* for cells with little cytoplasm with signs of squamoid differentiation (dense) often found in atrophic smears (see figure 2.7) and the term *reserve cells* for primitive cells with cytoplasm without signs of squamoid differentiation (hazy cytoplasm).

(2) *Basal and parabasal cells.*   These are round to oval cells. The nuclear area varies from 45 to 90 μm^2, the cell area from 105–1200 μm^2 (low N/C ratio) (figure 2.7 and 2.11). The nuclei occupy about one half of the cell (figure 2.11), which has a fine chromatin pattern. The staining reaction of the cytoplasm is usually blue and the cytoplasm is fairly dense (Graham, 1972).

If the cells are improperly prepared, for example, allowed to dry before fixation, the cytoplasm may stain pinkish red. The immature cells generally lie in sheets, while the more mature parabasal cells usually lie separately. Parabasal cells usually predominate in smears from older women; in young women they are seen only under abnormal conditions (for example, in inflammation or oestrogen dificiency) (Smolka and Soost, 1971).

(3) *Intermediate cells.*   Intermediate cells are larger than parabasal cells. The amount of cytoplasm with respect to the nucleus is increased (figure 2.11): the nuclear area is 25–75 μm^2 and the cellular area is 1200–3000 μm^2 (low N/C ratio) (figure 2.7). The nucleus is vesicular and has a fine chromatin pattern. The cell is polygonal. The staining reaction of the cytoplasm is blueish (cyanophilic intermediates) or pink (eosinophilic intermediates). The cells lie in tight groups or discretely in the smear, depending upon the hormonal stimulation. Under the influence of hormones, the intermediate cells can accumulate glycogen, so that the cells become bulbous and the nucleus is pushed to one side (*navicular cells*). Intermediate cells can also be folded on themselves.

(4) *Superficial cells.*   Superficial cells, like intermediate cells, are polygonal. They are slightly larger than intermediate cells: cellular area varies from 2500 to 4500 μm^2 (figure 2.7). Their nuclei are small (10–25 μm^2) and condensed (pyknotic); at a magnification of 400, no internal structure is

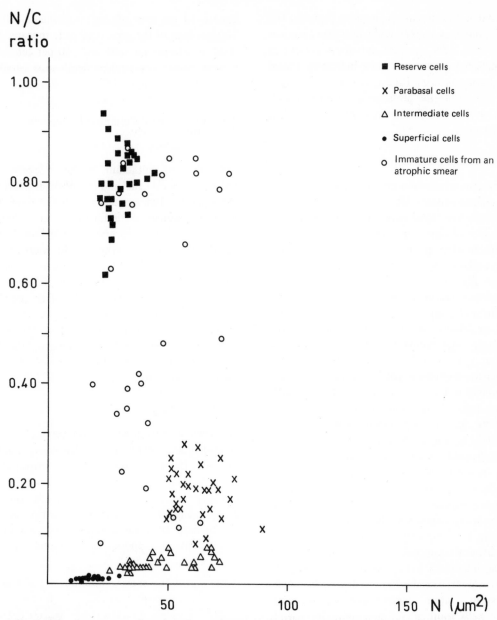

figure 2.7   Scattergram of nuclear size and nucleocytoplasmic ratio of the different cell types of stratified squamous epithelium. The nucleocytoplasmic ratio diminishes as the cell matures

visible. The staining reaction of the cytoplasm is either light blue (cyanophilic superficials) or pink (eosinophilic superficials). The superficial epithelial cells are almost always discrete and not in groups. They usually lie flat, in contrast to intermediate cells which may be folded on themselves. Cells

from the granular cell layer display small dark blue granules of various sizes in the cytoplasm. The granules, probably cytolysosomes (Gibb, 1969), are evenly distributed.

(5) *Anucleate squames.*   Anucleate squames are anuclear superficial squamous cells which are

polygonal and have pink to orange cytoplasm. The nuclear zone may appear as a lighter area ('nuclear ghost'). Anucleate squames are often present in combination with granular cells, indicating a final keratinisation process (Patten, 1978), for example, in the case of uterine prolapse (see section 7.4.4). Normally they are found only in a smear taken from the vulva.

2.3.1.3 Electron Microscopy

In transmission electron microscopy of Papanicolaou-stained smears (Ruiter *et al.*, 1979) the reserve cells with their bare nuclei look vital: the nucleus is blast-like with intact nuclear envelope, and mitochondria are present in the remnants of their cytoplasm. Because of its fragility the cytoplasm is often partly ripped away during smear preparation, resulting in bare nuclei.

In the cytoplasm of intermediate cells many loosely or densely packed tonofilaments are seen. Apart from some remnants of rough endoplasmic reticulum, cell organelles are almost absent and the nuclear envelope is partly lacking, both suggesting cellular death. Light microscopy, in which an intact and well-preserved nucleus is suggested, is misleading here. In most instances we are seeing dead nuclei in which the chromatin is condensed along a damaged nuclear membrane (see section 1.2.2). In superficial cells the cytoplasm contains many densely packed bundles of tonofilaments, providing cytoplasmic rigidity. There is no nuclear envelope or cell organelles. The nucleus is pyknotic. Thus, the fully matured squamous cell is like a dead leaf, well equipped to sustain mechanical and chemical influences from outside. The absence of intact plasmodia explains loose cellular attachment and easy exfoliation of superficial cells. In intermediate cells more intact plasmodia are found, resulting in exfoliation in clusters. The surfaces of both superficial and intermediate cells are covered with microridges (scanning electron microscope (SEM) photography). In intermediate cells these are less well-developed (Kjaergaard and Poulson, 1977). Nuclear degeneration is more pronounced in superficial cells than in intermediate cells. In a vitality test (tripane blue exclusion test) approxi-

mately 70 per cent of the intermediate cells and 100 per cent of the superficial cells appeared to be dead, in comparison with only 10 per cent of the reserve cells. Thus cellular death runs parallel to cytoplasmic maturation (Ruiter *et al.*, in the press).

2.3.2 Endocervical Columnar Epithelium

2.3.2.1 Histology

The columnar epithelium of the endocervix lines the endocervical canal and its glandular ducts from the squamocolumnar junction to the internal os, where it becomes continuous with the endometrial epithelium. The endocervical epithelium is made up of tall columnar epithelial cells, most of which are secretory and a few of which are ciliated (figure 2.8). One or more layers of reserve cells may also be found. The height of the epithelial cells depends upon the age of the subject and also varies to some extent with the phase of the menstrual cycle. The branching of the glandular ducts of the endocervix resembles a bunch of grapes (*racemose* pattern).

2.3.2.2 Cytology

(1) When seen from above, endocervical columnar epithelial cells have round nuclei; when seen from the side, the nuclei are oval or egg-shaped (figure 2.8). The nuclear area varies from $25-45 \ \mu m^2$, the cell area from $150-300 \ \mu m^2$. The nuclei usually lie eccentrically. The chromatin pattern is fine, and one or more small nucleoli sometimes are present. The cytoplasm of endocervical columnar epithelial

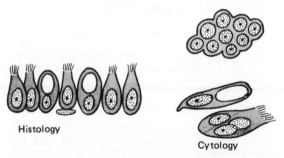

Histology

Cytology

figure 2.8   Schematic drawing of endocervical columnar epithelium

cells is usually pale blue. Occasionally cilia are visible, which may stain red. Ciliated columnar epithelial cells are more common in the post-menopausal smear (Reagan and Ng, 1973); the cell and nuclear size is usually smaller than in the reproductive period. The cytoplasm can be finely or coarsely vacuolated. Mucus from mucus-producing endocervical cells (goblet cells) stains blue. Depending upon the hormonal activity it will appear transparent and sparse of denser and striped. The endocervical columnar epithelial cells may be round and discrete when exfoliated spontaneously, but usually they form groups with the nuclei either in a honeycomb arrangement or in rows forming a palisade (figure 2.8), especially when abrasive sampling methods have been used (for example, Ayre spatula). Within a cell group variation in nuclear size (anisokaryosis) is possible. The endocervical cells which lie close to the internal os are of low columnar to cuboidal type and are difficult to distinguish morphologically from endometrial epithelial cells.

(2) The subcolumnar *reserve cells* show the same morphological pattern of exfoliation as described under squamous epithelium. The nuclei of the subcolumnar reserve cells are somewhat rounder. These cells can be seen in smears from sexually mature females, often, for example, after mechanical injury or in reserve cell hyperplasia (see section 7.4.1), or occasionally at the time of ovulation. In the event of inflammation or injury, multinucleate endocervical cells may also be present (see section 7.2.2.2). Moreover these cells may originate from the lining of a Nabothian cyst (see section 7.6.4).

Whether columnar endocervical cells will be encountered in the smear depends on

(1) the spatula (with or without an elongated tip which can reach the inner side of the endocervical canal).

(2) the position of the squamocolumnar junction and the area of metaplasia.

(3) hormonal contraceptives. Endocervical cells are less frequently found in smears of women using oral contraceptives (see section 14.2.1.2).

(4) pregnancy. In smears of pregnant women few columnar endocervical cells are found (see section 14.2.1.3).

2.3.2.3 Electron microscopy

The endocervical columnar cells in smear preparations may show various organelles: dilated rough

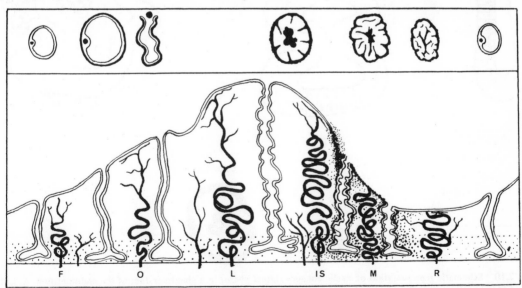

figure 2.9   Schematic representation of the cyclic changes in the ovary (above) and in the endometrium (below) (Bartelmez and Baltimore, 1957) F, follicular phase; O, ovulation; L, luteal phase; IS, premenstrual ischaemic phase; M, menstrual phase; R, regeneration

endoplasmic reticulum Golgi apparatus, mitochondriae, ribosomes. Many rounded vacuoles filled with a finely granular substance can be found, predominantly in the apical part of the cell. Occasionally a crystalline substance can be discerned. The apical side of the cells may display fine microvilli, as seen in the SEM photographs. The nucleus shows several indentations and an intact nuclear envelope (Ruiter *et al.*, 1979). In contrast to squamous epithelium, here cell maturation does not mean cellular death: the nuclear envelope and the mitochondria are intact.

2.3.3 Endometrium

2.3.3.1 Histology

The endometrium is a mucous membrane composed of stroma which is penetrated by glandular ducts. The surfaces of the epithelium and of the glandular ducts are covered with endometrial epithelial cells. The histological picture of the endometrium depends upon the hormonal stimulation and so varies at different periods of the menstrual cycle (figure 2.9). The first day of menstruation is considered as the first day of the cycle.

Day 5–14: *proliferative* phase or *follicular* phase. The endometrium is thin; the stroma is compact; the glands are sparse; the small lumens are lined with cuboidal epithelium. In the second half of this phase the glands are numerous, closely packed, and tortuous; the dilated lumens are lined with tall columnar epithelium. Mitoses are common.

Day 14–28: *Secretory* or *luteal* phase. After ovulation secretion is evident. Vacuoles are at first visible under the nuclei of the epithelial cells; but in the latter half of the secretory phase the vacuoles

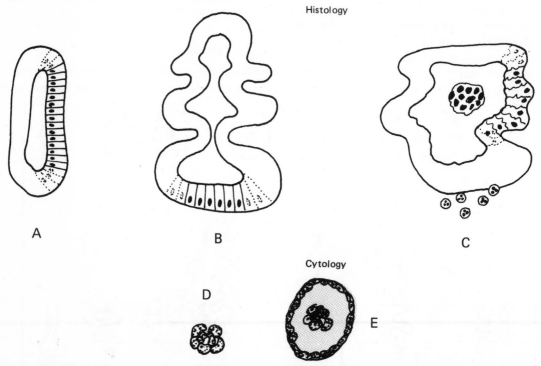

figure 2.10   Schematic representation of cyclic changes (luteal phase) in a glandular duct of the endometrium. A. Luteal phase. Central nucleus, vacuole underneath; B. luteal phase (late). Basally located nuclei, large vacuoles; C. menstrual phase. Schematic drawing of endometrial cells. Disorderly arrangement of endometrial nuclei (D); and a characteristic group of endometrial cells (E) in the early menstrual phase: packed nuclei in the centre surrounded by a lighter zone with relatively few nuclei.

are found above the nuclei (figure 2.10). The secretory products are discharged into the lumen. From day 21 onwards active secretion is less prominent. Involution of the epithelium begins, with shrinking of the nuclei. The stroma is oedematous. A reduction of the thickness of the endometrium follows prior to menstruation (premenstrual ischaemic phase).

Day 28–5: Menstrual phase. First necrosis and then haemorrhage takes place. Regeneration starts from the residual glands and stroma.

2.3.3.2 Cytology

Between the first and, at the latest, the fifteenth day of the menstrual cycle and just before the cycle restarts, endometrial cells can be found in the smear. These spontaneously exfoliated cells must travel a long distance through the endocervical canal so that the most vulnerable constituent, the cytoplasm, is often missing. The nuclei of exfoliated endometrial cells are kidney-shaped or round to oval; they are somewhat smaller than the nuclei

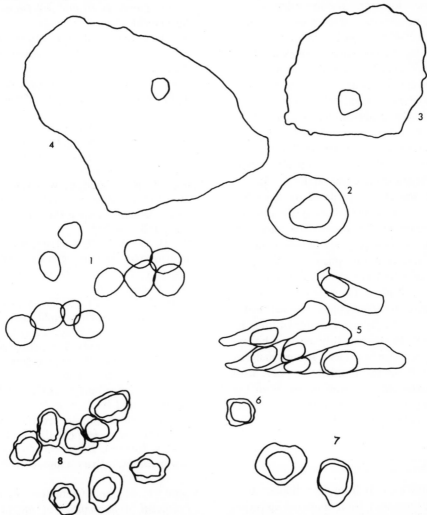

figure 2.11 Camera lucida drawings of various benign cell types. 1. Bare reserve cells; 2. parabasal cell; 3. intermediate cell; 4. superficial cell; 5. columnar endocervical cells in palissade arrangement; 6. endocervical cell (from honeycomb formation); 7. secretory endocervical cells (from honeycomb formation); 8. endometrial cells

of the endocervical columnar epithelial cells. The nuclear area varies from 20–40 μm^2 (see figure 2.7). Their chromatin pattern is granular and more coarse than that of endocervical columnar cells. Often one or two small chromocentres are seen. During menstruation endometrial cells are present in large irregularly shaped groups in which the nuclei lie close together and vary little in size (see figure 2.11). It is usually difficult, if not impossible, to discriminate epithelial cells from stromal cells. Both types are markedly influenced by hormones. Moreover, discriminating stroma cells from histiocytes may also cause a problem. At the end of menstruation the endometrial cells are accompanied by numerous histiocytes which lie in rows (the so-called 'exodus pattern'). Some of these histiocytes probably originate from the endometrium (Papanicolaou, 1953).

In menopausal and pregnant females, exfoliation of endometrial cells is abnormal. When an intra-uterine contraceptive device (IUD) has been inserted, endometrial cells can be found in the smear throughout the entire cycle (see section 14.3).

When the smears are prepared by *aspirating* material from the endometrial cavity the cells are arranged in strips or flat sheets. The nuclei are slightly larger because they are harvested in the proliferative and secretory phase of the cycle. The stromal cells have elongated nuclei and a tag of ill-defined cytoplasm (deep stromal cells) or resemble histiocytes (superficial stromal cells). Stromal cells also display size variations during the menstrual cycle; in the secretory phase a honeycomb arrangement can be evident. In such material endometrial cells in the proliferative phase with their dark nuclei can be distinguished from the larger cells in the secretory phase with their vacuolated cytoplasm (Koss, 1968).

2.3.4 Adnexa

Columnar epithelial cells from the fallopian tubes cannot be distinguished from columnar epithelial cells from the endocervix. Under normal conditions, no cells from the ovaries are seen in cervicovaginal smears.

References

Bartelmez, G. W. and Baltimore, P.D. (1957). The phases of the menstrual cycle and their interpretation in terms of the pregnancy cycle. *Am. J. Obst. Gynec.*, **74**, 931–55

Burghardt, E., (1970). Latest aspects of precancerous lesions in squamous and columnar epithelium of the cervix. *Int. J. Gyn. Obst.*, **8**, 573–80

Coppleson, M., Pixley, E and Reid, B. (1976). *Colposcopy. A Scientific and Practical Approach to the Cervix in Health and Disease*, Thomas, Springfield

Corey, R. B. and Pauling, L. (1955). *Proceedings of the Wool Textile Research Conference*, Australia, p. 249

Fawcett, D. W. (1966). *The Cell. Its Organelles and Inclusions*, Saunders, Philadelphia and London

Fitzpatrick, T. B., Arndt, K. A., Clark, W. H., Eisen, A. Z., Van Scott, E. J. and Vaughn, J. H. (1971). *Dermatology in General Medicine.* McGraw-Hill, New York

Franke, W. W., Schmid, E., Weber, K. and Osborn, M. (1979). HeLa cells contain intermediate-sized filaments of the prekeratin type. *Expl Cell Res.*, **118**, 95–109

Gibb, D. G. A. (1969). The histochemistry of hematoxylin staining granules (HSG) in the vaginal epithelium of the Proestrus Guinea Pig. *Acta Cytol.*, **13**, 89–93

Graham, R. M. (1972). *The Cytologic Diagnosis of Cancer*, Saunders, Philadelphia and London

Johnson, L. D., Easterday, C.L., Gore, H. and Hertig, A. T. (1964). The histogenesis of carcinoma in situ of the uterine cervix; a preliminary report of the origin of carcinoma in situ in subcylindrical cell anaplasia. *Cancer*, **17**, 213–29

Kjaegaard, J. and Poulson, E. F. (1977). Scanning electron microscopy of cotton swab smears from ectocervix. *Acta Cytol.*, **21**, 68–71

Koss, L.G. (1968). *Diagnostic Cytology and its Histopathologic Bases*, Lippincott, Philadelphia, pp. 96–109

Langley, F. H. and Crompton, A. C. (1973). *Epithelial Abnormalities of the Cervix Uteri*, Springer, Berlin

Osborn, M., Franke, W. W. and Weber, K. (1977). Visualisation of a system of filaments 7–10 nm thick in cultured cells of an epithelioid line (PtK$_2$) by immunofluorescence microscopy. *Proc. natn. Acad. Sci. U.S.A.*, **74**, 2490–4

Papanicolaou, G. N. (1953). Observations on the origin and specific function of the histiocytes in the female genital tract. *Fert. Steril.*, **4**, 472

Patten, S. F. Jr. (1978). *Diagnostic Cytopathology of the Uterine Cervix*, Karger, Basel

Reagan J. W. and Ng, A. B. P. (1973). *The Uterus* (ed. Norris, Hertig and Noell), Williams and Wilkins, Baltimore, pp. 320–47

Reagan, J. W. and Patten, S. F. jr. (1962). Dysplasia: a basic reaction to injury in the uterine cervix. *Ann. N.Y. Acad. Sci.*, **97**, 626–82

Rubio, C. A., Söderberg, G., Grant, C. A., Chi, C. and Krepler, R. (1976). The normal squamous epithelium of the human uterine cervix: a histological study. *Path. Europ.*, **11**, 157–62

Ruiter, D. J., Mauw, B. J. and Beyer-Boon, M. E. (1980). *Ultrastructure of normal cervical cells in Papanicolaou stained smear preparations*, in press

Smolka, H. and Soost, H. J. (1971). *Grundriss und Atlas der gynäkologischen Zytodiagonostik*, Thieme, Stuttgart, pp. 19–34

3

The Cervicovaginal Smear

Smears prepared by scraping the ectocervix or vagina contain epithelial and nonepithelial cells (red and white blood cells, histiocytes, etc.) and extraneous contaminants. In addition to these, cells from the placenta (though rarely seen) will be described.

3.1 Cells from Blood and Connective Tissue

3.1.1 Erythrocytes (Red Blood Cells)

Erythrocytes are found in smears when blood has passed through the external cervical os (menstruation, cervical ruptures, neoplasms) or as a result of scraping the ectocervix too roughly, or as a result of some abnormality of the ectocervix, for example, the presence of neoplasm.

Erythrocytes are small, round, orange-red or pink anucleate discs. Because of their biconcave shape, the centre is a lighter colour than the rim. When the bleeding has occurred some time in the past, the erythrocytes are somewhat pale and not as well defined. When there is much old blood in the smear the background may be orange-red. This may be seen during menstruation and also in the presence of some neoplasms (see section 10.2.3.3).

3.1.2 Leucocytes (White Blood Cells)

3.1.2.1 Polymorphonuclear Leucocytes (PMNs)

Leucocytes are approximately 1.5 times as large as erythrocytes. They are found in almost every smear, and are especially numerous in the second half of the menstrual cycle and during pregnancy. The number of leucocytes also increases when the cervix or vagina is inflamed. Leucocytes have segmented nuclei consisting of two or (usually) more dark blue lobes (figure 3.1). The cytoplasm, usually light grey, contains numerous granules. These granules are scarcely visible in neutrophil granulocytes stained by the Papanicolaou method. Eosinophil leucocytes are characterised by orange cytoplasmic granules.

3.1.2.2 Lymphocytes

Lymphocytes are found especially when there is a chronic inflammation. They are small round cells (slightly larger than an erythrocyte) with a dark nucleus which shows little structure with a small rim of cytoplasm (see figure 3.1).

3.1.3 Plasma Cells

Plasma cells are common in smears from chronically inflamed cervices. They have eccentric nuclei

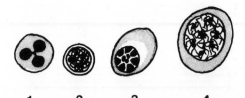

figure 3.1   Comparison of nuclear sizes. 1. Granulocyte; 2. lymphocyte; 3. plasma cell; 4. reticulum cell

(about the size of nuclei of lymphocytes) which have a typical radial structure (see figure 3.1). Next to the nucleus there is often a cytoplasmic clear zone, the perinuclear halo.

3.1.4 Histiocytes

Histiocytes generally have abundant, light grey, finely vacuolated cytoplasm. Their nuclei are often kidney-shaped with a fine, sometimes irregular, chromatinic pattern. A nucleolus may be present (figure 3.2). Histiocytes can be phagocytic so that their cytoplasm may contain blood pigment and other products of cell degradation. Sometimes multinucleate histiocytic giant cells are seen. When histiocytes are found in large numbers, they often form parallel rows. In contrast, epithelial cells are usually found in clusters. Histiocytes are encountered especially in healing processes such as on the seventh day of menstruation (*exodus* see section 2.3.3.2), after abortion, in association with chronic inflammation, neoplasms, or the wearing of a pessary, and after irradiation. In the case of intermenstrual bleeding or threatened abortion haematoidin crystals or 'cockleburrs' may be found in the cervical smear. The typical cockleburr is a rosette-shaped crystalline aggregate of radially arranged needles which stain either pinkish or orange-red. These structures are usually surrounded by or lie among histiocytes (Hollander and Gupta, 1974).

3.1.5 Reticulum Cells

Reticulum cells are found in a smear which manifests chronic lymphocytic cervicitis (section 7.2.3.1). They are accompanied by lymphocytes, plasma cells and histiocytes. Reticulum cells are moderately large cells with a small rim of cytoplasm. The nuclei have a fairly dark coarse chromatinic pattern; nucleoli are clearly visible.

3.1.6 Fibroblasts

Fibroblasts are young cells of fibrous connective tissue which are sometimes found in the smears when the epithelium has been injured due, for example, to ulcer (see section 7.5.1), chronic inflammation or trauma. They are closely related developmentally to histiocytes. These cells are elongated with a centrally situated oval nucleus and a fine regular chromatinic pattern.

3.1.7 Capillaries

Capillaries are the smallest blood vessels. One is sometimes found in the smear as a tubular structure usually containing erythrocytes.

3.2 Contaminants

A large and sometimes exotic variety of contaminants can 'pollute' the smear. As a result of a gynaecological examination just before the smear is taken, the smear can be contaminated with

(1) Petroleum or other lubricant jelly from the physician's glove. This appears as amorphous blue structures which are about the size of an intermediate cell.

(2) Glove powder (talc, starch) also from the examining glove. This is seen as small angular yellow-white structures (figure 3.3).

Cells from the male urogenital tract can frequently be found.

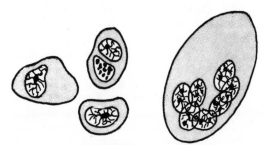

figure 3.2   Several histiocytes

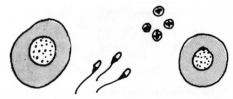

figure 3.3   Two parabasal cells, spermatozoa and talc

(1) Spermatozoa, which have ovoid heads with an anterior dark and a posterior light zone, and a tail (figure 3.3). When the smear is taken some time after coitus only the heads may be visible. The spermatozoa may be mingled with leucocytes and bacteria if the male sexual partner has urethritis or prostatitis.

(2) Cells from the seminal vesicle. These cells have hyperchromatic anisokaryotic nuclei and little cytoplasm (Meisels and Ayotte, 1976) which often contains the yellow-orange pigment lipofuscin.

Several contaminants may be encountered in the smear like pollen, vegetable cells (especially in the summer). *Penicillium*, *Alternaria* sp. or *Aspergillus* sp. conidia (fungi). Contamination by the intestinal parasites or their ova (*Enterobius vermicularis*, *Ascaris*) also occurs. Parts of a pubic louse (contaminant of the external genitals) stain orange-pink in the Papanicolaou stain. Contaminants from the urinary tract are, for example, *Schistosoma haematobium* or *Toxoplasma* pseudocysts. The various micro-organisms will be discussed in sections 7.3.1–7.3.5.

3.3 Cells from the Placenta

Under pathological conditions (abortion, placenta praevia) cells from the placenta may be found in a smear.

3.3.1 Syntrophoblast Cells

Syntrophoblast cells are multinucleate giant cells with an average of 50 nuclei per cell (Patten, 1978) and a characteristic coarse-grained chromatin pattern which resembles coarsely ground

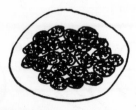

figure 3.4   Syntrophoblast cell. Compare with the multinucleate histiocytic giant cell in figure 3.2

pepper (Tweeddale *et al.*, 1968). The number of nuclei is large with respect to the amount of cytoplasm (figure 3.4). The cytoplasm appears granular, in contrast to the cytoplasm of a histiocytic giant cell.

3.3.2 Cytotrophoblast Cells

Cytotrophoblast cells are cuboidal cells with centrally situated nuclei. Cytologically, these cells cannot be identified as such. The cells may mimic cancer cells due to their prominent nucleoli, coarse chromatinic pattern and high nucleocytoplasmic ratio (Patten, 1978).

3.3.3 Decidual Cells

Decidual cells are stromal cells from the endometrium (in rare cases from the cervix) which are highly swollen due to their content of glycogen. Decidual cells have abundant cytoplasm with centrally situated nuclei which can be large. The nuclei often contain prominent multiple nucleoli. Decidual cells can be recognised by the fact that, in contrast to squamous epithelial cells, they are not flat but convex; moreover, the cytoplasm appears to be less dense (Danos and Holmquist, 1967).

References

Danos, M. and Holmquist, N. D. (1967). Cytologic evaluation of decidual cells: A report of two cases with false abnormal cytology. *Acta Cytol.*, **11**, 325–30

Hollander, D. H. and Gupta, P. K. (1974). Hematoidin Cockleburrs in cervico-vaginal smears. *Acta Cytol.*, **18**, 268–70

Meisels, A. and Ayotte, D. (1976). Cells from the seminal vesicles: contaminants of the V-C-E smear. *Acta Cytol.*, **20**, 211–19

Patten, S. F. (1978). *Diagnostic Cytopathology of the Uterine Cervix*, 2nd edn, Karger, Basel

Tweeddale, D. N., Scott, R. C., Fields, M. J., Roddick, J. W. and Ball, M. J. (1968). Giant cells in cervico-vaginal smears. *Acta Cytol.*, **12**, 298–304

Development and Physiology of the Female Genital Tract

4.1 Development of the Female Genital Tract

The primordia of the gonads (that is, the ovaries and the testes) and the other genital organs of the male and the female are morphologically alike at the earliest stage of embryonic development. Differentiation occurs in phases, with the gonads developing first, followed later by the other genital organs. The first signs of genital development appear in the 4–5-week-old embryo at the mesonephros (primitive kidney). This is called the area of the primitive sex or germ cells. The primitive germ cells migrate to this region from the yolk sac (which lies outside the actual embryo) and form the primordial oogonia (female) and spermatogonia (male) (Hamilton *et al.*, 1959).

The origin of these primitive germ cells is not certain but an attractive theory is that they are blastomeres, that is, cells which have separated from a fertilised ovum before the first differentiation (totipotent cells). If we now limit our discussion to the female genital tract, then two facts appear to be important.

(1) Differentiation of the gonads is determined by the sex chromosomes of the embryo. This differentiation occurs at about the seventh week of embryonic development.

(2) The development of the organs adjacent to the gonads is also determined by the sex chromosomes. These include the *wolffian ducts*, which in the male later develop into the genital tract and the urinary tract (kidney, ureter, bladder and urethra) and the *müllerian* ducts, which become the female reproductive tract (figure 4.1).

The development of both the internal and the external genitalia is determined by the sex chromosomes. The internal genitalia develop first, followed by the external genitalia, which are formed from the urogenital sinus. If the embryo carries no Y chromosome, the müllerian ducts develop leading ultimately to the formation of the female genital organs (see section 5.2).

4.1.1 The Development of the Ovary

The 'primary gonad' (also called the 'indifferent gonad'), consisting of primitive germ cells in the so-called 'germinal' epithelium and indifferent stroma, is found in embryos of 7–8 weeks. Female germ cells are termed oogonia until they enter the prophase of meiosis when they are termed *oocytes*. Oogonia proliferate by mitosis with diminishing frequency until the third month of foetal life. Meiosis commences before the primordial follicles are formed at 4.5–5.5 months. Just before ovulation, many years later, the first meiotic division is completed. Most of the ova degenerate, while about 400 are ovulated in the entire reproductive period.

After the fourth or fifth month primordial follicles appear, consisting of an oocyte enclosed by a layer of low cuboidal epithelium; they later become the *graafian follicles.* In the foetus several primordial follicles can ripen; sometimes follicles

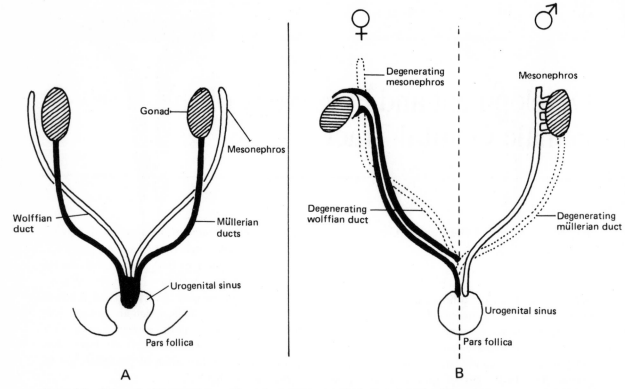

figure 4.1   Schematic diagram of the embryonic development of the gonads and other genital organs in the male and female. A. Before sex differentiation; B. after sex differentiation

even regress. The ovaries, which first form in the lumbar region, descend in the course of embryonic development to their final position in the pelvis.

4.1.2 The Development of the Other Organs of the Female Reproductive Tract

The other genital organs arise from the müllerian ducts. The ends of the müllerian ducts located in the abdominal cavity form the fallopian tubes including their fimbriae. The other section develops into the uterus and the upper two-thirds of the vagina (figure 4.2). Initially the uterus, as well as part of the vagina, develops as two symmetrical organs which later fuse. The müllerian ducts open into the urogenital sinus together with the wolffian ducts. The lower third of the vagina and the external genitalia develop from the so-called '*urogenital sinus*'.

In a newborn child, the genital tract is usually fully developed. The primary sexual characteristics by which male and female babies are distinguished consist of the vulva and vagina (female) and the penis and testes (male). Anomalies of these primary sexual characteristics are usually the result of abnormal growth, for example, failure of the müllerian ducts to fuse or incomplete migration of the ovaries. They can also be caused by chromosomal abnormalities, which are described in section 5.3. Cytological examination of the ovary of a newborn child shows that in general the primordial follicles predominate (about 400 000). Occasionally some secondary follicles and atretic follicles are also seen. It is not unusual to note signs of oestrogenic activity (see section 6.2.1) which generally can be attributed to oestrogenic stimulation from the mother; such signs are short-lived and temporary (vaginal spotting, witch's milk, etc.).

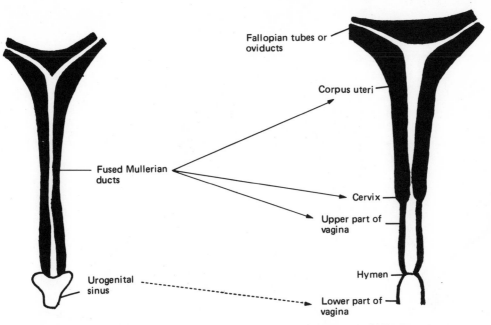

Fallopian tubes or oviducts

Corpus uteri

Fused Mullerian ducts

Cervix

Upper part of vagina

Urogenital sinus

Hymen

Lower part of vagina

figure 4.2   Schematic diagram of the development of the vagina, uterus and fallopian tubes

4.2 Neurohormonal Regulation of the Menstrual Cycle of Sexually Mature Females

Although the genital tract is morphologically complete at birth, it cannot function until the hypothalamus has matured. Only then are the *nuclei* of the hypothalamus (groups of cells which together have a specific function) capable of secreting substances (the so-called '*releasing factors*') which are transferred via a closed system of blood vessels to the anterior lobe of the pituitary. As a result, the pituitary secretes the hormones which are necessary for the functioning of the endocrine organs, such as the adrenal and thyroid glands, and the gonads. Such hormones, which in turn activate other hormonal systems, are called 'trophic hormones'. Each trophic hormone has a specific releasing factor. As far as gonadal function is concerned, there are two trophic hormones, follicle-stimulating hormone (FSH) and luteinising hormone (LH), as well as one common releasing factor, FSH–LH releasing factor (FSH–LH–RF).

If enough FSH–LH–RF is secreted, the ovaries will be stimulated to cause ripening of the follicles with subsequent endocrine function (secretion of oestrogen and later of progesterone) (figure 4.3). One of the functions of the ovary consists, therefore, of hormone production; another is the ability to ovulate, the generative function.

It has been found that FSH in particular affects the ripening of the primary follicle as well as proliferation of the granulosa cells. Under the influence of FSH oestrogen production begins. The oestrogen has two specific target organs, the genital tract and the hypothalamus. If a small amount of FSH–LH is secreted, then only follicle ripening will occur and only oestrogen will be secreted. It has been demonstrated that for ovulation to take place a combined FSH–LH *peak* is necessary. After ovulation the gonad will produce progesterone in addition to oestrogen. Progesterone influences the same target organs as oestrogen. Taking the above into account, how can the menstrual cycle be explained?

As long as the hypothalamus is not mature, the

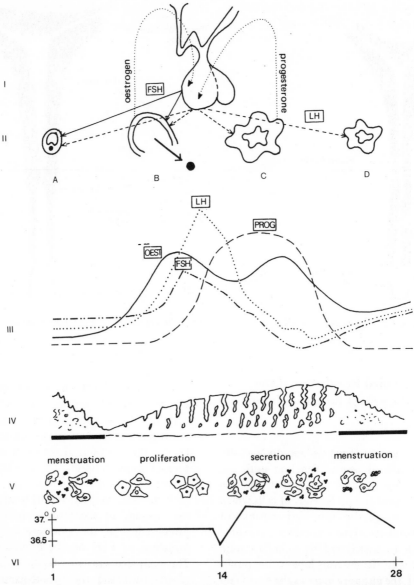

figure 4.3   **The menstrual cycle. I. Cyclic activity of the pituitary; II. egg ripening (A), ovulation (B), formation of the corpus luteum (C) and involution of the corpus luteum to the corpus albicans (D); III. blood levels of oestrogen, progesterone, FSH and LH; IV. endometrial cycle; V. cyclic changes in the vaginal epithelium as seen in a vaginal smear; VI. cyclic changes in the basal temperature**

amount of FSH–LH secreted will be such that sufficient oestrogen will be produced by the ovary to induce the mucous membrane of the uterus to proliferate. Usually the first cycle involves only this stage.

The oestrogen has another target organ: the hypothalamus. A high concentration of oestrogen has an inhibiting effect on those cells in the hypothalamus which produce the releasing factor, so that the secretion of the latter decreases or ceases. The result is a rather abrupt reduction in FSH–LH secretion and thus a decrease in ovarian activity, especially in oestrogen production. The result is disintegration of the mucous membrane of the uterus with consequent uterine bleeding. This first menstrual bleeding is called the '*menarche*'. The effect of the oestrogen on the hypothalamus is called a '*feedback*'. In fact the monophasic anovular cycle has now been described. This type of cyclic pattern is found especially at puberty and towards the end of the reproductive phase of life (see section 4.3.5).

When the hypothalamus is fully grown, sufficient FSH–LH–RF is secreted for a biphasic cycle. The degree of secretion, and therefore the amount of FSH and LH produced, fluctuates with each cycle. When the oestrogen concentration decreases the nuclei of the hypothalamus will no longer be inhibited and thus the releasing factor will be secreted freely. FSH and LH will then gradually be released, leading to ripening of a follicle in the first phase (follicular phase) of the menstrual cycle. Moreover, oestrogen production will again increase. At day 12 of the menstrual cycle there is a fairly sudden marked elevation in FSH–LH secretion (the so-called 'FSH–LH peak'). This leads to an ovulation 48 hours later. The mature oocyte leaves the follicle and is taken up by the fallopian tube. Under the influence of the FSH–LH peak the cells of the follicle that are left behind assume another endocrine function: progesterone secretion. This group of cells is now referred to as the *corpus luteum* (see section 2.2.4.2). Immediately after the FSH–LH peak, the secretion of FSH–LH drops rapidly to the old level. After the 14th day, the ovary produces not only oestrogen (with a proliferative effect) but also progesterone (with a secretory effect). This progesterone phase (*luteal phase*) lasts about 14 days. The mucous membrane in the uterus no longer proliferates. Instead it is secretory in character; moreover, glycogen is produced, which is a primary nutrient for the implanted ovum.

The combined concentration of oestrogen and progesterone inhibits the activity of the hypothalamic nuclei, that is, of the secretion of FSH–LH–RF and so reduction of the blood FSH and LH

levels occurs. Finally there is a decrease in the ovarian activity, resulting in a drop of oestrogen and progesterone levels. The endometrium, which is dependent upon oestrogen production, degenerates, with ensuing menstrual bleeding (Bartelmez and Baltimore, 1957). The biphasic cycle is now complete. The decrease in the oestrogen and progesterone concentrations in the blood counteracts the hypothalamic inhibition so that a new cycle can begin.

A similar relationship also exists between the hypothalamus and the thyroid gland, and between the hypothalamus and the adrenal glands. The term biphasic applies to the two phases of hormone concentration (first only oestrogen, later progesterone and oestrogen) as well as to the thermoregulation of the body. If the temperature is taken every day during a normal cycle, two phases can be distinguished: during the first phase (proliferative phase) the temperature is on average slightly lower than during the second phase (secretory phase) (see figure 4.3). This can be explained by the fact that progesterone causes a slight rise in terperature.

4.3 Endocrinology of the Various Life Phases of the Female

4.3.1 Childhood

Up until the eighth or ninth year there is little difference between the concentration of sex hormones in boys and girls. At this stage the hypothalamus in girls begins to secrete releasing factors periodically, resulting in oestrogen production in the ovaries (Turner, 1966).

4.3.2 Puberty

At puberty sexual maturity is achieved. It begins in girls when they are about 10 years old and is generally completed by the sixteenth year. The growth spurt in particular is striking; it usually starts around the tenth year. This is followed by breast development (10–11 years) and the growth of pubic hair (11–13 years). Finally the menarche (first uterine bleeding) occurs (11–13 years). The growth of the girl is influenced by oestrogenic gonadal activity as well as by other growth regulators.

In addition to the menarche, there is also an *adrenarche* which slightly precedes the menarche. This is characterised by an increase in the activity of the adrenal cortex, especially in the production of androgens, which are essential for the development of the external genitalia and the breasts. The uterine bleeding, which occurs more or less periodically after the menarche, is usually anovulatory at first. The girl is not considered sexually mature until the ovary has achieved both a generative function and an endocrine function.

4.3.3 Sexual Maturity

The period of sexual maturity is characterised by the ability to bear children. It begins with the first biphasic cycle and ends when the generative function of the ovary ceases. This period lasts about 30 years (between the fifteenth and forty-fifth years). The characteristics of the biphasic cycle in the period of sexual maturity have already been described. The essential feature is the generative function (the ability to ovulate) coexisting with the endocrine function. If, during the secretory phase, the oocyte is fertilised after ovulation by a spermatozoon and if implantation is successful, pregnancy will follow.

4.3.4 Pregnancy

When pregnancy occurs the biphasic cycle is suspended. In fact, a prolonged extension of the secretory phase follows under the influence of the progesterone. This is first produced in the corpus luteum and later by the placenta itself.

The endocrine activity in pregnancy is in fact regulated by the *foetoplacental unit* which is responsible for the marked elevation in the progesterone level. Pregnancy is terminated by abortion or by a delivery. The loss of the foetoplacental

unit is at this time the major endocrinic change. After delivery lactation begins. The main lactogenic hormone, prolactin, is also secreted by the pituitary gland. During lactation prolactin inhibits the nuclei of the hypothalamus so that the biphasic cycle usually will occur less frequently as long as the mother nurses her child.

4.3.5 Climacteric

At the climacteric gonadal function decreases. Usually biphasic cycles alternate with anovulatory monophasic cycles. In addition, oestrogenic activity gradually decreases, which induces bleeding. This phase is also called the 'premenopause'. It closely resembles the phase following the menarche.

Once ovarian endocrine function decreases to such an extent that bleeding no longer occurs, the term '*postmenopause*' is used. The final menstruation is called the '*menopause*'.

The climacteric is characterised by vasovegetative disturbances caused by irregularity of the cycle (Käser *et al.*, 1969). Because inhibition of the hypothalamus is irregular and sometimes absent, various releasing factors may be secreted in unequal proportions. As a result, thyroid dysfunction, obesity and vasovegetative abnormalities can develop. Irascibility, palpitations, excessive sweating and emotional upset are frequent symptoms. Once a new balance has been reached and the eventual climacteric complaints have disappeared the woman enters her last phase of life: old age.

4.3.6 Old Age

In old age a new equilibrium is established. The ovaries barely function. The adrenal cortex has assumed some functions of the ovary. It produces oestrogen in small quantities and an androsterone (a male sex hormone) which can be converted to oestrogen.

The main characteristic of old age is atrophy of the genitalia. A fairly common clinical picture is that of senile vaginitis as a result of oestrogen deficiency, where the patient complains of dryness or itching of the vagina and vulva. Sometimes there is a brown discharge due to tiny haemorrhages, which readily occur in the atrophic mucous membrane and are visible macroscopically as small dots.

References

Bartelmez, G. W. and Baltimore, Ph.D. (1957). The phases of the menstrual cycle and their interpretation in terms of the pregnancy cycle. *Am. J. Obstet. Gynec.*, 74, 931—55

Hamilton, W. J., Boyd, J. D. and Mossman, H. W. (1959). *Human Embryology*, Heffer, Cambridge

Käser, O., Friedberg, V., Over, K. G., Thomsen, K. and Zander, J. (1969). *Gynäkologie und Geburtshilfe*, Thieme, Stuttgart

Turner, D. C. (1966). *General Endocrinology*, Saunders, Philadelphia and London

5

Sex Differentiation and Sex Chromatin

5.1 Introduction

Every human cell has 44 autosomes (chromosomes which are not involved in sex differentiation) arranged in pairs and 2 single sex chromosomes, a fact which was not established with certainty until the last twenty years. During interphase the chromosomes cannot be identified individually, since they are 'unrolled'. When mitosis begins the chromosomes become visible as chromatids arranged in pairs (see section 1.4.2). In this phase, morphological differentiation of the chromosomes is possible. There are two different sex chromosomes in the male: the X and the Y chromosome. In females there are two X chromosomes. A morphological chromosomal analysis yields the karyotype of each individual. While the chromosomes are uncondensed in interphase, there is one exception — one of the two X chromosomes in the cells of females. This is the so-called 'inactive X chromosome' or 'Barr body' (Barr and Bertram, 1949). The Barr body may therefore be seen in cells with two X chromosomes, that is, cells from a normal female. The nuclei of the cells from males do not contain an inactive X chromosome; therefore there is no Barr body. The number of X chromosomes per cell is equal to n + 1 where n = the number of Barr bodies per cell. When there are three X chromosomes per cell, two Barr bodies will be seen. Some examples:

XXX (tri-X female) = 2 Barr bodies per cell

XXY (Klinefelter's   = 1 Barr body per cell
  syndrome)
XO (Turner's   = 0 Barr bodies per cell
  syndrome)

Since the work of Caspersson and his colleagues in the early 1970s it has become practical accurately and definitively to diagnose chromosomal disorders routinely by determination of the banding pattern of each chromosome. While some sex chromosome related diseases can be studied by determination of Barr bodies and neutrophil 'drumsticks', these methods are no longer the ones of choice and when the clinician is faced with a patient who appears to have a genetic disease there is little reason why such a patient should not have the benefit of a complete karyotype with banding pattern for all of the chromosomes.

Determination of sex is, however, a fascinating topic and we will describe below how sex chromosomes affect the outward appearance of individuals, especially in those instances where multiple sex chromosomes are involved. In order to understand this subject some knowledge of normal and abnormal sex differentiation is necessary.

5.2 Normal Sex Differentiation

The principle of sexual reproduction is the fusion of a spermatozoon and an oocyte. As a result of this there is a continuous exchange of genetic material ensuring a large (in fact unlimited) genetic variation. Nature strives to achieve bisexuality or a difference between the sexes. The significance of 'two types' (male and female) is difficult to comprehend, let alone explain, but it is found in all higher organisms. In man the two sexes can be distinguished by differences in

(1) chromosomal pattern: XX (female) and XY (male).

(2) production of gonadotropins (FSH and LH) and sex hormones (cyclic in females, non-cyclic in males).

(3) gonads (testes in males; ovaries in females).

(4) internal genital organs.

(5) external genital organs.

(6) physique (skeleton, fat distribution, musculature).

(7) psyche (interests, disposition, etc.).

(8) breast development, pattern of hair growth, voice level.

N.B. (3), (4) and (5) are the primary sex characteristics; (6), (7) and (8) are the secondary sex characteristics.

In the early embryonic stage there is no difference between a male and a female. Wolffian ducts and müllerian ducts are present in both (see section 4.1). Full expression of the Y chromosome (the Y chromosome, as the carrier of all specific male characteristics, is 100 per cent active) includes suppression of the development of the müllerian ducts and stimulation of the formation of the male genital organs from the wolffian ducts. In the absence of the Y chromosome the müllerian ducts will always develop. Also, in the absence of testes (or if the wolffian ducts should not react to testosterone), a female phenotype (having the outward appearance of a female) will develop. In contrast, the development of a female genital tract is not dependent on the presence of ovaries.

Between the second year and puberty there is very little sexual development. During puberty the primary and secondary sex characteristics become more pronounced. In girls the development is influenced by the production of oestrogen and progesterone (in the ovaries); in boys by the production of testosterone (in the testes). The secretion of the sex hormones is activated during puberty by the production of the pituitary hormones FSH and LH (see section 4.2). In girls, in the course of time, this secretion becomes cyclic whereas in boys it remains at a constant level.

5.3 Abnormal Sex Differentiation

Normally, sex differentiation proceeds without difficulties, resulting in time in an unmistakable 'man' or 'woman'. During the embryonic phase, however, something may go wrong, resulting in abnormalities of the secondary sex characteristics: insufficient sex differentiation (*hypogonadism*) or intermingling of the male and female characteristics (*intersexuality, hermaphroditism*).

5.3.1. Hypogonadism

In men as in women some types of hypogonadism, like several forms of intersexuality, can be attributed to an abnormal *number* of sex chromosomes. This abnormality can occur during meiotic division when the X and Y chromosomes are not divided equally between the daughter cells and one cell receives two and the other no sex chromosomes (Barr, 1961). Figure 5.1 illustrates which gametes (paired cells) may then develop, as well as the abnormal number of chromosomes which can result after fertilisation. Of the many possibilities,

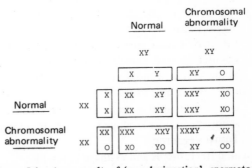

figure 5.1 **As a result of 'non-dysjunction', spermatogenesis or oogenesis can produce gametes which have either too many or too few sex chromosomes. After fertilisation many various combinations may result. XO and XXY are the most common; XXX is not seen very often; YO is never encountered**

XO and XXY are the most common. An XO karyotype causes *Turner's syndrome*, a type of female hypogonadism (agenesis of the ovaries); the XXY type leads to *Klinefelter's syndrome*, a form of male hypogonadism (underdeveloped testes without spermatogenesis). There are many rare variants, such as XXX, XXXX, etc.

Another important type is the so-called '*mosaicism*', where there is an unequal distribution of the sex chromosomes; this takes place during one of the first divisions of the fertilised egg cell. For instance, some of the cells may have a 46—XX pattern and other cells a 45—XO pattern (XX/XO mosaicism). The possibilities and variations are legion. The abnormalities of these men and women may be such that they fall between those individuals with a 'true' Klinefelter's syndrome or a 'true' Turner's syndrome and a normal individual. As the chromosomal abnormality increases, the intelligence quotient usually decreases. Several clinical examples of hypogonadism are described below.

5.3.1.1 Turner's Syndrome (women)

Clinical picture: short stocky stature, webbed neck, cubitus valgus, shield-like chest.

Chromosomes: 44 + XO (no Barr bodies). If some of the cells have 45 chromosomes and some 46 (XX), this is called a mosaic Turner's syndrome; in these cases the percentage of Barr bodies is smaller than that of a normal female. In other words, in patients with *mosaic* Turner's syndrome, the percentage of Barr bodies in the left buccal smear will differ from the percentage in the right buccal smear. For this reason it is essential to take a smear from the right as well as the left cheek and to evaluate them separately.

Gonads: streak ovaries (bands of connective tissue at the site of the ovaries) in 'true' Turner's syndrome; underdeveloped ovaries in mosaic Turner's syndrome.

Genital tract: uterus and vagina are present.

Therapy: patients with Turner's syndrome visit the clinician because of delayed puberty and primary amenorrhoea. Since these patients have underdeveloped ovaries or none at all, treatment is limited to hormonal therapy. Pregnancy is impossible.

5.3.1.2 Klinefelter's Syndrome (men)

Clinical picture: slim graceful stature, underdeveloped testes, sterility due to azoospermia, sparse body hair, possible mental retardation.

Chromosomes: 44 + XXY (1 Barr body). Patients with mosaic Klinefelter's syndrome, as well as individuals with more than two X chromosomes and one Y chromosome (XXXY), are all classified under Klinefelter's syndrome. The more X chromosomes present, the lower the intelligence quotient.

Gonads: underdeveloped testes without spermatogenesis.

Therapy: none, or testosterone. The sterility cannot be remedied.

5.3.1.3 Tri-X (XXX) Female (super female)

Clinical picture: female, sterility, mental retardation.

Chromosomes: 44 + XXX (2 Barr bodies); or 44 + XXXX (3 Barr bodies). Again, the more X chromosomes present, the more pronounced mental retardation will be.

Gonads: normal ovaries.

5.3.1.4 'True' Gonodal Dysgenesis

Clinical picture: the outward appearance of a girl in childhood; no puberty; final development into eunuchnoidal type; no menstruation, sterility.

Chromosomes: 44 + XX (1 Barr body).

Gonads: streak ovaries.

5.3.2. Intersexuality

In this type of individual the external genital organs show male as well as female characteristics. The types are classified in various ways. A distinction can be made between '*pseudohermaphroditism*', where the gonads are either totally male (testes) or totally female (ovaries), and 'true' hermaphroditism, where the external genital organs as well as the gonads are bisexual, that is, both testicular and ovarian tissue can be discerned.

Male 'pseudohermaphrodites' have 'ambivalent characteristics' (see section 5.2, numbers 1–8), an XY karyotype and gonads in the form of testicles; female 'pseudohermaphrodites' have an XX karyotype and therefore possess ovaries. The following classification is practical rather than scientific.

5.3.2.1 Female Pseudohermaphroditism (karyotype XX; ovaries)

(1) Adrenogenital syndrome. This is found in girls who have undergone virilisation before birth as a result of overproduction of male hormones in the adrenal cortex. Virilisation is limited to the external genitalia; usually there is only slight enlargement of the clitoris, but sometimes it may resemble a penis with hypospadias (see section 5.3.2.2). The internal genital organs are normal so that pregnancy is possible later. Early diagnosis and treatment are essential.

(2) Intrauterine virilisation. This can develop as a result of the maternal ingestion of male hormones (androgens) or a hormone-producing neoplasm in the mother.

N.B. female pseudohermaphrodites are fertile; male pseudohermaphrodites are almost always sterile.

5.3.2.2 Male Pseudohermaphroditism (karyotype XY; testes)

(1) Dysgenetic male pseudohermaphroditism. In general this develops as follows: in the embryo the testes do not produce enough androgens for total masculinisation of the external genitalia. In a mild form this causes only slight *hypospadias*. This is a congenital abnormality in which the urethra opens on the underside of the penis due to incomplete closure of the urogenital canal. In its most severe form dysgenetic male pseudohermaphroditism is characterised by almost total feminisation of the external genital organs with clitoral hypertrophy as the only macroscopic abnormality. Many transitional forms exist. Moreover, it is also possible that degeneration of the müllerian ducts was incomplete

so that a vagina or a (tiny) uterus, or both, may be present.

(2) Syndrome of testicular feminisation. This is a rare phenomenon, worth considering because of the unusual manner in which it develops. These individuals are in principle 'males', thus the karyotype is 46–XY and the gonads are testes. The testes produce testosterone but because of a defect in the receptor organs (which should react to this male hormone) there is no reaction at all. Physical development proceeds as if no male hormone has been secreted; the external organs are therefore female. These individuals are phenotypic females with strikingly well-shaped breasts, a small vagina (that part which arises from the urogenital sinus) and little pubic hair. However, the development of the müllerian ducts has been suppressed by the Y chromosome; therefore there is no uterus, menstruation does not occur and a pregnancy is impossible.

5.4 Identification of the Sex Chromatin

Many nuclear stains can be used to demonstrate chromatin structures and nuclear membranes. In the nuclei of some intermediate squamous epithelial cells, a small biconcave mass of chromatin can be seen lying against the inner side of the nuclear membrane; it is larger than the chromocentres of the same nucleus and appears as a part of the nuclear membrane (figure 5.2). This is the inactive X chromosome or *Barr body*. It is observed best at a magnification of about x 1250. Occasionally a stray clump of chromatin may be identified as a Barr body: therefore normal males also appear to have a few cells with 'Barr bodies' although the percentage of nuclei with these false Barr bodies is usually small. Since Barr bodies cannot be seen in all cells, the percentage of visible Barr bodies in a normal female never reaches 100. Fluctuations of the percentage of Barr bodies with the menstrual cycle is reported (Blanco del Campo and Ramirez, 1965). Pansegrau and Peterson (1964) found Barr bodies in 30–70 per cent of the cells in specially stained smears taken from the mucous membrane of the cheek (buccal smears) of normal

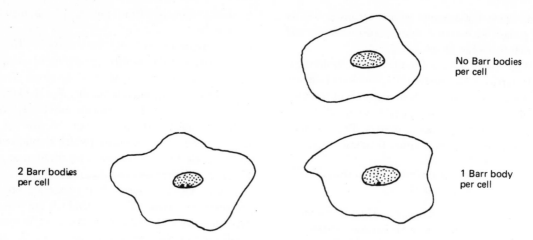

figure 5.2   **Barr bodies in an intermediate cell**

women. In general 0–9 per cent of the cells in normal males contain bodies that look like Barr bodies. The percentage may vary from laboratory to laboratory, depending upon the smear preparation technique or the staining method.

5.4.1 Technique for Evaluating Barr Bodies

To determine the percentage of Barr bodies, a smear taken from the mucous membrane of the cheek (left and right) or the vagina is used. The preparations may be stained according to the Papanicolaou method. The Barr bodies stain dark blue like the rest of the chromatin. Also the Cresyl-Echt Violet staining method can be used (see section 15.5.4).

To determine the percentage of Barr bodies, at least 100 clearly visible nuclei must be evaluated. In the report the number of cells with Barr bodies is reported as a percentage.

If more than 20 per cent of the cells contain sex chromatin and the individual is a phenotypic female, then the report is: 'Results consistent with a normal phenotypic female'. If Barr bodies are found in 5–10 per cent of the cells and the individual is a phenotypic female, then new smears from the left and the right cheek must be requested. If there is a noticeable difference between the results of the right and left buccal smears, then the

probable finding is 'mosaic Turner's syndrome'. If less than 5 per cent of the cells contain Barr bodies and the individual is a phenotypic female, then the report must be: 'Sex chromatin less than 5 per cent, results indicate Turner's syndrome'.

If Barr bodies are seen in 0–5 per cent of the cells from a phenotypic male, then the results confirm that the individual is a normal phenotypic male. If 5–20 per cent of the cells contain Barr bodies and the individual is a phenotypic male, then new smears from the left and the right cheek must be requested. If there is a noticeable difference in the results, this can indicate a mosaic Klinefelter's syndrome.

If more than one Barr body per cell is found, this must be stated clearly (for example, tri-X female).

N.B. Demonstration of the Y chromosome is possible in interphase cells by means of fluorescent microscopy. If the atebrine stain is used, the Y chromosome will be seen because of its vivid fluorescence.

References

Barr, M. L. (1961). *Das Geschlechtschromatin in die Intersexualität*, Thieme, Stuttgart

Barr, M. L. and Bertram, E. G. A. (1949). Morphological distinction between neurones of the male and female and the behaviour of the nucleolar satellite during accelerated nucleoprotein synthesis. *Nature,* **163**, 676–7

Blanco del Campo, M. S. and Ramirez, O. E. G. (1965). Fluctuations of the sex-chromatin during the menstrual cycle. *Acta Cytol.,* **9**, 251–6

Pansegrau, D. G. and Peterson, R. E. (1964). Improved staining of sexchromatin. *Am. J. clin. Path.,* **41**, 266–72

6

Hormonal Cytology

6.1 Introduction

The epithelia of the female are influenced by the sex hormones. To study hormonal effects the evaluation of squamous epithelial cells either scraped from the vaginal or buccal mucosa, or exfoliated from the urinary tract is most convenient.

An assessment of vaginal or buccal epithelial cells is called a vaginal or buccal cytogram, of squamous epithelial cells in urinary sediments a urocytogram. Either method can be repeated daily if necessary, thus enabling study of the effect of changing hormone levels in the menstrual cycle or the effect of the administration of hormonal drugs. As early as 1925 Papanicolaou reported the potentialities of cytohormonal evaluation (Papanicolaou, 1925) in vaginal smears. In 1944 the urocytogram was used by Biot and Beltran Nunez, followed by Papanicolaou in 1948 (Papanicolaou, 1948). The main bulk of spontaneously exfoliated cells in urinary sediments are derived from the squamous epithelium of the urethra and the trigonum of the bladder; a negligible number of cells are of true urothelial origin. The vaginal, urethral and trigonal epithelia have a common embryonic origin, the sinus urogenitalis. In the light of this common embryological source the parallel reactions to the sex hormones become comprehensible.

Hormonal cytology is a bioassay, which means that it is not the concentration of circulating hormone which is being determined; rather it is the effect of the hormone on the target organ (the stratified squamous epithelium in this case) which is being evaluated. One problem here is that the sensitivity of the target organ to the sex hormone varies from person to person. Moreover, it is usually not the sole effect of one hormone that is registered but the combined effect of several hormones. Also the administration of hormonal drugs can influence the hormonal pattern. It is essential to keep these facts in mind if a correct cytohormonal evaluation is to be achieved.

6.1.1 The Influence of Sex Hormones on the Squamous Epithelium

6.1.1.1 Oestrogens

Oestrogens promote the growth and maturation of the stratified squamous epithelium up to and including the superficial layer. The smear will contain many *superficial epithelial cells* when the oestrogen level is high and unopposed by progesterone, as in the first half of the cycle. These cells lie quite flat and are generally discrete.

A small dose of oestrogens can cause atrophic squamous epithelium to develop into epithelium with several layers of intermediate cells. When the dose of oestrogens is increased, the intermediate cells will mature into superficial cells. The concept of 'oestrogen effect' should only be used when oestrogens alone circulate in the bloodstream, thus exerting a monohormonal effect (Pundel, 1957).

6.1.1.2 Progesterone

Once the stratified squamous epithelium has matured under the influence of oestrogens, progesterone causes a rapid desquamation of the topmost layers. The intermediate cells can have curled edges (*folding*); they exfoliate as compact groups of cells (*clusters*, that is, a cell group in which the margins of the individual cells have become indistinct). Many Döderlein's bacilli (see section 7.3.1.1) and leucocytes can appear in the smear; as a result of *cytolysis* (dissolution or destruction of cells) of the intermediate cells, numerous naked vesicular nuclei are present. Progesterone also promotes the storage of glycogen in the squamous epithelial cells. The smear then contains many *navicular* (boat-shaped) cells in which the nucleus is pushed aside by the glycogen.

When the progesterone level is high (for example, in pregnancy) many large clusters of navicular cells appear in the smear.

When there is a mild oestrogen deficiency, as may be encountered at the time of the menopause, the cytological pattern cannot be distinguished from that characteristic of progesterone or androgen stimulation (Pundel, 1957). However, the clusters are usually slightly smaller (no more than 10 cells).

If progesterone is administered to patients with an atrophic epithelium, maturation of the squamous epithelium, including the superficial layers, is the result. Upon administration of progesterone to patients with a mature epithelium the superficial layer disappears and no superficial cells are found in the smear.

6.1.1.3 Androgen

Administration of this hormone when the stratified squamous epithelium is atrophic (smears with exclusively parabasal cells) results in smears with predominantly intermediate cells. These smears are rich in cells (Boschann, 1956). If androgens are administered to patients with a fully matured stratified squamous epithelium, the opposite effect is seen: the superficial cells disappear from the cell pattern and are replaced by intermediate cells (Wied et al., 1958). Prolonged administration of androgens produces a smear pattern with cytolysis.

6.1.2 Description of the Cytohormonal Patterns

The hormonal patterns identified in the smear can be described in different ways. Various indices have been proposed for this purpose (Wied, 1968).

6.1.2.1 Karyopyknotic Index (K. I.)

To determine the K. I. the number of pyknotic nuclei per 100 intermediate and superficial epithelial cells is established (Pundel, 1957). The K. I. can vary from 0 (atrophy, pregnancy) to 100 (oestrogen therapy, oestrogen-producing neoplasms).

During the menstrual cycle the K. I. varies from 0–32 in the follicular phase, to 12–90 at the ovulatory peak, and 0–47 in the luteal phase (Lencioni, 1975). There is a large individual variation in the K. I. (Castellanos and Sturgis, 1963) (figure 6.1).

6.1.2.2 Maturation Index (M.I.)

In this case 100 squamous epithelial cells are counted and classified as parabasal, intermediate or superficial cells. Thus, for example, if the count is 0 parabasal cells, 50 intermediate cells and 50 superficial cells, then the M. I. is 0:50:50. The term 'shift to the left' is used when many parabasal cells are counted; a 'shift to the right' indicates the presence of many superficial cells.

6.1.2.3 Eosinophilic Index (E. I.)

The number of squamous epithelial cells with eosinophilic cytoplasm per 100 squamous epithelial cells is counted. However, factors such as the pH of the vagina and involuntary air-drying of the cells prior to a wet fixation (see section 15.4) influence the cytoplasmic colouring so markedly that a reliable vaginal cytogram is practically impossible. In contrast, with the urocytogram the most commonly used index is the E. I.

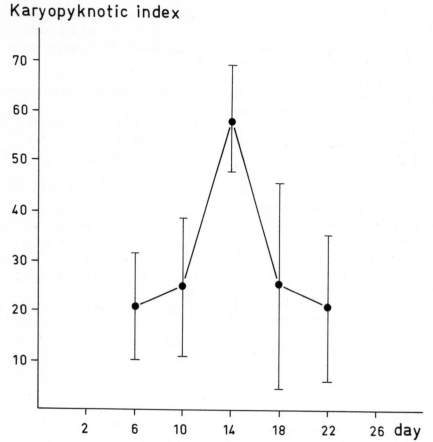

figure 6.1   Variation of the K.I. during the normal menstrual cycle with standard
deviations

Changes in oestrogen level are best described by the K. I. in both the vaginal cytogram and the urocytogram (Lencioni, 1975). At ovulation there is a peak in both the eosinophilic and in the karyo-pyknotic index, followed by a decrease in both.

6.1.2.4 The Number of Cells

In urinary sediments we deal, not with cell scraping, but with spontaneous exfoliation of squamous cells, so the number of cells can be taken into account. The number of epithelial cells per ml is dependent on the day of the cycle (Biot and Beltran Nunez, 1944).

6.1.2.5 Description of the Pattern

The cell pattern (cell crowding, exfoliation pattern, presence of navicular cells, etc.) should be described. In this way the oestrogen effect as well as the progesterone effect can be taken into account (Koss, 1968).

6.2 Cytohormonal Patterns

Since the epithelial lining is influenced by the concentration of circulating hormones, the cytological make-up of vaginal smears or urinary sediments will vary in different periods of life.

6.2.1 Physiological Cytohormonal Patterns

6.2.1.1 Birth to 7 Days

Since the maternal sex hormones can penetrate the placenta they exert an influence on the epithelia of the baby. The vaginal epithelium of a newborn child is therefore fully mature.

6.2.1.2 From the First Week to Puberty

In this period the production of sex hormones is very low. The vaginal smear will normally manifest atrophy (many parabasal cells).

6.2.1.3 Puberty

At puberty production of the sex hormones begins. The vaginal epithelium slowly reaches maturity. At first many intermediate epithelial cells are seen in the vaginal smear; when the (anovulatory) menstrual cycles begin, many superficial cells are also present. In the second half of these cycles, however, a true progesterone pattern is not yet seen (see section 6.2.1.4).

6.2.1.4 Sexual Maturity

When the menstrual cycles become ovulatory, the following consecutive patterns can be expected.
(1) *Menstrual phase* (1st–5th day). The smear contains erythrocytes, leucocytes, endometrial cells, superficial and intermediate epithelial cells.
(2) *Proliferative or follicular phase* (6th–10th day). First the 'clean-up crew' appears: a large number of histiocytes. There are also many intermediate squamous epithelial cells (without folding), polymorphonuclears, and endometrial cells (figure 6.2). Towards the end of the proliferative phase, the number of superficial squamous epithelial cells increases (Papanicolaou, 1933).
(3) *Ovulation* (11th–13th day). During this phase there are numerous superficial epithelial cells; the cells lie flat and are obviously discrete. The pattern is 'clean', that is, practically without leucocytes and with very few bacteria (figure 6.3). In air-dried smears, a fern-pattern of the endocervical mucus can be discerned.

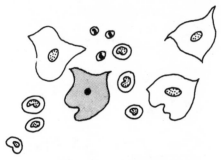

figure 6.2   **Early proliferative phase**

(4) *Secretory or luteal phase* (14th–28th day). The pattern changes abruptly after ovulation: now the intermediate squamous epithelial cells predominate. Within several days the *characteristic progesterone pattern* appears: folding and clustering of intermediate cells, navicular cells, polymorphonuclears, and many Döderlein's bacilli (figure 6.4).

Towards the end of the cycle, marked cytolysis may develop accompanied by many polymorphonuclears. Just before menstruation the K. I. increases once again. In some women endometrial cells are also seen in the smear several days before menstruation. In some women with normal ovulatory cycles, the characteristic progesterone pattern is absent and only the midcycle peak of K. I. and E. I. points to ovulation.

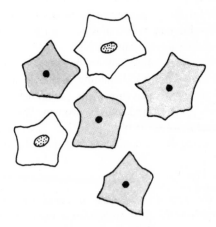

figure 6.3   **Ovulation**

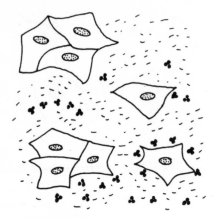

figure 6.4   Secretory phase

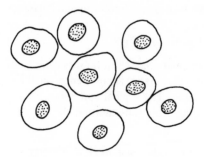

figure 6.5   Post-partum pattern

6.2.1.5 Pregnancy

In the event of pregnancy the corpus luteum does not involute but instead grows larger, producing increasing amounts of progesterone and oestrogen. The cytological pattern of pregnancy is the progesterone pattern (clustering and folding of squamous epithelial cells and the presence of navicular cells). In the first trimester it is not as pronounced as in the third, when numerous Döderlein's bacilli and the accompanying cytolysis are seen. The K. I. is less than 5.

About three months after conception, the placenta takes over from the corpus luteum the task of producing progesterone and oestrogens. If this change does not proceed smoothly, then the progesterone level may drop, sometimes even far enough for the pregnancy to be threatened. Cytologically this may be manifested as an increase in the K. I. (see also section 6.2.2.3).

In the week preceding confinement the K. I. may increase to 30, heralding a change in the function of the placenta. This phenomenon is, however, not observed in every woman. Therefore hormonal cytology is of little value in determining the expected day of confinement (Lencioni, 1975).

6.2.1.6 Post Partum

With the expulsion of the placenta the most important producer of progesterone and oestrogen disappears. The smear pattern changes to one chiefly composed of parabasal epithelial cells, which contain glycogen and are somewhat angular. The typical M. I. will be about 80:20:0. The cytoplasm of some of the parabasal cells will be pinkish red. Such cells are called 'lactational' or 'post-partum cells' (figure 6.5). They are derived from the parabasal epithelial layer which becomes hypertrophic during pregnancy and exfoliates after delivery (Boschann 1956). These cells appear in the smear until the ovarian cycle has resumed, even as long as nine months after delivery (MCLennan and McLennan, 1975). One third of the women in the post-partum period do not show these typical post-partum cells; highly divergent patterns are seen.

6.2.1.7 Lactation

If the mother nurses her child, the post-partum pattern may persist for as long as the ovarian cycle is suppressed.

6.2.1.8 Climacteric

In the climacteric the cycles may become anovulatory and irregular. In this period persistent follicles may be encountered (figure 6.6): the graafian follicle remains intact and ovulation does not occur. As a result haemorrhage or withdrawal bleeding (but not a true menstruation) may take place (see section 6.2.2.5).

During the climacteric the following cytological patterns can be encountered.

(1) In the event of ovulatory cycles: the same pattern as in sexually mature females.

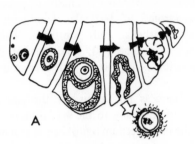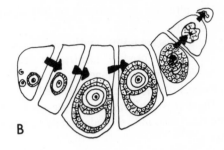

figure 6.6 Schematic drawing of the ovary with a ripening follicle. A. Ovulatory cycle; B. anovulatory cycle with persistent follicle

(2) In the event of anovulatory cycles: in the second half of the cycle there is either a high K. I. (especially if there is a persistent follicle) or a pattern of intermediate epithelial cells without glycogen storage (Symposium, 1960).

In both ovulatory and anovulatory cycles the following may also be seen.

(3) A progesterone pattern with many Döderlein's bacilli and cytolysis.

(4) The cytological pattern of early atrophy, that is, both parabasal and intermediate cells as well as some superficial epithelial cells ('mixed picture').

6.2.1.9 Postmenopause and Old Age

When ovarian cycles no longer occur the stratified squamous epithelium no longer undergoes cyclic change. A highly variable cellular pattern can be seen (Symposium, 1960).

(1) Early postmenopause: many intermediate epithelial cells which generally lie flat and separately.

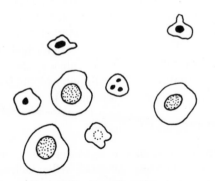

figure 6.7 Atrophic pattern

(2) Mixed pattern: all three cell types are present, for example, M. I. 30:30:40. This pattern is seldom seen except postmenopausally.

(3) Postmenopause and old age: atrophy. Parabasal cells predominate (figure 6.7). If there are many parabasal cells with reddish orange cytoplasm and a pyknotic nucleus, the pattern is called 'red atrophy'. In 75 per cent of these smears there are also reserve cells in rows or in syncytia.

6.2.2 Pathological Hormonal Patterns

In some cases deviations from the normal hormonal levels are reflected in the cytological patterns. Several examples of the abnormalities which can produce a specific cytogram are listed below.

6.2.2.1 Insufficient Corpus Luteum

A luteal insufficiency can occur in anovulatory or ovulatory cycles. In the former the K. I. remains low during the cycle; in the latter the cytogram of the first half of the cycle is normal with an ovulatory peak, but in the second half 'progesterone patterns' with cellular clustering, folding, etc., are subnormal and, in addition, the K. I. remains high.

6.2.2.2 Amenorrhoea

Amenorrhoea is the absence of menstruation in the sexually mature female. There is a distinction between primary amenorrhoea (the woman has never menstruated) and secondary amenorrhoea (the woman has menstruated at least once). The causes of amenorrhoea are highly divergent.

(1) The pituitary is inhibited by the central nervous system.

(2) The ovaries are insufficiently stimulated.

(3) The ovaries produce insufficient sex hormones or secrete male hormones.

(4) Normal ovaries have not developed.

(5) The uterus is missing, or it is present but the endometrium does not react adequately to ovarian hormones.

(6) The adrenal glands produce an excess of male hormones.

(7) The Stein–Leventhal syndrome.

(1) The pituitary can be inhibited by the brain (for example, as a result of strong emotions or stress). Consequently the ovaries are not stimulated by the pituitary gland so that the menstrual cycle does not take place. As soon as the inhibition is removed, the menstrual cycle will recur.

Cytogram: no specific pattern; no cyclic changes Barr body (+).

(2) Insufficient quantities of FSH and LH may be produced either due to a lesion in the pituitary itself or as a result of reduced stimulation of the pituitary by the hypothalamus. The ovarian follicles do not reach full maturity so that ovulation cannot take place. This is the case, for example, in Sheehan's syndrome (haemorrhage in the pituitary after delivery).

Cytogram: 'dormant pattern', that is, mainly intermediate epithelial cells without a pronounced progesterone effect; no cyclic changes; atrophy in severe cases. Barr body (+).

(3) The ovaries produce insufficient oestrogen or progesterone, for instance after damage due to irradiation; it is also possible that there is an ovarian neoplasm which secretes male hormones (arrhenoblastoma, hilus cell tumour).

Cytogram: dormant pattern, not cyclic; if there is an androgen-producing tumour, the pattern includes angular parabasal cells. Barr body (+).

(4) Normal ovaries have not developed. Some of these patients do not have a chromosomal abnormality ('true' ovarian dysgenesis, see section 5.3.1.4); others have Turner's syndrome (see section 5.3.1.1) or the syndrome of testicular feminisation (see section 5.3.2.2).

Cytogram: atrophy in patients with Turner's

syndrome or ovarian dysgenesis; in patients with the syndrome of testicular feminisation intermediate epithelial cells are seen. Barr body: Turner's syndrome (−); syndrome of testicular feminisation (−); patients with ovarian dysgenesis (+).

(5) There is no uterus, or the endometrium reacts pathologically to the sex hormones. In both cases the endometrium is not shed so that menstruation does not occur.

Cytogram: normal cyclic pattern. Barr body (+).

(6) The adrenal cortex may secrete many male hormones, for example, in congenital adrenal hyperplasia and Cushing's disease. The overproduction can be due to either hyperplasia or neoplasia of the adrenal cortex.

Cytogram: atrophic or many intermediate cells. Barr body (+).

(7) Stein-Leventhal syndrome. These patients appear virile; they generally have secondary amenorrhoea and polycystic ovaries.

Cytogram: not cyclic; many intermediate cells of the androgenic type. Barr body (+).

6.2.2.3 Abortion and Miscarriage

Abortion is the expulsion of the products of pregnancy in the first three months of pregnancy. Abortion may have many causes, including a relative shortage of progesterone. This shortage may occur especially during the third month of pregnancy when the placenta should take over hormonal production (progesterone and oestrogen) from the ovary. If this process is disturbed or fails to develop, the level of progesterone will drop so that the oestrogen predominates, expressed in the cytogram by an elevation of the K. I. and E. I. If abortion can no longer be averted, endometrial cells may be found in the smear (Wachtel, 1969). Moreover, cells from the placenta may also be seen, such as syntrophoblast cells, cytotrophoblast cells and decidual cells (see section 3.3).

6.2.2.4 High-risk Pregnancy

When the pregnancy is in danger the smear may contain numerous parabasal cells, indicating a decrease in both progesterone and oestrogen levels, or the K. I. may increase. In some cases the change is qualitative: the intermediate cells do not exfoliate in clusters but as discrete cells and there is no glycogen storage, that is, the navicular cells disappear. The hormonal levels during pregnancy can be studied in cytograms (Lencioni *et al.*, 1973). The diagnosis of disturbed pregnancy should never be made on one specimen but on repeated examinations to establish a curve of cytohormonal indices (figure 6.8).

In 62 per cent of all abnormal pregnancies the K. I. curves were abnormal; in normal pregnancies only 6 per cent of the urocytograms were classified as pathological (Lencioni, 1975). An abnormal curve means an insufficient foetoplacental unit (death of foetus, placental insufficiency, etc.). The abnormal indices may return to normal (favourable prognosis) or may get worse (unfavourable prognosis) (figure 6.8). The use of urocytograms in combination with amnioscopy can help discover an inadequately functioning placenta. If pregnancy is so far advanced that the foetus is viable, then delivery should be induced (Nyklicek, 1972).

In patients with abnormal pregnancies a small dose of oestrogen can be administered with a prognostic significance. If the K. I. was in the normal range, the result may be (1) increase of K. I. This is a bad prognostic sign. It may point to foetal death or an insufficient placenta. (2) The K. I. is not influenced. This is a good prognostic sign. It indicates an active, well-functioning foetoplacental unit. If the K. I. was already elevated the reaction may be as follows. (1) The K. I. is unchanged or is lowered. This is correlated with a favourable course of the pregnancy. (2) The K. I. increases. This is a bad prognostic sign.

The vast literature concerning the use of urocytograms in the follow-up of pathological pregnancies is surveyed in Lencioni's book (1975).

6.2.2.5 High Karyopyknotic Indices in Climacteric and Postmenopausal Women

In general it can be stated that a smear containing many superficial cells taken from a woman who is climacteric or postmenopausal is indicative of an abnormality. The chief source of oestrogen production in menopausal women is the adrenals where the precursor steroid is produced (see section 3.4.6). When the adrenals are stimulated (by anxiety for instance) all adrenal hormone levels are elevated resulting in an increased pyknotic index. A high K. I. can also be caused by the following.

(1) Persistent follicle. This is a graafian follicle which, instead of rupturing on the 14th day of the cycle, persists and continues to produce oestrogen (see figure 6.6). This is common in the climacteric and rare in sexually mature women. The cytogram shows a high K. I. (> 75). Once the follicle deteriorates bleeding can occur even though ovulation has not taken place (withdrawal bleeding). The K. I. will then decrease. However, it is also possible that bleeding will occur while the follicle is still intact; then the K. I. remains high.

(2) Oestrogen-producing ovarian neoplasms. Some ovarian neoplasms produce sex hormones, such as hilus cell tumours and arrhenoblastomas, which may secrete male sex hormones, and granulosa cell tumours, which may produce oestrogens (see section 13.1.2). The vaginal smear from postmenopausal women with a granulosa cell tumour will show a high K. I., and often small groups of endometrial cells are seen.

(3) Oestrogen-containing drugs and cosmetics can produce some oestrogen effect, resulting in a maximum K. I. of 50, and no parabasal cells.

(4) Several other pharmaceutical products such as digitalis and anticoagulant drugs also cause a high K. I.

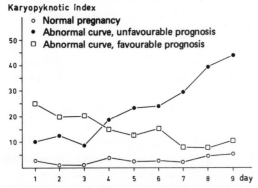

Karyopyknotic index
○ Normal pregnancy
● Abnormal curve, unfavourable prognosis
□ Abnormal curve, favourable prognosis

figure 6.8   KI curves of high-risk pregnancies. The urocytograms were made in the 34th and 35th weeks of pregnancy

6.2.2.6 Castration

When both ovaries of a sexually mature female have been excised the ovarian cycle will stop abruptly. Immediately after surgery the vaginal smear will become atrophic. Some time· later the adrenal glands may start to secrete increased amounts of oestrogen and androgen, so that the vaginal smear may contain intermediate cells, sometimes even with glycogen.

In postmenopausal women the adrenal glands are the main source of oestrogen. Stimulation of the adrenals (as in anxiety) may result in high levels of all adrenal hormones, resulting in an increased K. I.

N. B. iatrogenic influences on the cytohormonal patterns are discussed in chapter 14.

6.3 Preparatory Techniques for Cytohormonal Evaluation

The preparations for cytohormonal evaluation can be made in various ways.

(1) *Vaginal cytogram.* Swabs are taken from the lateral wall of the vagina on various days of the menstrual cycle. The patient can learn to do this herself. The smears can be stained according to the Papanicolaou or the Shorr method (see sections 15.5.1–3) (Shorr, 1941). In unstained smears the cell shape, cell size and nuclear pyknosis can be evaluated with phase contrast microscopy (Wied, 1956) but not the staining characteristics of the cytoplasm (eosinophilic or cyanophilic).

(2) *Urocytogram.* Urinary smears contain many squamous epithelial cells that can be evaluated (Lencioni and Staffieri, 1969). The preparatory technique of urinary sediments is described in section 15.3.6.

The differences between urocytograms and vaginal cytograms include (a) a smaller percentage of glycogen-containing cells in urinary sediments than in vaginal smears (25 and 50 per cent respectively) during pregnancy: (b) a lower E. I. in urinary sediments than in vaginal smears, amounting to a constant difference of approximately 10 per cent (Lencioni, 1975). The indices of urocytograms run parallel with those of vaginal cytograms

(figure 6.9). Lencioni states that the sensitivity of the two methods does not differ.

Advantages of the urocytogram are (a) the patient can provide the urine herself; (b) there is no contamination with immature (metaplastic) cells from the transformation zone at the portio; (c) there is no influence of vaginal pH; (d) there are less disturbing inflammatory changes.

Disadvantages are (a) there is more work involved; (b) the urine has to be prefixed or a bacteriostatic agent has to be added to prevent the detrimental effect of bacterial growth (see section 15.3.6).

(3) *Buccal cytogram.* Swabs are made of the mucous membrane of the cheek (Anderson et al., 1969). This mucous membrane also reacts to changes in the hormone levels.

These three examinations can be repeated daily if necessary. The indices of buccal cytograms run parallel with those of vaginal cytograms (figure 6.9).

(4) *Endometrial aspiration.* The secretory activity of the endometrial cells in the luteal phase of the menstrual cycle can be evaluated.

6.3.1 Prerequisites for a Reliable Cytohormonal Evaluation of the Stratified Squamous Epithelium

In order to be able to evaluate a cytogram properly, the best possible well-fixed smears must be available. Air-drying prior to wet fixation makes the staining characteristics of the cytoplasm unreliable (see section 15.4). In addition, whoever evaluates the smears must have the following data at hand: (1) age of the patient; (2) date the smear was taken; (3) date of the last menstrual period; (4) hormone therapy (contraceptive, etc.); (5) reason for examination.

In order to be able to evaluate the menstrual cycle (for example, has ovulation occurred?), several smears (at least three) must be taken during one cycle, preferably for 2–3 cycles. The following points must be taken into consideration.

(1) Infection. A smear cannot be evaluated if trichomoniasis, mycotic infections or bacterial infections exist.

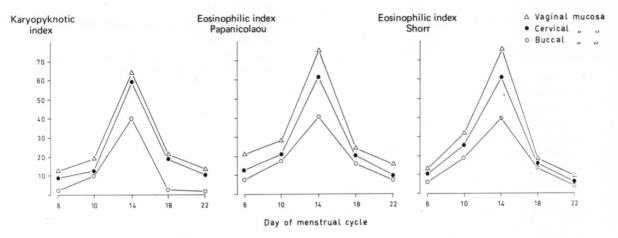

figure 6.9 K.I. and E.I. curves of the same patient during one menstrual cycle

(2) Exogenous hormone effects cannot be distinguished from the endogenous ones.

(3) Drugs can affect the pattern of the vaginal smear; for example, tetracycline causes a shift towards intermediate cells (Koss, 1968) and digitalis and anticoagulants generally induce a shift towards superficial cells (see section 6.2.2.5).

(4) In general anucleated superficial epithelial cells are not the result of a high oestrogen level but are due to contamination from the vulvar skin, infection, the presence of a pessary or prolapse.

(5) Döderlein's bacilli can complicate the smear evaluation by causing marked cytolysis. Such patterns are seen when the progesterone level is high (for example, during pregnancy), in the climacteric and when certain contraceptive drugs are used. Cytologically these can be differentiated by first destroying the Döderlein's bacilli with an antibiotic (Symposium, 1962).

6.3.2 Application of Cytohormonal Evaluation

(1) Assessment of ovulation. The day of ovulation is the day of the peak of the eosinophilic and karyopycnotic indices (see figure 6.9). The duration of the follicular and luteal phases can thus be calculated. In fertility studies, when ovulation is induced by drugs, hormonal cytology can help evaluate the effect of the drug.

(2) Analysis of amenorrhoea (see section 6.2.2.2).

(3) Monitoring high-risk pregnancies such as diabetic pregnancies (Lencioni *et al.*, 1973).

(4) Assessment of the effect of hormonal drugs (for example, treatment of breast cancer with hormones). The oestrogenic potency of the drugs is expressed by the elevation of the K. I.

(5) Treatment of climacteric complaints. Some postmenopausal women with widely fluctuating K. I.s may profit from a low dose of oestrogen to stabilise the hormonal status (Lencioni, 1975). In women under oestrogen treatment the E. I. of the urocytogram should not surpass 30, and the K. I. should not be over 60 (Lencioni, 1975).

(6) Epidemiological studies. In patients with carcinoma *in situ* of the cervix the K. I. is high compared with patients of a control group of the same age (Rubio, 1973) (see section 10.2.3.2).

References

Anderson, W. R., Belding, J. and Pixley, E. (1969). Oral cytology: a hormonal evaluation. *Acta Cytol.*, **13**, 81–3

Biot, R. and Beltran Nunez, N. (1944). Modificaciones periodicas del sedimento urinario en relación con el ciclo menstruel. Su posible aplicación como test de ovulación. *Sem Méd. Buonos Aires*, **2**, 532

Boschann, H. W. (1956). Cytologische Unter-suchungen über die Wirkung von Androgenen am atrofischen Vagina-epitheel in Abhängigkeit von Dosierung und Applikationsakt. *Arch. Gynäk.*, **187**, 39

Castellanos, H. and Sturgis, S. H. (1963). Urinary cytology in the endocrine evaluation of the normal female. *Progr. Gynaec.*, **IV**, 98

Koss, L. G. (1968). *Diagnostic Cytology and its Histopathologic Bases*, Lippincott, Philadelphia, p. 131

Lencioni, L. J. (1975). *L'Urocytogramme*, Maloine, Paris

Lencioni, L. J., Martinez Amézaga, L. A., Alonso, C. and Hungria de Camargo, L. A. (1973). Urocytogram and Pregnancy II: correlation with fetal condition at birth in high risk preg-nancies. *Acta Cytol.*, **17**, 125–7

Leneioni, L. J. and Staffieri, J. J. (1969). Urocyto-gram diagnosis of sexual precocity. *Acta Cytol.*, **13**, 382–8

McLennan, M. T. and McLennan, C. E. (1975). Hormonal patterns in vaginal smears from puerperal women. *Acta Cytol.*, **19**, 431–3

Nyklicèk, O. (1972). Vaginal cytology and amnio-scopy in prolonged pregnancies. *Acta Cytol.*, **16**, 48–50

Papanicolaou, G. N. (1925). The diagnosis of early pregnancy by the vaginal smear method. *Proc. Soc. exp. Biol. Med.*, **22**, 436

Papanicolaou, G. N. (1933). The sexual cycle in the human female as revealed by vaginal smears. *Am. J. Anat.*, **52**, 519

Papanicolaou, G. N. (1948). Diagnosis of preg-nancy by cytologic criteria in catheterized urine. *Proc. Soc. exp. Biol. Med.*, **67**, 247

Pundel, J. P. (1957). *Acquisitions Récentes en Cytologie Vaginale Hormonale*, Masson, Paris, pp. 143–7

Rubio, C. A. (1973). Estrogenic effect in vaginal smears in cases of carcinoma in situ and micro-invasive carcinoma of the uterine cervix. *Acta Cytol.*, **17**, 361–5

Shorr, E. (1941). A new technique for staining vaginal smears. A single differential stain. *Science*, **94**, 545

Symposium on effects of endogenous estrogens on the vaginal epithelium (1960). *Acta Cytol.*, **4**, 9–154

Symposium on effects of progestational agents (1962). *Acta Cytol.*, **6**, 211–310

Wachtel, E. G. (1969). *Exfoliative Cytology in Gynaecological Practice*, Butterworths, London, pp. 55–145

Wied, G. L. (1956). Phase contrast microscopy, an office technique for prescreening of cytological vaginal smears. *Am. J. Gynec.*, **71**, 806

Wied, G. L. (1968). The cytologic indices for hormonal assessment. Symposium on Hormonal Cytology. *Acta Cytol.*, **12**, 87–127

Wied. G. L., del Sol, J. R. and Dargan, A. M. (1958). Progestational and androgenic substances tested on the highly proliferated vaginal epithelium of surgical castrates. II. Androgenic substances. *Am. J. Obst. Gynec.*, **75**, 289

Benign Changes in the Vagina, Cervix and Endometrium
Part I: Infection and Inflammation

7.1 Introduction

Infection is the invasion of the body by micro-organisms which may lead to inflammation. The agent causing the infection may come from outside the body (exogenous) or it may have been a commensal microorganism in the host which, for some reason, multiplied suddenly and spread within the host (commensal infection).

Inflammation is a local reaction to tissue injury caused by microorganisms, physical agents (irradiation, cauterisation), mechanical factors (trauma) or chemical (caustic) agents. The development and cause of infection depend on

(1) the virulence of the microorganism;

(2) the resistance of the body;

(3) the growth-inhibiting effect of other microorganisms present;

(4) the condition of the tissue at the relevant site.

The resistance of the body is highly dependent upon the constitution and state of health of the individual.

7.2 Infection and Inflammation in the Vagina, Cervix and Endometrium

There are several types of commensal microorganism which live in the vagina and the cervix of their hostess; it can be said that they exist together in an equilibrium. If this equilibrium is disturbed, these microorganisms can multiply. A commensal infection then develops (that is, an infection caused by microorganisms which were already present in the body) which can lead to inflammation.

The natural protection of the vagina and the cervix against infections is determined by

(1) the stratified squamous epithelium in the vagina and ectocervix;

(2) the acidity (pH) in the vagina;

(3) the equilibrium between the various microorganisms present;

(4) a good state of general health.

Thus the chance that invasion from outside or a commensal infection will cause inflammation depends upon whether one or more of the following has occurred.

(1) Damage to the squamous epithelium by mechanical or chemical factors (trauma, change in pH, use of vaginal sprays, etc.).

(2) Ectopy (see section 2.2.3.2). Endocervical columnar epithelium can more easily be penetrated by bacteria.

(3) Decrease in the thickness of the squamous epithelium (atrophic epithelium is only a few cell layers thick).

(4) Change from acidic to neutral or alkaline environment. During the menstrual cycle the pH varies from 6.8 during menstruation to 3.9 during the second half of the cycle. The bacterium *Haemophilus vaginalis* grows best in a neutral environment, trichomonads in an alkaline environment.

(5) Rapid increase in or abundant supply of microorganisms.

(6) Deterioration of the general condition of the woman.

Most patients with (endo)cervicitis complain of a 'white discharge' (leucorrhoea). Sometimes it will contain blood. Leucorrhoea implies an excessive amount of usually whitish discharge from the cervix. It can be caused by (1) microorganisms; (2) hormones. The discharge caused by hormones is a clear mucus. (3) allergy. Discharge can develop, for example, as an allergic reaction to rubber condoms.

In vaginitis the main complaints are burning and dryness of the vagina. Spread of the infection, causing endometritis and salpingitis, can give rise to pain in the lower abdomen. Acute endometritis may develop after delivery or abortion, and is usually due to bacterial infection.

7.2.1 Histology of Inflammation

An inflammatory process develops primarily in the stroma in close proximity to the capillaries. The local reaction to inflammation includes hyperaemia, escape of fluid (exudation), escape of polymorphonuclear neutrophilic leucocytes (leucopedesis) and later also changes in the stroma. Leucocytes and macrophages (including histiocytes) are involved in phagocytosis. Eosinophilic granulocytes are found, particularly when the inflammation is due to allergy or parasites. In addition to local inflammatory reactions, regional reactions (involvement of the lymphnodes causing lymphadenitis) and general phenomena (fever, leucocytosis) can develop. When inflammation persists, it becomes chronic. The cellular infiltrate then changes in character: instead of polymorphonuclears, lymphocytes, plasma cells and histiocytes now predominate.

7.2.2 Cytology of Inflammation

The smear will contain histiocytes and many polymorphonuclears. In the event of chronic inflammation, plasma cells and lymphocytes may also be found. The epithelial cells show inflammatory changes and epithelial breakdown products may be found in the background. In addition, many different microorganisms may be observed such as trichomonads, fungi and various bacteria. Culture is necessary to determine whether the bacteria are pathogenic, that is, whether they are capable of causing the observed inflammatory changes in the epithelium. In addition to the changes in the squamous epithelium, the *composition of the cell population* will also change. When the upper layers of the epithelium have been affected, cells from the lower layers of the epithelium (parabasal cells) will be seen. This phenomenon is even more pronounced when there is marked regeneration of already injured epithelium (see section 7.5.2) (Bibbo and Wied, 1973). The inflammatory irritation, on the other hand, may increase the maturation of the squamous epithelium, leading to a smear pattern with predominantly superficial cells and sometimes with anucleate squames.

In general a pattern is identified as inflammatory only when the smear reveals that

(1) there is a marked leucocytosis (mild and moderate leucocytosis are physiological);

(2) the epithelial cells are completely covered with leucocytes or leucophagocytosis has developed;

(3) plasma cells and/or lymphocytes are present;

(4) changes can be seen in the epithelial cells or in the composition of the cell population, or both;

(5) virocytes are present (see section 7.3.5.1);

(6) pathogenic microorganisms are present (for example, trichomonads, fungal filaments or spores, etc.).

7.2.2.1 Inflammatory Changes in Squamous Epithelial Cells

Both the cytoplasm and the nucleus can undergo changes in the presence of inflammation.

The *cytoplasm* can show the following abnormalities.

(1) *Vacuolisation.*   Small vacuoles may appear in the cytoplasm; sometimes they will merge into one large vacuole which pushes the nucleus to one side.

The thin border of cytoplasm can usually be identified as that of a squamous epithelial cell because it retains its compact appearance. Sometimes leucocytes are seen in the epithelial cells, usually in a vacuole; this is leucophagocytosis.

(2) *Cytolysis.* The cytoplasm first appears ragged, and finally dissolves completely. Only the nucleus is left. This occurs in particular when Döderlein's bacilli are present.

(3) *Perinuclear halo.* The cytoplasm at the nuclear membrane is lighter in colour. The boundary between the light and dark zones of cytoplasm is vague (figure 7.1A).

figure 7.1 Changes in squamous epithelial cells due to inflammation. A. Perinuclear halo; B. cytoplasm appears compact; C. karyorrhexis; D. pyknosis; E. enlarged nucleus; F. karyolysis

(4) *Changes in staining reaction.* When a certain type of inflammation is involved, the intermediate cells may be stained pink (eosinophilia). In senile vaginitis (inflammation of atrophic squamous epithelium) the basal cells may be stained red; the cytoplasm then appears more dense than normal (figure 7.1B). The change to a cytoplasmic eosinophilic staining reaction is due to ischaemia or degeneration.

The following changes can be seen in the *nucleus.*

(1) The nucleus can be enlarged and pale due to fluid absorption (figure 7.1E). This results in *anisonucleosis* or *anisokaryosis* (the nuclei vary in size).

(2) Multinucleation is common.

(3) There can be wrinkling of the nuclear membranes and selective condensation of the chromatin at the nuclear margin with clearing of the nuclear centre. There is retention of nuclear symmetry, and the nucleolus disappears (Gondos, 1974).

(4) Degeneration may cause nuclear shrivelling or *pyknosis*, disintegration of the nucleus into fragments or *karyorrhexis*, or dissolution of the cell or *karyolysis* (figure 7.1D, C, F) or any combination of these.

Characteristics of degenerating cells shared with dysplastic and malignant cells include nuclear enlargement, chromatin condensation, hyperchromasia and cytoplasmic vacuolisation. Dysplastic and malignant cells, however, usually exhibit *diffuse* chromatin clumping (in contrast to the 'empty' nucleus with marginal chromatin condensation in inflammation), irregular nuclear borders (polymorphism) and enlarged irregular nucleoli (Gondos, 1974) (see section 9.5.2.1).

Atrophic smears may contain cyanophilic bodies ('blue blobs'), similar in size and shape to parabasal cells. At the centre of these bodies the remains of a shrunken nucleus can almost always be found. These cells must not be mistaken for nuclei of cancer cells or trichomonads. 'Blue blobs' will be found in smears from postmenopausal women, containing predominantly parabasal cells in various stages of degeneration. Ultimately the 'blue blobs' disintegrate to form granular background material. No inflammatory reaction is present (Ziabkowski and Naylor, 1976).

7.2.2.2 Inflammatory Changes in Endocervical Columnar Epithelial Cells

(1) *Changes in the cytoplasm.*   The cytoplasm of endocervical glandular cells is no longer well defined, but lies in tatters around the nucleus. The vacuoles in the cytoplasm may contain one or more polymorphonuclears or the remains thereof. In a small number of cases numerous anucleate small ciliated tufts are found (terminal plate and pink or red cilia) in the smear next to endocervical columnar cells without cilia but with vacuolated cytoplasm, resembling histiocytes. This phenomenon, called ciliocytophthoria (CCP), originally thought to be caused by a virus, is probably a degenerative change (Muller Kobold-Wolterbeek and Beyer-Boon, 1975).

(2) *Changes in the nucleus.*   The nuclei can vary markedly in size (anisonucleosis) but the shape is always round to oval. The nucleus sometimes has a large nucleolus, occasionally even two. The chromatin may be somewhat coarsened but never markedly so. Nuclear overlapping (as occasionally seen in malignant columnar cells) does not occur. Multinucleation is common in endocervicitis; in a multinucleate endocervical cell, nuclear overlapping can be encountered. In the event of regeneration, mitotic figures are seen in the endocervical epithelium.

7.2.2.3 Inflammatory Changes in Endometrial Cells

The cervical smear will contain groups of endometrial epithelial cells with slightly swollen nuclei and sometimes small nucleoli. Often there are polymorphonuclears between the epithelial cells. In chronic endometritis, plasma cells or lymphocytes may appear among the endometrial epithelial cells.

7.2.2.4 Background of the Preparation

If there is an inflammatory process the background of the smear may consist of fibrin (pink granular material), protein, leucocytes and cellular debris. Protein stains a smooth pink, in contrast to mucus which is streaked. In section 10.2.3.2 the background encountered when a malignant neoplasm is present is discussed in detail.

7.2.3 Special Types of Cervicitis, Vaginitis and Endometritis

7.2.3.1 Chronic Lymphocytic Cervicitis (Follicular cervicitis)

Chronic lymphocytic cervicitis is characterised histologically by subepithelial (cervical or vaginal mucosa) collections of lymphocytes admixed with reticulum cells (Roberts and Ng, 1975). In some cases follicle formation is noted. By ulceration or by scraping the cervix firmly, elements of a follicle may be found in the smear, such as:

(1) small or mature lymphocytes characterised by a round hyperchromatic nucleus with an uniformly dense chromatin and no nucleoli. A thin rim of cytoplasm may be present (see section 3.1.2.2).

(2) large or immature lymphocytes, 1.5–3 times the size of the small lymphocytes with less hyperchromatic nuclei.

(3) reticulum cells with pale nuclei and prominent nucleoli (see section 3.1.5). There is often evidence of phagocytosis. Mitotic figures are often observed.

(4) Plasma cells, histiocytes and polymorphonuclear leucocytes may also be present.

All the cells occur *singly* and aggregates are not observed. If this pattern is not recognised the cells can erroneously be interpreted as malignant undifferentiated cells. These small malignant cells are less anisokaryotic and exfoliate in cell groupings (Roberts and Ng, 1975). Also the smear pattern is easily mistaken for malignant lymphoma. In malignant lymphoma, however, the pattern is usually monotonous consisting of only one type of cell, whereas various cells are seen in chronic lymphocytic cervicitis (Eisenstein and Battifora, 1965).

7.2.3.2 Senile Vaginitis

Senile vaginitis is inflammation of the atrophic epithelium of the cervix and vagina. It is characterised by parabasal cells with pycnotic or fragmented nuclei or both, a change in the staining reaction of the cytoplasm (red instead of blue, which is the reason for the term 'red atrophy'; Koss, 1968) and a tendency to form syncytia (Smolka and Soost, 1971). These smears often have dark purple streaks composed of nuclei that have been streaked out by the spatula when the smear was made. The cytological picture of senile vaginitis may be difficult to interpret. The pycnotic nuclei in particular may cause problems in evaluation. It is essential to remember that these nuclei are dark and homogeneous without a clearly defined chromatin pattern.

When interpretation of a smear from a patient with senile vaginitis is difficult, the clinician can be requested to treat the patient with oestrogen, either vaginally or by mouth. A new smear taken 2–3 days later will have a 'clean' background and mature epithelial cells. If carcinoma cells are present they should be easily recognisable because they do not react to oestrogen.

7.2.3.3 Specific Inflammations

The term specific inflammation is used whenever a specific pathogenic agent gives rise to a specific morphological picture. One such example is *tuberculosis.*

Almost always tuberculous endometritis or cervicitis is secondary to tuberculosis of the fallopian tubes (which results from a primary tuberculosis of the lung or intestine). Histological examination reveals that the stroma of the endometrium or cervix contains caseous necrosis surrounded by epithelioid cells (tubercles), histiocytes and Langhans' giant cells. The cervical smears include elements of the granulomas such as: (1) epithelioid cells. These cells have slender nuclei, a fine chromatin pattern and ill-defined cytoplasm; (2) histiocytes; (3) lymphocytes and plasma cells; (4) Langhans' giant cells, with their character-

istic location of the nuclei towards the periphery of the cytoplasm. They resemble histiocytic giant cells, whose nuclei are more central and whose cytoplasm may contain digested material.

If epithelioid cells and Langhans' giant cells are found in the smear then tuberculosis should be considered (Highman, 1972). The final diagnosis can only be established on the basis of histological and bacteriological studies (Ziehl Neelsen stain for acid-fast bacilli). The pattern of tuberculous endometritis or cervicitis must be distinguished from that of tissue repair and ulceration (see sections 7.5.1 and 2). The cytological pattern of tuberculous vaginitis is the same as that of tuberculous endometritis (Coleman, 1969). One should realise, however, that tuberculous endometritis or cervicitis is now rare in Western society.

7.3 The Microbacteriological Flora of the Vagina and the Cervix

7.3.1 Bacteria

Bacteria are unicellular organisms which are fairly small (about 2 μm in diameter) with a barely differentiated structure. They consist of nuclear material or karyoplasm (there is no nuclear membrane) and cytoplasm with a cytoplasmic membrane. This is enclosed by a cell wall. Some bacteria also have a capsule (for example, pathogenic streptococci and pneumococci) and flagella or whiplike processes which provide the bacteria with a means of locomotion (figure 7.2). All nutritional elements necessary for the growth of the bacteria must be present in the environment and physico–

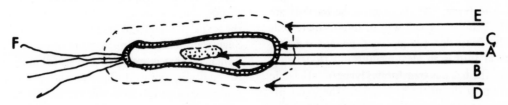

figure 7.2   Schematic drawing of a bacterium. A. Karyoplasm; B. cytoplasm; C. cytoplasmic membrane; D. cell wall; E. capsule; F. flagella

chemical factors (temperature, osmosity, etc.) must meet specific requirements. This dependence upon the environment is used to identify bacteria: a specific type of bacteria will multiply rapidly in a certain medium whereas the same bacteria will just be able to remain in equilibrium or will die out in a different medium.

Bacteria can fulfil a useful function; however they may also be pathogenic either in a restricted sense (that is, under certain circumstances) or without restrictions (that is, their mere presence is sufficient). The term pathogenic means 'capable of inducing sickness'. An example of an unrestricted pathogenic bacterium is *Pasteurella pestis*. Restricted pathogenic bacteria induce sickness only under certain circumstances, such as superabundance of microorganisms, lowered resistance of the host, a change in the environment favourable to the microorganism, destruction of the autochthonous flora, changes in or damage to the protective epithelium, etc.

Bacteria are classified according to their morphological characteristics, such as rod-shaped (bacilli), spherical (cocci), spiral-shaped (spirochetes), as well as their biochemical and physiological characteristics, such as an affinity for a certain stain (Gram-negative and Gram-positive), growth capacity and growth pattern in a specific medium, dependence on oxygen (aerobe, facultative aerobe, and anaerobe) and resistance to specific antibiotics.

In routine cytology it is only possible to establish the shape of the bacteria; further identification must be left to a bacteriologist.

7.3.1.1 Autochthonous Flora of the Vagina

(1) *Döderlein's bacilli or lactobacilli.*   Döderlein's bacilli are rod-shaped; they can be connected in chains (figure 7.3). The bacteria vary in length from 3 to 6 μm. The *enzymes* of the bacteria are able to dissolve the cell wall of intermediate cells (cytolysis) so that the glycogen present is freed, which in turn is an ideal medium for Döderlein's bacilli. The bacillus transforms glycogen into lactic acid causing the pH to be lowered. The lower pH provides an optimum environment for Döderlein's bacilli, which now multiply rapidly.

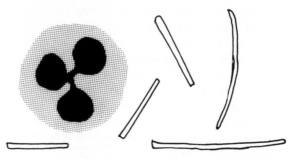

figure 7.3   Long and short Döderlein's bacilli. For comparison purposes a leucocyte is also shown

A vaginal flora predominantly composed of Döderlein's bacilli is found under the following conditions: during pregnancy, during the second half of the menstrual cycle, when progesterone-containing contraceptive drugs are used, and sometimes during the menopause, especially in diabetic patients.

(2) *Corynebacterium.*   These Gram-positive rods can be discriminated from lactobacilli by their arrangement in groups. It is almost impossible to identify them in the cervical smear. These bacteria can proliferate in the vagina because the mucous membrane functions as culture medium. Decaying epithelial cells ensure a continuous supply of nutrients in the form of amino acids and glycogen.

7.3.1.2 Flora from Outside

Bacteria from the surrounding environment (skin, towels, etc.) can enter the vagina. If the autochthonous flora is poorly developed, as in a young girl with atrophic glycogen-poor epithelium, they can dominate the field. In the sexually mature female, most of the microorganisms from outside (from the skin or the peritoneum) are introduced during coitus. Semen can contain pathogenic microorganisms from the prostate or urethra of the sexual partner (who has prostatitis or urethritis). Such transmission of microorganisms is said to be 'venereal', that is, pertaining to sexual intercourse. In addition, coitus influences the pH and the protein concentration in the vagina (the ejaculate is very rich in protein) which can affect bacterial growth. For example, we found that if Döderlein's bacilli are observed in the smear of the female partner before coitus, they will have disappeared about 12 hours after coitus and be replaced by cocci (the peritoneal flora). About 16 hours after coitus this phenomenon is at its maximum; the preparation may be covered entirely by a cloud of bacteria without any sign of a leucocytic reaction or inflammatory changes in the epithelial cells ('coitus effect'). In these smears the pattern is more 'mature' (many superficial epithelial cells) than before coitus, when the glycogen-containing intermediate cells predominate. Thirty-two hours after coitus, Döderlein's bacilli reappear and the glycogen-containing intermediate cells are once again dominant. When a condom is used the vaginal flora does not change.

In general, one has to be very cautious when reporting on the bacterial flora seen in smears. The cytological picture of a bacterial infection is characterised by a general eosinophilia of the cells, and nuclear pyknosis. The bacteria cover the smear, flocking together at the cell margins of epithelial cells, giving them a frailed appearance. Inflammatory changes of the epithelial cells (see section 7.2.2) are noted. Large numbers of polymorphonuclears and bacteria may hide the epithelial cells. In that case a repeat smear after adequate therapy should be made.

The flora from outside include

(1) *Perineal bacteria.*   Bacteria in the intestine and on the skin are a heterogeneous group consisting of large and small rods, and cocci which lie adjacent to one another and can be confused with diplococci. This flora can also include staphylo-

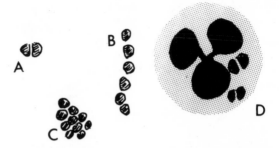

figure 7.4   A. Diplococci; B. streptococci; C. staphylococci; D. intracellular diplococci in a polymorphonuclear leucocyte

cocci (in groups resembling a bunch of grapes) and streptococci (in chains) (figure 7.4). Staphylococci and streptococci are only pathogenic in the vagina when the epithelium is damaged. The perineum flora can be introduced into the vagina during coitus but also, for example, during vaginal examination.

(2) *Haemophilus vaginalis.*   *Haemophilus vaginalis* is a small rod-shaped bacterium. It is probably the most common inflicting agent in the vagina. It is transmitted by sexual intercourse. In the smear these bacteria are seen mainly *on* squamous epithelial cells which, as a result, stain dark purple and appear cloudy (figure 7.5). In the North American literature these cells are called 'clue cells'. These clue cells must be discriminated from epithelial cells covered with Döderlein's bacilli (clearly defined, not cloudy) or with perineal bacteria (frailed cell margins).

(3) *Leptothrix.*   *Leptothrix* is a nonpathogenic

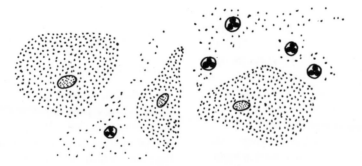

figure 7.5   Clue cell with *Haemophilus vaginalis*

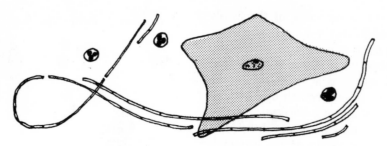

figure 7.6   *Leptothrix*

thread-like bacterium which can lie in loops and sometimes in pairs (figure 7.6). *Leptothrix* are much longer than Döderlein's bacilli and the latter never lie in loops. *Leptothrix* is often found with trichomonads; however, they can also be encountered in the smear without trichomonads or other organisms.

(4) *Gonococci. Gonococcus* is the organism which causes gonorrhoea. The bacteria are shaped like coffee beans and are found in a characteristic pattern of pairs (diplococci) whereby the round sides of the two beans face outwards (see figure 7.4). They are slightly larger than the cocci in the perineal flora. In most cases the intracellular diplococci can be found in routine screening of the Papanicolaou-stained cervical smears (Arsenault *et al.*, 1976). If such bacteria are found in a leucocyte (intracellular), this must be reported and a bacteriological culture must be recommended. *Gonococci* may be found in cervical smears although the infection is not always suspected clinically.

(5) *Mycobacterium tuberculosis* (see section 7.2.3.3)

(6) *Actinomyces. Actinomyces* belong to the 'higher' bacteria. They can be found in women with an IUD in situ (Gupta *et al.*, 1976). When the Papanicolaou stain is used, they appear as bales of wool with thin threads protruding outwards. At a high magnification the threads sometimes resemble strings of beads with branches at right angles.

In addition to the above groups, many other bacteria may be present in the cervico-vaginal smears which cannot be distinguished morpho-logically with the Papanicolaou stain. The names of the various microorganisms inhabiting the genitalia are found in table 7.1.

7.3.2 Mycoplasma

Mycoplasmas are microorganisms which are so small that they pass through bacterial filters. They can barely be seen with the light microscope. Mycoplasmas are not classified as viruses because, in contrast to viruses, they can grow in a cell-free medium, contain both DNA and RNA and are sensitive to antibiotics (Märdh *et al.*, 1971). It is presumed that a certain type of mycoplasma, the so-called 'T-strain', is responsible for urethritis and vaginitis (Taylor-Robinson *et al.*, 1969).

Cytological pattern: the epithelial cells are covered by a blue cloud of ill-defined structures. There are numerous polymorphonuclears; trichomonads are also often found. The epithelial cells sometimes have perinuclear halos which can be caused by either the mycoplasma or the trichomonads (Meisels *et al.*, 1971).

7.3.3 Protozoa

7.3.3.1 Trichomonas vaginalis

Trichomonas vaginalis is a protozoan which is found in the vagina, either as a saprophyte or as a pathogenic organism (Bridland, 1962). This unicellular microorganism moves by means of a trailing flagellum which is not seen in Papanicolaou-stained preparations.

table 7.1: Classification of the genital microorganisms (Dunlop, 1975)

(1) Autochthonous vaginal strains without aetiological significance
Lactobacillus acidophilus (Döderlein's bacilli)
Corynebacteria
Streptococcus

(2) Perineal flora
Enterococci
Escherichia coli
Proteus sp.
Pseudomonas aeruginosa
Corynebacteria
Staphylococcus albus
Streptococci

(3) Causative agents of vaginal discharge and endometritis
Haemophilus vaginalis
Corynebacteria
Neisseria gonorrhoeae (gonococcus)
Bacteroides
Mycobacterium tuberculosis
Nocardia
Mycoplasmas
Trichomonas vaginalis
Candida sp.
Viruses

The staining reaction of trichomonads is grey, bluish grey or greenish grey. It is pear-shaped to triangular or rounded. It can vary from 8 to 20 μm in diameter. An oval, faintly stained nucleus and fine red granules may be seen in the organism (figure 7.7).

In the event of a pronounced inflammatory reaction, the characteristic purple colour of the smear is striking; it is caused by the combination of the pinkish red colour of the mature epithelial cells and the blue polymorphonuclears. The polymorphonuclears are often arranged as an agglomeration around the parasite. The nuclei of the squamous epithelial cells are enlarged and hyperchromatic; the chromatin pattern can be irregular and a perinuclear halo may be seen. Secondary

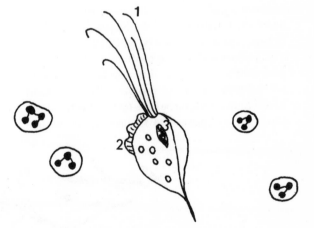

figure 7.7   Schematic drawing of a *Trichomonas*.
1. Flagella; 2. undulating membrane; 3. nucleus

organgeophilia of parabasal and intermediate cells is common. Sometimes the epithelial changes are such that a mild dysplasia is suspected. For this reason it is recommended that a second smear be taken after treatment of the infection to be certain that the changes seen were indeed caused by infection with the trichomonad.

In atrophic smears, mucus, cell fragments and parabasal cells showing karyolysis are often incorrectly identified as trichomonads.

An infection due to *Trichomonas vaginalis* can produce the following clinical phenomena; (1) foamy vaginal discharge or leucorrhoea;(2) dryness of the vagina; (3) post-coital bleeding or inter-menstrual bleeding or both. Trichomoniasis can, but need not, give rise to inflammation.

Some authors believe that trichomoniasis gives an increased risk of developing squamous carcinoma *in situ* (Meisels, 1969). Prolonged trichomoniasis which has not been treated does indeed occur in the same socioeconomic classes as carcinoma *in situ*; however, a *causal* relationship has never been demonstrated (Collette, 1976). According to Koss (1959), it is possible that epithelium which has undergone malignant changes is more susceptible to trichomoniasis than normal epithelium.

7.3.3.2 Entamoeba histolytica

Entamoeba histolytica infection is widespread in (sub)tropical areas. Amoebiasis outside of the gastrointestinal tract is infrequent, but has been observed, for instance, in the female genital tract. It produces a wide variety of clinical symptoms and findings and can be confused with malignant disease. The cytological diagnosis is based mainly on the presence of the protozoa. The organisms have a round—oval shape $(15-60\ \mu m^2)$ with faintly basophilic cytoplasm and frequent erythrophago-

cytosis. The nucleus is small. The background of the smear may contain many polymorphonuclears and necrotic granular material. With the aid of the PAS stain the parasite can be readily identified because of its high glycogen content (Fentanes de Torres and Benitez-Bribiesca, 1973).

7.3.4 Fungi

Fungi are microorganisms which multiply through spore formation or division. The spores grow into long filaments (hyphae) which in turn form branches to become a mycelium. The rudimentary part derived from the spore is the thallus. For classification of fungi, the nature and the presence or absence of the mycelium and the method of spore formation are important. The simplest forms of colony and spore formation are seen in the unicellular fungi: the *Saccharomyces* (baker's yeast) and the *Cryptococcus*. These reproduce by bud formation (gemmation) and do not produce a mycelium. The mother cell develops a bud which breaks off and grows into a mature cell which in turn also produces a bud. A slightly more complicated type of fungus is *Candida* in which several germinal ducts develop from the spore. The germinal ducts form long branching hyphae in which cell division occurs. New spores develop on the hyphae.

Cytological pattern: with the Papanicolaou stain the filaments of *Candida* become pinkish red, sometimes light blue; they have an obvious structure (resembling a bamboo cane) in contrast to structureless threads of mucus (figure 7.8). Sometimes the branches can be seen clearly. The epithelial cells often lie in clusters (progesterone pattern, see section 6.1.1.2) from which the fungal

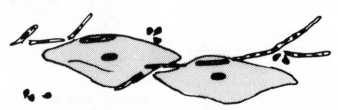

figure 7.8   Filaments and spores of *Candida*

filaments protrude like spider's legs. The *fungal spores* resemble grape seeds. Usually, but *not* always, numerous polymorphonuclears are seen, many of which may be fragmented.

In the case of a *Torulopsis* infection (Criptococcaceae family) spores of variable size (2–8 μm) with unilateral gemmation are seen in small groups or isolated. Filamentation is absent. The spores may surround the epithelial cells. Döderleins bacilli are often present. Cellular alteration is slight; eosinophilia is frequently encountered (Boquet-Jiménez and Alvarez San Cristóbal, 1978).

Most of the fungal infections in the vagina are caused by *Candida* (also called *Monilia*), a few by *Geotrichum candidum* (Dunlop, 1975) and *Torulopsis*. Vaginal *Torulopsis* produces few clinical symptoms such as a slight pruritus or burning. Leucorrhoea is scarce. In contrast, the clinical picture of a *Candida* infection is (1) vaginal discharge: white, cheesy, placque-like, not odiferous; (2) redness of the mucous membrane; (3) marked itching of the vulva or vagina, or both.

Candida infections occur predominantly (1) when the progesterone level is high (during pregnancy and when contraceptive drugs are used); (2) when the bacterial equilibrium is disturbed, for example, by broad-spectrum antibiotics or chemotherapeutic drugs; (3) in women who often wash the vagina with soap. Soap disrupts the equilibrium of the normal bacterial flora; (4) in diabetics.

7.3.5 Viruses

A virus is a submicroscopic organism which is characterised by the absence of independent metabolism and by reproduction that is possible only in living healthy cells of man or animals, in embryonic tissue (chicken eggs) or in cells of a tissue culture. Many viruses are smaller than bacteria and can therefore pass through bacteria filters. Viruses contain only one nucleic acid, either DNA or RNA; otherwise they consist of protein. In addition some viruses contain fats and carbohydrates. Many viruses can remain for long periods in human cells without causing signs of illness (latent). In this period the virus is undetectable. Under certain conditions (stress, for instance)

the virus can multiply and the infection will then pass from 'latent' to 'clinically manifest', and the virus becomes again detectable.

Early in this century Ellerman and Bang demonstrated that the chicken leukaemia virus is oncogenic, that is, induces cancer. The oncogenicity of the virus is derived from the fact that the DNA of the virus can be incorporated in the chromosomes of the host cells; these then change in such a manner that the daughter cells escape the growth-regulating mechanism of the body. Ultimately the daughter cells, usually after several mutations, can become true carcinoma cells (see also section 9.4).

In gynaecological oncology it is mainly the herpes genitalis or herpes type II and the condyloma virus which are considered as possibly oncogenic and are therefore the centre of attention (see section 10.4.1).

7.3.5.1 Herpes simplex virus Type II (HSV type II)

The herpes simplex type II virus or herpes genitalis is closely related to the herpes simplex type I virus or herpes facialis virus, which causes blisters on the lips. Serological cross-reactions between these two viruses do exist (Teplitz *et al.*, 1971). The symptoms of a herpes genitalis infection can be: blisters or tiny ulcers on the vulva, vagina or cervix, redness as a result of hyperaemia and occasionally swelling of the lymph nodes in the groin due to infection; it may also cause a vaginitis. Herpes genitalis infection is asymptomatic in 0.09 per cent of females (Jordan *et al.*, 1972). The disease is self-limiting and after an attack the virus may assume a state of latency, possibly in the neurones of the sacral ganglia.

The herpes genitalis is transmitted mainly venereally but is (strangely enough) also encountered in children and nuns (Langley and Crompton, 1973).

Cytology: The changes in epithelial cells in the various stages of the infection are as follows.

1st stage: increased granularity in the nucleus and fine intranuclear vacuolisation. It may be difficult to distinguish these changes from those seen in degenerate cells.

2nd stage: the chromatin pattern has faded in

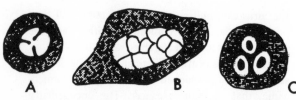

figure 7.9 Cytological pattern of herpes. A. Virocyte with ground glass aspect in nucleus and condensation of the chromatin at the nuclear border; B. virocyte (a multinucleate giant cell); C. multinucleate virocyte with inclusion bodies in the nucleus

its entirety (so-called 'ground glass' appearance of the nucleus). This is caused by swelling of the viral material in the nucleus (Langley and Crompton, 1973). A distinct nuclear membrane is visible; the cytoplasm becomes dense and basophilic.

3rd stage: the nucleus contains an acidophilic inclusion body which is surrounded by a clear zone (figure 7.9) (Ng *et al.*, 1970). The inclusion bodies have been described by virologists as 'tombstones', because they reveal the death of the cell, and they are not, as some authors suggest, a sign of recurrent infection.

In the second and third stages many multinucleate giant cells are found. In fact, when these preparations are screened it is these multinucleate giant cells which are first noted. They can contain 20 or more nuclei lying close together, moulding against each other without overlapping, in contrast to those in a multinucleate endocervical gland cell or histiocyte. The shape of the cell can be abnormal (tadpole, etc.; Koss, 1968). In these giant cells the same nuclear changes are seen as in the mononuclear cells. The multinucleate giant cells are characteristic for a herpes infection.

The virocytes (cells with virus-induced morphological changes) can come from the ectocervical as well as the endocervical epithelium. We diagnosed herpes virocytes in 1 out of 10 000 smears, one tenth of the frequency reported by Patten (1978). Naib *et al.*, (1966) reported an incidence of 1.6:1000. The prevalence of herpes infection is almost twenty times higher in women attending venereal disease clinics than in women attending antenatal and gynaecological clinics (Coleman *et al.*, 1977). Many women have a combination of two or more venereal diseases.

The diagnosis of a herpes infection is important for several reasons. Women with herpes infection ought to be screened for gonorrhoea. Herpetic lesions of the uterine cervix as necrotic cervicitis may macroscopically mimic invasive cancer. Babies from mothers with genital herpes infection can be infected during vaginal delivery; this infection can be fatal. Finally women with herpes infection may have a concomitant carcinoma *in situ* or invasive cervical cancer (see section 10.4.1) (Rawls *et al.*, 1969).

Except for multinucleate giant cells in herpes infection, cytological changes induced by viruses are not pathognomonic for a particular virus. For this reason the cytological diagnosis is only tentative. For a conclusive diagnosis virus identification can be performed by transmission electron microscopy in Papanicolaou-stained routine smears (Coleman *et al.*, 1977), and by virus isolation. Virus isolation is not always possible, due to the interval between the cytological and virological investigation. In a prospective study of 197 women at St Mary's Hospital, London, only 3 out of 11 women with successful virus isolation had giant cells in the smear taken at the same clinic attendance (Coleman *et al.*, 1977). In an additional 5 patients clinical evidence of genital herpes was established, and the concurrent smears contained giant cells, although virus isolation was negative. In conclusion one may remark that some cases can be picked up by virus isolation alone (a very expensive procedure), and other cases by exfoliative cytology.

7.3.5.2 Condylomata acuminata

Condylomata acuminata or genital warts are hystologically defined as a focal papillary outgrowth of squamous epithelium, supported by projecting cores of fibrovascular tissue. When such a growth occurs alone, the term squamous papilloma (see section 7.6.1) is used; when they are multiple and/ or multifocal (vulva and vagina, vagina and cervix) they are referred to as condylomata acuminata (Marsh and Brooklyn, 1952).

Condylomata acuminata are acquired by venereal contact, and are associated with other venereal diseases and high promiscuity (Stormby, 1974).

Recently, the term 'flat condyloma of the cervix' has been introduced (Meisels *et al.*, 1977). These authors distinguish three different types of condylomata: warty lesions ('papillary type'), flat lesions and endophytic lesions. In the native stratified squamous epithelium of the vulva, vagina and ectocervix the warty lesions predominate, whereas in the metaplastic epithelium flat and endophytic lesions are common (Metzelaar-Venema, 1978). Viral particles of the human papilloma virus type have been identified in the cell nuclei of these flat condylomatous lesions (Laverty *et al.*, 1978). The association of condylomata with nuclear atypia and cancer is discussed in section 10.2.2.1.

Histology. Histologically all varieties of condylomata display elongation of rete pegs, acanthosis, koilocytosis, multinucleation, parakeratosis and hyperkeratosis. However, these phenomena differ in quantity: in the flat lesions the parakeratosis and hyperkeratosis are minimal or absent altogether, and in the warty lesions they dominate the picture.

Cytology. In smear preparations, the presence of koilocytotic cells is the main diagnostic criterion for condylomata. These cells (koilocytes) were first described by Papanicolaou in 1960, and many other reports followed (Stormby, 1974; Meisels and Fortin, 1976; Purola and Savia, 1977). Koilocytotic cells are defined as cells with a well-demarcated clear perinuclear halo surrounded by a dense cytoplasmic zone. The shape of the clear zone is either oval or scallopped. A koilocytotic cell can be distinguished from a glycogen-laden navicular cell by three features: (1) a navicular cell has a spherical central part, whereas a koilocytotic cell is flat: (2) a navicular cell often has a nucleus that is pushed aside by the glycogen, whereas the position of the nucleus of a koilocytotic cell is not influenced by the halo; (3) the clear zone of the navicular cell is ill defined and pillow shaped, against a well-demarcated oval or scallopped clear zone of the koilocytotic cell. The halo in squamous cells in cases with trichomonas infestation is small and ill defined.

Besides koilocytosis multinucleation is a striking feature. The cells may contain as many as 25 nuclei. Nuclear moulding does not occur (see herpes simplex virus, section 7.3.5.1). The cytoplasm of these giant cells can be koilocytotic, dense or granular. In the koilocytotic cells papilloma virus particles have been observed in routine smear preparations (Hills and Laverty, 1979).

The characteristic koilocytotic cells are found in all flat lesions, but usually in the warty lesions only nondiagnostic anucleate squames and parakeratotic cells are found. Thus cytology is a highly sensitive test in identifying flat condyloma, but an insensitive test in specifying the macroscopically visible warty lesions.

7.3.5.3 Less Frequent Viral Infections

(1) *Lymphogranuloma venereum.* This infection is rare in Europe and the USA. It may induce granulomas with caseous necrosis. The smear contains histiocytes containing small blue cytoplasmic inclusion bodies (Donovan bodies).

(2) *Cytomegalovirus infection.* The endocervical epithelium in particular is suspectible to cytomegalovirus (CMV) infection (Vesterinen *et al.*, 1975). In an infected cell at first small irregular inclusion bodies are observed. Later the enlarged nuclei contain a very large, usually single inclusion body surrounded by a halo which gives the cells an 'owl eye' appearance. The cytoplasm may contain fine, granular, basophilic inclusions. Electron microscopy of the inclusion-bearing cells may verify the presence of the cytomegalovirus (Coleman *et al.*, 1977).

Cytomegalovirus infection is common, and is often symptomless in women of childbearing age. Reactivation of latent cytomegalovirus occurs in 2–4 per cent of pregnant women (probably due to the disturbance of steroid metabolism) (Coleman, *et al.*, 1977). Cytological screening of cervical smears is not a practical way of detecting cytomegalovirus. The number of affected cells is often very low (Morse *et al.*, 1974). However, if inclusion-bearing cells are detected in the smear of a pregnant woman, it is important to investigate the possibility. of an active cytomegalovirus infection, because this may threaten the health of the baby.

(3) *Infection caused by adenovirus.* Cells with

features suggesting adenovirus infection can be of endocervical, metaplastic or parabasal type. Early in the infection they contain about 3 or 4 small eosinophilic nuclear inclusions with peri-inclusion halos; later a large eosinophilic nuclear inclusion with an irregularly lobulated contour develops. Some chromatin deposition on the nuclear membrane may be found. Multinucleated virocytes are not found (Laverty *et al.*, 1977).

(4) *Inclusion cervicitis.*   The virus is related to the lymphogranuloma virus. In these patients physical examination reveals that the portio has a characteristic bright red colour. In the smear clusters of perinuclear basophilic inclusion bodies are seen in the cytoplasm of both endocervical and metaplastic cells, which creates a granular appearance to the cytoplasm (Naib, 1970). This infection is as common as HSV infection (Dunlop, 1975), although it does not seem to be recognised as readily.

(5) *Chlamydia infection.*   Formerly classed with the viruses Chlamydiae have been removed from this group. It is often associated with vaginitis, cervicitis of endometritis. In the smear, characteristic inclusion bodies, containing coccoid bodies, are seen in the metaplastic cells. In addition, multinucleation and intracytoplasmic perinuclear vacuolation can be seen. Epithelial atypia may be present. In some cases lymphoid cells and plasma cells were also present (Gupta *et al.*, 1979).

References

Arsenault, G. M., Kalman, C. F. and Sorensen, K. W. (1976). The Papanicolaou smear as a technique for gonorrhoea detection: a feasibility study. *J. Am. Vener. Dis. Ass.*, 2, 35–8

Bibbo, M. and Wied, G. L. (1973). Identification of inflammatory reactions, tissue repair, viral infections and microbiologic classifications in cytologic specimens of the female reproductive tract. *Tutorials Cytol.*, 9, Chicago

Boquet-Jiménez, E. and Alvarez San Cristóbal, A. (1978). Cytologic and microbiological aspects of vaginal *Torulopsis*. *Acta Cytol.*, 22, 331–4

Bridland, R. (1962). Trichomoniasis. *Tskr. Nörske Laegoforg.*, 82, 441

Coleman, D. V. (1969). A case of tuberculosis of the cervix. *Acta Cytol.*, 13, 104–7

Coleman, D. V., Russell, W. J. I., Hodgson, J., Tun Pe and Mowbray, J. F. (1977). Human Papova virus in Papanicolaou smears of urinary sediment detected by transmission electron microscopy. *J. clin. Path.*, 30, 1015–20

Collette, H. J. A. (1976). *Epidemiologische Aspecten van het Cervixcarcinoom*, Drukkerij Boeijinga, Apeldoorn

Dunlop, S. J. C. Goes. (1975). Personal communication.

Eisenstein, R. and Battifora, H. (1965). Lymph follicles in cervical smears. *Acta Cytol.*, 9, 344–6

Fentanes de Torres, E. and Benitez-Bribiesca, L. (1973). Cytologic detection of vaginal parasitosis. *Acta Cytol.*, 17, 252–7

Gondos, B. (1974). Cell degeneration: Light and electron microscopic study of ovarian germ cells. *Acta Cytol.*, 18, 504–10

Gupta, P. K., Hollander, D. H. and Frost, J. K. (1976). Actinomycetes in cervicovaginal smears: an association with IUD usage. *Acta Cytol.*, 20, 295–7

Gupta, P. K., Lee, E. F., Erozan, Y. S., Frost, J. K., Geddes, S. T., Donovan, P. A. (1979). Cytologic Investigations in Chlamydia infection. *Acta Cytol.*, 23, 315–20

Highman, W. J. (1972). Cervical smears in tuberculosous endometritis. *Acta Cytol.*, 16, 16–20

Hills, E. and Laverty, C. R. (1979). Electron-microscopic detection of papilloma virus particles in selected koilocytotic cells in a routine cervical smear. *Acta Cytol.*, 23

Jordan, S. W., Evangel, E. and Smith, N. L. (1972). Ethnic distribution of cytologically diagnosed Herpes Simplex genital infections in a cervical cancer screening program. *Acta Cytol.*, 16, 363–5

Koss, L. G. (1968). *Diagnostic cytology and its histopathologic bases*, Lippincott, Philadelphia, pp. 143–64

Koss, L. G. and Wolkinska, W. H. (1959). Trichomonas vaginalis cervicitis and its relationship to cervical cancer, a histocytological study. *Cancer*, 12, 1171–93

Langley, F. H. and Crompton, A. C. (1973).

Epithelial Abnormalities of the Cervix Uteri, Springer, Berlin

Laverty, C. R., Russell, P., Black, J., Kappagoda, N., Benn, R. A. V. and Booth, N. (1977). Adenovirus infection of the cervix. *Acta Cytol.*, **21**, 114–17

Laverty, C. R., Russell, P., Hills, E. and Booth, N. (1978). The significance of non-condylomatous wart virus infection of the cervical transformation zone. A review with discussion of two illustrative cases. *Acta Cytol.*, **22**, 195–201

Märdh, P. A., Stormby, N. and Weström, L. (1971). Mycoplasma and vaginal cytology. *Acta Cytol.*, **15**, 310–15

Marsh, M. and Brooklyn, N. Y. (1952). Papilloma of the cervix. *Am. J. Obstet. Gynec.*, **64**, 281–91

Meisels, A. (1969). Microbiology of the female reproductive tract as determined in the cytology specimen in the presence of cellular atypias. *Acta Cytol.*, **13**, 64–71

Meisels, A., and Fortin, R. (1976). Condylomatous lesions of the cervix and vagina I. *Acta Cytol.*, **20**, 64–71

Meisels, A., Fortin, R. and Roy, M. (1977). Condylomatous lesions of the cervix II. *Acta Cytol.*, **21**, 379–90

Meisels, P. A., Stormby, N. and Weström, L. (1971). Mycoplasma and vaginal cytology. *Acta Cytol.*, **15**, 310–15

Metzelaar-Venema, A. (1978). Correlation study between macroscopy and cytology of condylomatous lesions of the cervix *8th European Congress of Cytology*, Szczecin

Morse, A. R., Coleman, D. V. and Gardner, S. D. (1974). An evaluation of cytology in the diagnosis of herpes simplex virus infection and cytomegalo virus infection of the cervix uteri. *J. Obstet. Gynec. Br. Commonw.*, **81**, 393–8

Muller Kobold-Wolterbeek, A. C. and Beyer-Boon, M. E. (1975). Ciliacytophthoria in cervical cytology. *Acta Cytol.*, **19**, 89–91

Naib, Z. M. (1970). *Exfoliative Cytopathology* 2nd edn, Little Brown, Boston

Naib, Z. M., Nahmias, A. J. and Josey, W. E. (1966). Cytology and histopathology of cervical herpes simplex infection. *Cancer*, **19**, 1026–31

Ng, A. B. P., Reagan, J. W. and Lindner, E. (1970). The cellular manifestations of primary and recurrent herpes genitalis. *Acta Cytol.*, **14**, 124–9

Papanicolaou, G. N. (1960). *Atlas of Exfoliative Cytology, Supplement 2*, Harvard University Press, Cambridge, Mass

Patten, S. F., Jr. (1978). *Diagnostic Cytopathology of the Uterine Cervix*, 2nd edn, Karger, Basel

Purola, E. and Savia, E. (1977). Cytology of gynecologic condyloma acuminatum. *Acta Cytol.*, **21**, 26–31.

Rawls, W. E., Tompkins, W. A. F. and Melnick, J. L. (1969). The association of Herpes virus type 2 and carcinoma of the uterine cervix. *Am. J. Epidemiol.*, **89**, 547–54

Roberts, T. H. and Ng, A. B. P. (1975). Chronic lymphocytic cervicitis: cytologic and histopathologic manifestations. *Acta Cytol.*, **19**, 235–43

Smolka, H. and Soost, H. J. (1971). *Grundriss und Atlas der Gynäkologischen Zytodiagnostik*, Thieme, Stuttgart, pp. 111–16, 138–43

Stormby, N. (1974). Morphology of virus induced changes. *4th European Congress of Cytology*, Ljubljana

Taylor-Robinson, D., Addey, J. P., Hare, M. J. and Dunlop, E. M. C. (1969). Mycoplasmas and 'non-specific' genital infection. *Br. J. vener. Dis.*, **45**, 265–73

Teplitz, R. L., Valco, Z. and Rundall, T. (1971). Comparative sequential cytologic changes following in vitro infection with Herpesvirus types I and II. *Acta Cytol.*, **15**, 455–9

Vesterinen, E., Leinikki, P. and Saksela, E. (1975). Cytopathogenicity of cytomegalovirus to human ecto- and endocervico-epithelial cells in vitro. *Acta Cytol.*, **19**, 473–81

Ziabkowski, T. A. and Naylor, B. (1976). Cyanophilic bodies in cervico-vaginal smears. *Acta Cytol.*, **20**, 340–2

Part II: Proliferation and Regeneration

7.4 Proliferative Lesions

7.4.1 Reserve Cell Hyperplasia

In the transition zone the bipotential reserve cells underneath the columnar endocervical epithelium can proliferate without maturation. That is, the reserve cells or their progeny do not become keratinised and die, as the squamous epithelial cells do. A proliferation of reserve cells without maturation is called *reserve cell hyperplasia*. Reserve cell hyperplasia can develop into metaplasia (see section 7.4.2) in the course of time (Reagan and Patten, 1962).

Haam and Old (1964) observed that foci of reserve cell hyperplasia are common in post-menopausal women.

7.4.1.1 Histology

The histological pattern of reserve cell hyperplasia has been described in detail in the literature (Haam and Old, 1964; Song, 1964; Burghardt, 1970). In reserve cell hyperplasia there can be 5–12 (in extreme cases) layers of primitive cells (reserve cells). Underneath the columnar epithelium maturation and stratification do not occur; the cellular boundaries are vague. The cytoplasm of these primitive cells is fragile without visible signs of maturation (Beyer-Boon and Verdonk, 1978). The cells have round to oval nuclei and finely granular chromatin. The bipotential character of these cells is discussed in section 7.4.2 (metaplasia).

7.4.1.2 Cytology

Near the columnar epithelial cells, sometimes even up against them, are numerous oval nuclei. The nuclei resemble to some extent the nuclei of columnar epithelial cells but are slightly smaller, and some may have a pointed tip at one end. A honeycomb pattern is never seen. Limited aniso-karyosis may be observed. The chromatin pattern is always fine; a small nucleolus may be present. Occasionally there will be a small amount of poorly defined sparse cytoplasm. Most of the nuclei are, however, naked, having lost their fragile cyto-plasm due to the smear procedure (see section 2.3.1.3). The stripped nuclei display a characteristic exfoliation pattern: they lie in rows (sometimes with branches), in dense clumps or side by side in pairs. The nuclei lie with one tip over the next nucleus (like shingles). In the dense clumps and rows nuclear moulding can occur (figure 7.10).

7.4.1.3 Transmission Electron Microscopy
see section 2.3.1.3

7.4.2 Metaplasia

Metaplasia is a process in which the cells differentiate in an abnormal direction. When columnar

figure 7.10 Reserve cells. From left to right: reserve cells with pointed tip; mutual indentation of reserve cells (moulding); reserve cells which resemble endocervical columnar cell nuclei

epithelium is replaced by stratified squamous epithelium, the term *squamous metaplasia* is used. It probably develops via a chain of events.

When the columnar endocervical epithelium is damaged the reserve cells may proliferate. These undifferentiated bipotential cells can mature into metaplastic epithelial cells so that metaplastic epithelium is found where columnar epithelium is expected. Sometimes the metaplastic epithelium is still partly covered by the original columnar epithelium (figure 7.11).

Whenever maturation of the metaplastic epithelium is not yet completed, two junctions can be seen: the transistion between squamous epithelium and metaplastic epithelium, and the transition between metaplastic epithelium and columnar epithelium (figure 7.12). Metaplasia can also occur in the glandular ducts.
ition between squamous epithelium and metaplastic epithelium, and the transition between metaplastic epithelium and columnar epithelium (figure 7.12). Metaplasia can also occur in the glandular ducts.

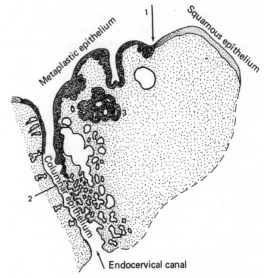

figure 7.12 Thin section of the transition zone. 1. Squamo-squamous junction; 2. squamocolumnar junction; 3. metaplastic epithelium is also present in the glandular ducts

Squamous metaplasia is a common surface in the uterine cervix and serves as protection. It is often a reaction to external stimuli (tissue injury, change of vaginal pH) or hormonal stimule (von Haam and Old, 1964; Song, 1964; Coppleson and Reid, 1966) and is influenced by the use of oral contraceptives (see section 14.2.1.3).

7.4.2.1 Histology

Various histological patterns can be seen depending upon the stage of maturation. The term *immature*

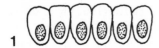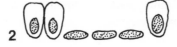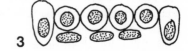

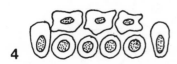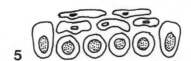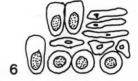

figure 7.11 Histological patterns in the various stages of the development of metaplasia. 1. Columnar epithelium; 2. damaged columnar epithelium with reserve cells; 3., 4., 5. maturation of bipotential reserve cells into squamous epithelial cells (metaplastic cells); 6. mature squamous epithelium, partly covered with endocervical epithelial cells

metaplasia is used when the uppermost layer consists of immature metaplastic epithelial cells or columnar cells. Mature metaplastic epithelium can be distinguished from native squamous epithelium only by its location: metaplastic epithelium is always found above underlying glands and in the endocervical glands.

7.4.2.2 Cytology

Morphologically cells from metaplastic epithelium lie between (parabasal) squamous and columnar epithelial cells; the size of the nucleus is slightly smaller. The nuclei often have a clearly visible nucleolus. The amount of cytoplasm and the shape of the cell depend upon the degree of maturation. Sometimes mucus vacuoles may appear in the cytoplasm. When the metaplastic cells have not been spontaneously exfoliated but were scraped, the cells will have thin cytoplasmic tails (figure 7.13). In the immediate neighbourhood of a group of metaplastic cells columnar epithelial or squamous epithelial cells may be found. Metaplastic cells are often encountered next to reserve cells in the same smear. When the metaplastic epithelium has fully matured the number of columnar and metaplastic cells in the smear decreases and an increasing amount of squamous epithelial cells is found (figure 7.14).

Immature metaplastic cells are round or oval with little cytoplasm (figure 7.16). They often exfoliate in sheets. As the cells mature the amount of cytoplasm increases and the shape becomes polygonal. The cells tend to be isolated. Mature metaplastic cells strongly resemble normal squamous epithelial cells; their origin, however, may be betrayed by the fact that the cytoplasm has a dark

outer zone and a lighter inner zone (Patten, 1978) (see figure 7.13).

Immature metaplastic cells cannot always be distinguished from parabasal cells. In the reproductive period the presence of these cells points either to the existence of a zone of metaplasia (in most cases) or to the presence of an erosive lesion. Many mature metaplastic cells cannot be differentiated cytologically from normal squamous epithelial cells.

Occasionally the pattern of *keratinising metaplasia* may be encountered. The smear will then contain small cells with the typical shape of metaplastic cells and orange cytoplasm. This can be due to degeneration or keratinisation of the cytoplasm. If the latter is assumed then there is a discrepancy between the differentiation of the cytoplasm and the amount of cytoplasm. When minimal nuclear alteration occurs (that is, nuclear enlargement) the term *atypical metaplasia* is used (Patten, 1978), representing an early stage of development for dysplasia (Coppleson and Reid, 1966; Patten, 1978). In these cells the cytoplasm is abundant and the nucleocytoplasmic ratio remains normal (figure 7.15) These large cells with large nuclei may represent vitamin dificiency (as in old age). When the chromatin abnormalities increase we use the term dysplasia (see section 10.2.2).

7.4.2.3 The Relationship Between Reserve Cell Hyperplasia, Metaplasia and Squamous Carcinoma *in Situ*

Studies by Reagan and Patten (1962) have shown that reserve cell hyperplasia and metaplasia both occur in the same part of the cervix, namely, proximal to the squamocolumnar junction. Most

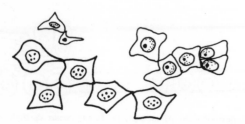 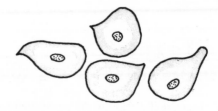

figure 7.13   Metaplastic cells

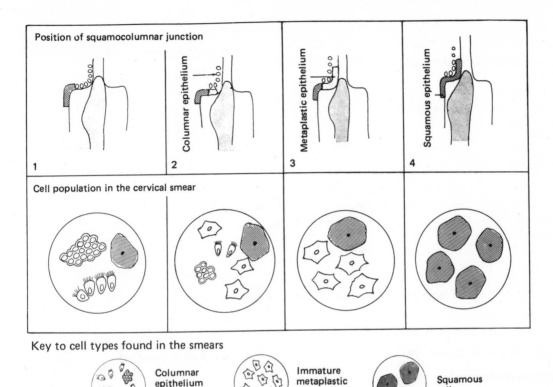

figure 7.14 Schematic drawing of the ectocervix and the various cell patterns. 1. Squamocolumnar junction on the ectocervix. The smear contains squamous and columnar epithelial cells. 2. A small area of metaplasia (transformation zone) can be discerned. The smear contains columnar cells, metaplastic cells and squamous epithelial cells. 3. A large area of metaplasia is present. The smear contains metaplastic and squamous epithelial cells. 4. The metaplastic area has fully matured. In the smear only squamous epithelial cells can be discerned

carcinomata *in situ* also arise in the same area (Patten, 1978).

Coppleson and Reid (1966) demonstrated that the transition from columnar epithelium to metaplastic epithelium takes place within a relatively short time. Via colposcopic examination they established that large areas of metaplastic epithelium develop in foetal life, in early adolescence (Pixley, 1971) (probably associated with the onset of sexual activity) and during the first pregnancy (Coppleson *et al.*, 1976).

The process of metaplasia may be arrested at any stage, to persist in an immature state. Even in postmenopausal women immature metaplastic epithelium is identified (Coppleson *et al.*, 1976). The normal metaplastic process, having reached maturity, does not seem subject to the development of squamous cancer. On the other hand, in the initial phases of the process the primitive epithelial cells are vulnerable to genetic change (see also mutuation, section 9.4), and so neoplastic potential may be acquired (Coppleson *et al.*, 1976).

In this context it is interesting to mention that we found immature metaplastic cells twice as often in dysplastic lesions progressing to cancer than in lesions regressing to normal (see section 10.3.2 and table 10.9) and reserve cells ten times as often.

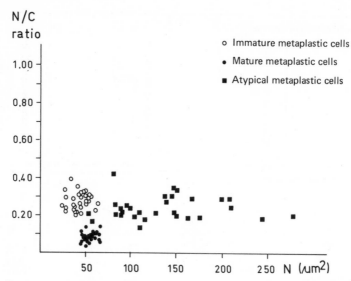

figure 7.15   Scattergram of immature, mature and atypical metaplastic cells

7.4.2.4 Electron Microscopy

In transmission electron microscopy the cytoplasm of a metaplastic cell shows the same characteristics as the intermediate squamous epithelial cell (see section 2.3.1.3). The nuclear envelope may or may not be intact. At the SEM level squamous metaplasia is characterised by a mosaic arrangement of the cells (as in native squamous epithelium) covered with microvilli (as the native columnar epithelium) although rudimentary (Rubio and Kranz, 1976).

table 7.2 The presence of metaplastic and columnar cells in normal smears and smears from carcinoma *in situ*

	C	M	A	n
Normal smears	63%	48%	23%	80 000
Positive smears (carcinoma *in situ*)	73%	86%	8%	150

C = Columnar cells; M = Metaplastic cells; A = neither columnar nor metaplastic cells; n = number of smears

7.4.3 Basal Cell Hyperplasia

In basal cell hyperplasia the number of basal cells in squamous epithelium may increase. If the top layers of the epithelium are mature, there will be no signs of this abnormality in the smear. Only when the uppermost layers of the epithelium are missing (for example, in the event of inflammation) will the smear contain many basal cells, often with a prominent nucleolus (Naib, 1970). The post-partum pattern is caused by hyperplasia of the basal cell layer (see section 6.2.1.6).

7.4.4 Leucoplakia

Leucoplakia is in essence a clinical concept. The clinician understands leucoplakia to mean 'white patches'. Excessive keratin production may result in the appearance of leucoplakia. This is sometimes observed when a pessary is worn or when there is a marked prolapse of the uterus. The main goal of the epithelial change is protection against external stimuli. This can be achieved by an increase in overall thickness (acanthosis) or further differentia-tion, that is, the formation of a layer of keratinised

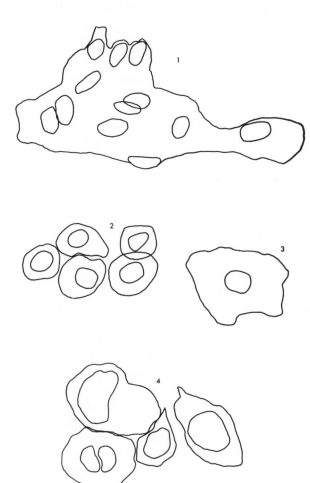

figure 7.16   Reserve cells and metaplastic cells. Camera lucida drawings. 1. Sheet of reserve cells; 2. immature metaplastic cells; 3. metaplastic cell; 4. atypical metaplastic cells

cells (hyperkeratosis). The degree of keratin formation is often proportional to the thickness of the granular cell layer (Patten, 1978). The following histological and cytological patterns can be expected.

7.4.4.1 Leucokeratosis or Hyperkeratosis

Instead of nonkeratinising squamous epithelium, keratinising squamous epithelium is observed. This epithelium usually has an obvious layer of granular cells covered with a layer of anucleated squamous cells (squames). The cytological pattern is characterised by these anucleated squames (figure 7.17) and, in some cases, also epithelial cells from the granular layer; the latter are intermediate or superficial squamous cells with granules in the cytoplasm.

7.4.4.2 Leucoparakeratosis

The epithelium is covered partly with squames and with squamous cells which show definite signs of keratinisation but have retained their nuclei (parakeratosis). Sometimes the keratinised layer is missing and then several layers of parakeratotic cells will be seen. The smear will contain a large number of these parakeratotic cells. They are fairly small polygonal cells with bright orange cytoplasm and round hyperchromatic nuclei (about as large as the nucleus of an intermediate cell).

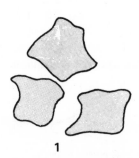

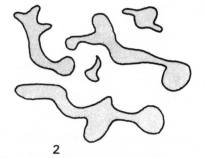

figure 7.17   Leucoplakia. 1. Anucleate superficial cells (squames) in leucokeratosis; 2. squames with abnormal shape from keratinising squamous cell carcinoma

7.4.4.3 Atrophy with Keratinisation

Atrophic epithelium can sometimes be covered with a layer of parakeratotic cells and squames. The cytological pattern cannot be distinguished from that of leucoparakeratosis: in addition to anucleated squamous cells there are also small parakeratotic cells. The nuclei are markedly hyperchromatic or pyknotic. Karyorrhexis is often seen.

7.4.4.4 Keratinising Squamous Cell Carcinoma

This lesion, which is discussed in chapter 10 (section 10.2.4.2), can appear as a leucoplakia and be covered with a layer of squames. The squames are often abnormal in shape (figure 7.17). The presence of these abnormal squames in the smear indicates that further examination is necessary.

7.5 Repair and Regeneration

7.5.1 Ulcer

An ulcer is a local defect in the covering epithelium and underlying stroma with only a slight tendency towards healing. The continuous pressure of a pessary can, for example, often lead to ulceration. The histological pattern is dominated by the inflammatory reaction, which is often accompanied by necrosis. The smear will contain numerous lymphocytes, granulocytes, histiocytes, fibroblasts and, in some cases, multinucleated giant cells (granulation tissue).

7.5.2 Tissue Repair

7.5.2.1 Histology

Whenever stratified squamous epithelium or columnar epithelium is damaged and the surface consists of stroma, re-epithelialisation will take place. The cells that will cover the denuded area originate from the columnar epithelium, the squamous epithelium (Gonzàlez-Merlo *et al.*, 1973) or from reserve cells (Epstein, 1972). Tissue repair is encountered particularly in patients with a pronounced cervicitis, after a biopsy is taken, after surgery or immediately after irradiation.

7.5.2.2 Cytology

In the smear there will sometimes be easily recognised fibroblasts, parabasal cells and groups of so-called *repair cells* (figure 7.18). The origin of the latter is not clear (Bibbo *et al.*, 1971); most probably they originate from epithelia of either columnar or squamous type (Geirsson *et al.*, 1977). These cells, in reacting to external stimuli, have an increased metabolic activity as reflected by nuclear and nucleolar enlargement, as well as increased mitotic activity (Geirsson *et al.*, 1977).

Repair cells have oval nuclei which vary somewhat in shape; multinuclearity is striking. The cells often lie in syncytia, that is, within the groups of cells the cellular boundaries cannot be identified. The chromatin pattern is rather fine and regular. Large, often multiple, nucleoli can be present; these large nucleoli are indicative of active protein synthesis. The nucleolar/nuclear ratio remains low (large nucleolus in large nucleus). The cytoplasm has ragged edges and is usually abundant (figure 7.19). Leucocytophagy is frequently seen. In addition to repair cells, several reserve cells and metaplastic epithelial cells are also often present. In addition, atypical reserve cells of the monomorphic type (see section 10.2.1.2) may be observed (Epstein, 1972), arranged in syncytia. Epstein assumes that these cells are derived from regenerating cells at the base of the ulcer.

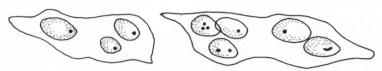

figure 7.18   Cytological pattern of tissue repair: syncytia with large nuclei. Note the large, sometimes multiple, nucleoli and the ragged boundaries of the cytoplasm. The nucleolar/nuclear ratio is low

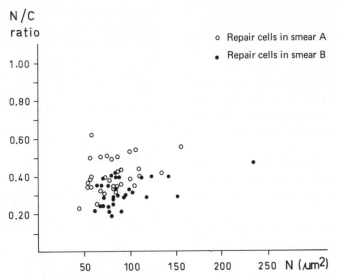

figure 7.19   Scattergram of two examples of tissue repair

Cells arising from benign reparative reactions involving the uterine cervix have many features of cancer cells (see section 9.5), such as cells from a large-cell nonkeratinising squamous cell carcinoma or adenocarcinoma of the uterine cervix. However, it is rare to identify these so-called repair cells in isolated form (Patten, 1978). Also the chromatin pattern is important: in contrast to carcinoma cells, the nuclei of the cells in tissue repair have a fine chromatin pattern. Differentiation from adenocarcinoma can be difficult. In tissue repair neither nuclear stacking nor three-dimensional cell groups are seen. There may be a striking resemblance between tumour cells from soft-tissue sarcomas of the uterus and repair cells. In the presence of a sarcoma, however, many isolated cells may be encountered (Geirsson *et al.*, 1977). Long-term follow-up studies over a period of 1–6 years revealed that in very few patients did the repair reaction antedate carcinoma *in situ* (Geirsson *et al.*, 1977).

N.B. when the tissue repair cells appear to have a slightly coarsened chromatin pattern, it is recommended that a second smear be taken ±6 months later.

7.5.3 Erosion

Erosion is both a clinical and a pathological concept; the sense of the term can, however, vary. The clinician understands erosion to mean a more or less sharply defined red spot on the cervix. The pathologist, on the other hand, speaks of erosion

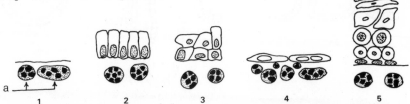

figure 7.20   Several histological patterns which fit the clinical concept of 'erosion'. 1. True erosion; 2. ectopia; 3. metaplasia; 4. tissue repair (repair cells); 5. mature squamous epithelium for the purpose of comparison. a, capillary with erythrocytes

when a superficial ulceration exists in the mucous membrane limited to the epithelium. When a clinician uses the word erosion, therefore, various histological and cytological patterns can be expected, such as (figure 7.20):

(1) True erosion. The superficial layers of the epithelium are missing so that the surface of the uterine cervix consists of basal epithelial cells and stroma cells. The smear will contain many (para) basal cells.

(2) Ectopia. Part of the ectocervix is covered with columnar epithelium. In the smear there will be numerous columnar epithelial cells often with prominent nucleoli.

(3) Metaplasia. Metaplastic epithelium may be thinner than mature squamous epithelium so that it appears red.

(4) Ulcer (see section 7.5.1).

(5) Tissue repair (see section 7.5.2).

(6) Macroscopically a carcinoma can also appear red (see section 10.5.2).

7.6 Other Conditions

7.6.1 Squamous Papilloma of the Cervix

A squamous papilloma is a benign tumour of squamous epithelial origin with supporting stroma.

In contrast to the multifocal condylomatous papillomata (see section 7.3.5.2) a squamous papilloma is an unifocal growth and cannot be transmitted (Marsh, 1952). In our experience, koilocytosis is not seen in 'true' squamous papillomas, and, therefore, these are not detected by exfoliative cytology.

7.6.2 Cervical Polyps

A polyp is a benign pedunculated tumour covered with glandular epithelium (figure 7.21). The diagnosis of a cervical polyp cannot be established cytologically. However, it is possible to encounter micropolyps which have been scraped from the cervix in their entirety. They are covered with low columnar to cuboidal epithelium which encloses a cell-rich stroma and sometimes a cellular infiltrate with round nuclei (plasma cells, lymphocytes).

7.6.3 Endometrial Polyp

An endometrial polyp has a pedunculated structure, extends from the endometrium and is covered with endometrial epithelium. The diagnosis of an endometrial polyp cannot be established by

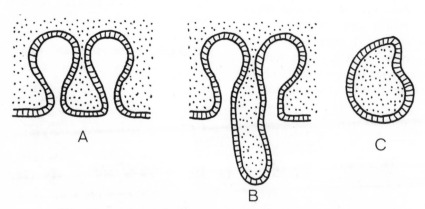

figure 7.21   Formation and exfoliation of an endocervical polyp. A. Endocervical glandular ducts; B. endocervical polyp; C. endocervical polyp (cross-section)

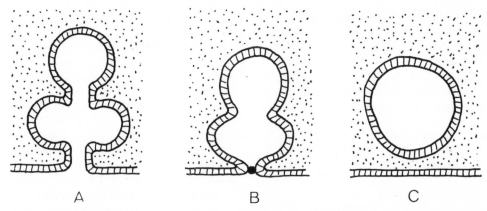

figure 7.22   Formation of nabothian cyst. A. Endocervical glandular duct; B. closed endocervical glandular duct, some accumulation of secretion in the lumen; C. nabothian cyst filled with mucus

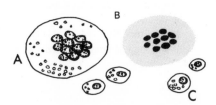

figure 7.23   Cells from nabothian cysts. A. Multinucleate endocervical cell with foamy cytoplasm and vesicular nuclei; B. multinucleate cell with smooth orange cytoplasm and small pycnotic nuclei (changes due to degeneration); C. endocervical cell with foamy cytoplasm which is difficult to distinguish from a histiocyte

cytology. Sometimes small groups of endometrial epithelial cells are found during the second half of the cycle. Moreover, it is possible to encounter very large groups of endometrial cells — larger than normally seen in a smear.

7.6.4 Nabothian Cysts

The endocervical glandular ducts can become plugged as a result of inflammation or formation of metaplastic epithelium (figure 7.22). Small cysts may then develop as a result of the accumulation of secretions; macroscopically, the cervix will appear blue and rough in such a case. When a nabothian cyst is broken during scraping the smear will contain a streak of necrotic material with many multinucleate giant cells with abundant foamy cytoplasm (figure 7.23). The nuclei of these giant cells are larger than the nuclei of histiocytic giant cells (Tweeddale and Ball, 1968). There will be no phagocytosed material in the pink cytoplasm of these multinucleate endocervical cells, in contrast to histiocytes. Nuclear overlapping may be seen. When the multinucleate endocervical cells degenerate the nuclei become pycnotic and the cytoplasm stains a smooth orange (figure 7.23). These cells can be mistaken for dysplastic cells (see section 10.2.2).

References

Beyer-Boon, M. E. and Verdonk, G. W. (1978). The identification of atypical reserve cells in smears of patients with premalignant and malignant changes in the squamous and glandular epithelium of the uterine cervix. *Acta Cytol.*, 22, 305—11

Bibbo, M., Keebler, C. M. and Wied, G. L. (1971). The cytologic diagnosis of tissue repair in the female genital tract. *Acta Cytol.*, 15, 133—7

Burghardt, E. (1970). Latest aspects of precancerous lesions in squamous and columnar epithelium of the cervix. *Int. J. Gynec. Obstet.*, 8, 573—80

Coppleson, M. and Reid, B. A. (1966). A colposcopic study of the cervix during pregnancy and the puerperium. *J. Obstet. Gynaec. Br. Commw.*, 73, 575—85

Coppleson, M., Pixley, E. and Reid, B. (1976). *Colposcopy. A Scientific and Practical Approach to the Cervix in Health and Disease*, 3rd edn. Thomas, Springfield

Epstein, N. A. (1972). The significance of cellular atypia in the diagnosis of malignancy in ulcers of the female genital tract. *Acta Cytol.*, **16**, 483–9

Geirsson, G., Woodworth, F. E., Patten, S. F. Jr. and Bonfiglio, T. A. (1977). Epithelial repair and regeneration in the uterine cervix I. An analysis of the cells. *Acta Cytol.*, **21**, 371–8

Gonzàlez-Merlo, J., Ausín, J., Lejárcegui, J. A. and Márguez, M. (1973). Regeneration of the ectocervical epithelium after its destruction by electrocauterization. *Acta Cytol.*, **17**, 366–71

Haam, E. von and Old, J. W. (1964). Reserve cell hyperplasia, squamous metaplasia and epidermidization. In: *Dysplasia, Carcinoma in situ and Microinvasive Carcinoma of the Cervix Uteri* (ed. L. A. Gray), Thomas, Springfield, pp. 41–82

Marsh, M. R. (1952). Papilloma of the cervix. *Am. J. Obstet. Gynec.*, **64**, 281–91

Naib, Z. M. (1970). *Exfoliative Cytology*, 2nd edn, Little Brown, Boston

Patten, S. F. (1978). *Diagnostic Cytology of the Uterine Cervix*, 2nd, Karger, Basel

Pixley, E. (1971). *Colposcopy*, Thomas, Springfield

Reagan, J. W. and Patten, S. F. (1962). Dysplasia: a basic reaction to injury in the uterine cervix. *Ann. N. Y. Acad. Sci.*, **97**, 662–82

Rubio, C. A. and Kranz, I. (1976). The exfoliating cervical epithelial surface in dysplasia, carcinoma *in situ* and invasive squamous carcinoma I. Scanning electron microscopic study. *Acta Cytol.*, **20**, 144–50

Song, J. (1964). *The Human Uterus: Morphogenesis and Embryological Basis for Cancer*, Thomas, Springfield

Tweeddale, J. W. and Ball, M. J. (1968). Giant cells in cervico-vaginal smears. *Acta Cytol.*, **12**, 298–304.

Tumours

8.1 Introduction

A tumour (growth) or neoplasm (new formation) is an abnormal autonomous mass of tissue which originates in cells in the body. A neoplasm grows more rapidly than normal tissue and its growth is not coordinated with that of the surrounding tissue. In contrast to so-called reactive processes, such as hyperplasia or an inflammatory reaction, tumour growth is continuous, even when the stimuli leading to proliferation disappear (Willis, 1960).

8.2 Classification of Tumours

Tumours can be classified as benign or malignant; they can also be grouped according to their cell type and degree of differentiation.

8.2.1 Benign and Malignant Tumours

Benign tumours are characterised by slow growth and well-defined margins with respect to the surrounding tissue. Growth is self-limiting. In contrast to malignant tumours they do not metastasise (Anderson, 1976).

In general, their histological pattern is characterised by a regular architecture, absence of nuclear abnormalities and normal maturation of the cells; thus the structure usually resembles that of the tissue from which the tumour originated. Cytologically it is difficult or impossible to distinguish

these tumour cells from normal cells. An example of a benign tumour is a myoma of the uterus.

Malignant tumours (cancers), on the other hand, grow rapidly, invade the surrounding tissues and can become disseminated (metastasise). Histologically, the architecture of the tissue is disrupted and the cells are often immature and have abnormal nuclei. Thus a malignant tumour can easily be distinguished from the original tissue. When the malignant cells reach a high degree of maturity it may be difficult to classify them as either benign or malignant.

In the following table (table 8.1) some of the characteristics of benign and malignant tumours are compared. It will be clear that the clinical significance of malignant tumours is much greater than that of benign tumours.

8.2.2 Classification according to Cell Type

Microscopic examination may indicate the tissue in which the tumours originated or at least the tissue that most closely resembles the tumour. The classification of tumours parallels that of normal tissues (epithelial tumours, connective tissue tumours, etc.)

A tumour can be well, moderately or poorly differentiated. A well-differentiated tumour is characterised by a high degree of differentiation of the constituent cells, which means that their structure and shape closely correspond to those of the tissue from which the neoplasm originated

table 8.1 Some characteristics of benign and malignant neoplasms

	Benign	Malignant
Rate of growth	Slow	Rapid
Mitotic figures	Few	Many
Abnormal mitotic figures	Not present	Present
Chromatin pattern	Normal	Abnormal
Local growth	Expansive	Invasive
Encapsulation	Clearly present	Not or barely present
Destruction of surrounding tissue	Nonexistent or slight	Pronounced
Invasion of vessels	Usually non-existent	Often present
Metastasis	None	Often present
Effect on host	Slight	Obvious
Death (when untreated)	Rare, only as a result of local effect	Frequent

(the parent tissue). Tumour cells occasionally retain the secretory function of the parent cells, such as hormone production (for example, an oestrogen-producing granulosa cell tumour of the ovary). Sometimes the neoplasm is 'better' differentiated than the parent tissue: well-differentiated squamous cell neoplasms of the cervix may form anucleate squames in contrast to normal squamous epithelium of the cervix.

A poorly differentiated tumour consists of immature cells so that it may be barely possible to identify the tumour according to tissue type. Another word for undifferentiated is anaplastic or immature.

8.2.3 Nomenclature

A tumour is designated by the suffix -oma following the name of the cell type.

fibroma – neoplasm of fibrous connective tissue

myoma – neoplasm of muscular tissue

Malignant epithelial tumours are called carcinomas, for example, squamous cell carcinoma (originating in squamous epithelium), adenocarcinoma (originating in glandular epithelium).

Malignant mesenchymal tumours are called sarcomas; a fibrosarcoma originates in fibrous connective tissue, a myosarcoma in muscular tissue.

8.3 Metastasis and Invasive Growth of Malignant Neoplasms

Epithelial tumours are said to show invasive growth when they extend through the basal membrane into the underlying tissue. The neoplastic growth can be spear-like or club-shaped.

When a malignant neoplasm invades a blood vessel, neoplastic cells may be shed; these cells are subsequently transported to another site where they *may* become implanted and multiply. When this occurs the tumour is said to have metastasised. The word metastasis is used to indicate this process; the phrase metastatic deposit refers to the secondary lesion which has developed. A metastatic deposit generally exhibits the same structure as the original tumour. Dissemination of tumour cells usually occurs via lymphatic channels, blood vessels or serous cavities.

When the epithelium consists entirely of morphologically malignant cells but the basal membrane has not yet been penetrated, the term *carcinoma in situ* or intraepithelial carcinoma is used. Proliferation of the tumour cells then occurs within the boundaries of the epithelium. Carcinoma *in situ* may develop in any epithelial tissue (squamous epithelium of the ectocervix, glandular epithelium of the endometrium, etc.).

8.4 Premalignant Abnormalities

A premalignant lesion implies that there is a high risk that a malignant neoplastic cell population will develop in the lesion. Examples include atypical endometrial hyperplasia and squamous epithelial dysplasia (see sections 12.2.1 and 10.2.2).

8.5 Prognosis

Prognosis is the prediction of the probable course of a specific disease. The prognosis is determined by the following factors.

(1) The nature of the tumour (benign or malignant).

(2) The cell type of the tumour.

(3) The differentiation of the tumour.

(4) The extent of the tumour; in this respect metastasis of the tumour is very important.

(5) The reaction of the host to the tumour. Since this reaction cannot be measured as yet, it is not taken into consideration when the prognosis for a particular patient is given. The fact that this biologically determined host reaction (including immunological defence reaction) is significant has been indicated by the results of studies of untreated carcinoma patients.

(6) The site of the tumour.

8.6 The Cause of Cancer

For decades scientists have been searching for the cause of cancer. In 1775 the English surgeon Pott reported that soot might contain an agent which induces cancer (that is, a carcinogenic factor) after he discovered that chimneysweeps showed a high incidence of skin cancer (of the scrotum). Later this same phenomenon was observed among coaltar workers in Germany.

By means of animal experiments many carcinogenic substances have been discovered. In addition to chemical substances it was also found that ionising rays, viruses and hormones can induce cancer. In general the development of a neoplasm cannot be attributed to one agent alone but is often due to an interaction of several agents (Hiatt *et al.*, 1977).

In the literature, carcinogenic agents (those agents which can induce carcinomas) and co-carcinogenic agents (those agents which alone cannot induce cancer but in combination with other substances enhance the risk of cancer) are discussed.

There are many people who come into contact with carcinogenic and co-carcinogenic agents through occupational or environmental circumstances; these individuals fall in the so-called 'high-risk' groups. It is worthwhile to include these people in periodic screening programmes for cancer.

References

Anderson, W. A. D. (1976). *Pathology*, 4th edn, Mosby, St. Louis

Hiatt, H. H., Watson, J. D. and Winsten, J. A. (1977). *Origins of Human Cancer*, Cold Spring Harbor Laboratory

Willis, R. A. (1960). *Pathology of Tumours*, 4th edn, Butterworth, London

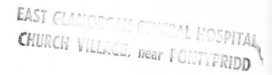
EAST GLAMORGAN GENERAL HOSPITAL CHURCH VILLAGE, near PONTYPRIDD

Morphogenesis and Morphology of Tumour Cells

9.1 Introduction

One of the characteristics of a mammalian cell is the presence of a constant number of chromosomes during interphase. In man the chromosome complex is made up of two identical sets, each consisting of 23 chromosomes (haploid number = n = 23), or a total of 46 chromosomes. Such cells are called diploid ($2n$) or euploid (a balanced set or sets). The number of chromosomes differs for each animal species (for example, 40 for the white mouse, 17–18 for the field mouse). Although the number of chromosomes differ, it appears that the total amount of genetic material, that is, DNA, is practically the same (Vendrely and Vendrely, 1949; Atkin *et al.*, 1959). In general it can be stated that the function of the cell is determined by the genetic information of the DNA in the nucleus.

> A *polyploid* cell is one containing a multiple of the diploid chromosome complex ($4n$, $8n$, etc.). The term *aneuploidy* is used when the number of chromosomes in a cell is not an exact multiple of the diploid number of chromosomes ($5n$, $7n$, etc.). A *hyperploid* cell contains more (x) than $2n$ chromosomes or a multiple thereof, ($2n + x$, $4n + x$, etc.); a *hypoploid* cell has less than $2n$ chromosomes or a multiple thereof ($2n - x$, $4n - x$, etc.) (Böhm and Sandritter, 1975).

The terms polyploid, etc., are used to indicate both the number of chromosomes and the DNA content of the cell. It is essential to remember this when reading the literature on this subject. In fact,

it is possible that the number of chromosomes, but not the amount of DNA, in the cell will be normal (Atkin *et al.*, 1959). The contrary is also possible. 'DNA-ploidy' need not therefore be the same as 'chromosome-ploidy'. In one individual, when the number of chromosomes is constant, the total amount of DNA in a nondividing diploid cell will be constant. During the S phase of the cycle (see section 1.4.1), which precedes cell division, the amount of DNA doubles (replication). During this process the cell exhibits 'DNA-hyperploidy'; at the end of the process the cell is 'DNA-polyploid'. During the subsequent mitosis, the number of chromosomes doubles (duplication). The cell first shows 'chromosome hyperploidy' and later 'chromosome polyploidy'. Therefore dividing tissue, that is, tissue with a high rate of mitosis, will contain nuclei with a high DNA content. In general, the amount of DNA will not exceed the tetraploid DNA value.

Regenerating tissue (for example, gastric ulcer), ageing tissue (liver), viral-infected tissue and malignant neoplasms can also contain cells with $8n$, $16n$, etc., chromosomes. Such highly polyploid cells can develop after abnormal mitosis or when nuclear fusion follows abnormal mitosis (see sections 9.3.1 and 4).

9.2 DNA and Chromosomes of Tumour Cells

Tumour cells often have an abnormal chromosome pattern, an abnormal amount of DNA, or both (Böhm and Sandritter, 1975).

The morphology of the chromosomes of a tumour cell can be studied by means of karyotyping. In most malignant tumour cells, not only the number but also the structure of the chromosomes is aberrant. Such chromosomes can be ring-shaped, or the arms may be too long, too short or unequal in length. The chromosomal abnormalities are usually the result of chromosome breakage and/or *recombination* of broken chromosomes which can occur during either the interphase or in mitosis (Stadler, 1931).

If a tumour contains an abnormal characteristic chromosome, then this chromosome to is called a *marker chromosome*. A well-known example is the 'Philadelphia chromosome' (abnormal chromosome 22) in chronic myeloid leukaemia (Baikie *et al.*, 1960).

Moreover, the DNA content of the tumour cells can be established and a histogram of the cell population can be made (figure 9.1). For determination of nuclear DNA the specific Feulgen staining method is used (see section 9.5.2.3). The term *DNA stemline* is used to denote the most common DNA value per cell in a tumour cell population. Since a tumour cell population is subject to division, there will also be cells with a multiple of the DNA stemline value. This is called a 'bimodal distribution'. A histogram of such a cell population is seen in figure 9.1. Strictly speaking the term 'stemline'

may only be used when such a bimodal distribution exists (Böhm and Sandritter, 1975).

The *chromosome stemline* is the most common number of chromosomes per cell in a tumour cell population (Makino and Kano, 1951). An aberrant chromosomal pattern and an abnormal amount of DNA can, for example, be caused by abnormal mitosis, endoreduplication or nuclear fusion (Brodsky and Uryvaeva, 1977).

9.3 Normal and Abnormal Mitosis, Endoreduplication and Nuclear Fusion

The number of mitotic figures per microscopic field plays an important role in establishing the histological diagnosis, 'malignancy'; this is not so in cyto-diagnosis since mitotic figures are not seen as often. Abnormal mitotic figures can occur in normal tissue; in malignant tumours, however, they are fairly common. In addition, various types of abnormal mitosis, endoreduplication and nuclear fusion are often found together in characteristic combinations (Oksala and Therman, 1974).

9.3.1 Abnormal Mitosis

9.3.1.1 The Original Nuclear Membrane remains Intact

During the normal prophase (B) the chromosomes duplicate (C) but the nuclear membrane does not dissolve. After completion of the division (E) the nucleus is tetraploid (polyploid), that is, a nucleus with twice the number of chromosomes (2 x 46). This is called endomitosis (figure 9.2).

9.3.1.2 Changes in the Duration of the Various Phases of Mitosis

(1) The prophase can be shorter than the metaphase (Scarpelli and von Haam, 1957). In such a case multipolar nuclear division often takes place.

(2) The prophase can be much longer than the metaphase. This is not as common as (1). Many

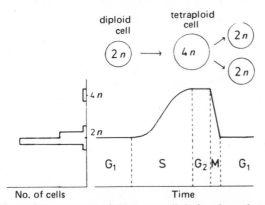

figure 9.1   Amount of DNA per cell during the various phases of the cell cycle. To the left is a histogram showing the distribution of the diploid and tetraploid cells. The diagram above the figure shows a diploid cell (2*n*) which yields two diploid cells after DNA synthesis (from: van Vloten, 1974)

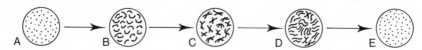

figure 9.2   Endomitosis

endomitoses (see section 9.3.1.1) are seen, whereas multipolar division is not as frequent (Oksala and Therman, 1974).

9.3.1.3 Abnormal or Missing Spindles

(1) *Abnormal spindles* (figure 9.3).   These consist for example of three centrosomes (B) which form a tripolar spindle (C). The result of such an abnormal mitotic division is three hypoploid nuclei (E), that is, three nuclei each with less than *2n* chromosomes. Quadripolar mitosis and ring-shaped metaphase configurations are also possible. In addition, during metaphase the chromosomes may adhere together, which often causes chromosome breakage. This is followed by recombination or loss of the broken chromosomes.

(2) *Missing spindles* (figure 9.4).   If the chromosomes remain in the equatorial plane (C, D), one tetraploid daughter cell will develop; in the telophase, constriction does not occur. This is called *restitution.* Another abnormal type of division (figure 9.5) is characterised by the absence of the spindle after the prophase (B) so that the chromosomes spread throughout the cell (D). During telo-

phase (E) micronuclei are formed with fewer chromosomes than the mother cell. The chromosomal patterns of the daughter cells differ. In mitotic divisions with abnormal or missing spindles chromosomes or parts of chromosomes can be lost, sometimes resulting in aneuploidy.

9.3.2 Endoreduplication

In endoreduplication the chromosomes duplicate without subsequent mitosis (figure 9.6). After endoreduplication the nucleus is tetraploid (B). This tetraploid cell may yield two tetraploid daughter cells (E) after mitosis (C, D). The process of endoreduplication can also repeat itself so that tetraploid nuclei will produce octoploid nuclei.

9.3.3 Amitosis

Amitosis is nuclear division without DNA replication and without mitosis. The cell splits apart into two daughter cells with unequal chromosomal patterns and hypodiploid nuclei. Nuclear frag-

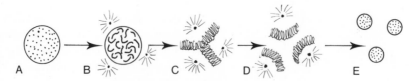

figure 9.3   Tripolar spindle

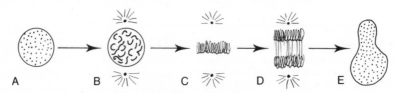

figure 9.4   Restitution

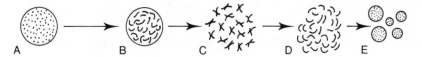

figure 9.5 Development of micronuclei

mentation can also be called amitosis. In such a case a new nuclear membrane forms around each fragment. Endoreduplication and amitosis cannot in fact be considered 'true' mitosis, since mitosis does not actually take place.

9.3.4 Cellular and Nuclear Fusion

Cellular fusion (figure 9.7) is a common phenomenon in malignant cells, particularly after abnormal mitosis (Hirono, 1951). Two fused (diploid) nuclei (C) together form one tetraploid nucleus, etc. Nuclear fusion takes place after cellular fusion (Harris, 1971).

The influence of a virus can also cause nuclear fusion. This has been demonstrated in in-vitro tests; with the Sendai virus, it was possible to bring about the fusion of cells from different animal species (Wiener *et al.*, 1971).

9.4 Development of Cancer

In normal tissue the dividing cells are to some extent subject to mutations, that is, changes in the genetic characteristics. These mutations can develop during the phase of mitosis as well as interphase (Comings, 1972). A mutation can occur spontaneously but can also be induced by, for example, exposure to ionising radiation, chemotherapeutic agents, viruses, or any combination of these. The chromosomal changes may be very tiny so that they cannot be observed with the light microscope, or coarser and recognisable as duplication of the chromosomes, breakage, recombination of broken chromosomes, etc. It is also possible that '*repair*' will occur, so that the chromosomal aberrations are corrected (Evans, 1974).

In the course of time more mutations may develop, until finally a cell will appear which has changed genetically with respect to the original cell to such an extent (it has a new set of genes)

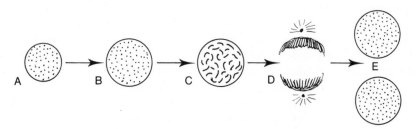

figure 9.6 Endoreduplicaton

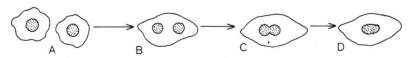

figure 9.7 Cellular and nuclear fusion

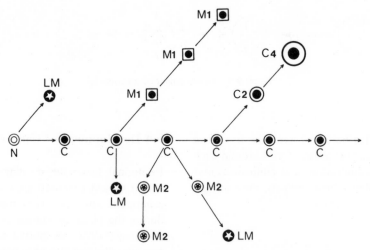

figure 9.8   Schematic diagram of the origin of cancer cells (symbols from Nowell, *Chromosomes and Cancer*, 1974). N, normal cell; LM, lethal mutant; C, clonal cancer cell; M1, mutant of cancer cell; M2, another mutant of cancer cell; C2, cancer cell after division with replication of DNA; C4, cancer cell after division of C2 resulting in 4 times as much DNA as in C

that it becomes independent of the regulatory mechanisms of the body. This cell will now be able to divide without being inhibited and, partially through abnormal mitosis, will also be able to form new mutants (figure 9.8). In this manner a cell population ultimately develops with obvious morphological nuclear anomalies (Macfarlane, 1974).

9.4.1 The Development of a Neoplastic Cell Clone

Through mutation a normal cell (N) can ultimately give rise to a cell (C) in which the number and/or the structure of the chromosomes is abnormal (figure 9.8). After division this tumour cell (C) will form daughter cells which in turn will divide, producing a population of cells which closely resemble the original cell. Such a population is called a clone. In this tumour cell population various new mutations can develop which either die out (LM) or are capable of proliferation (C, C2, M1, M2; figure 9.9). Each of these cells has a characteristic chromosomal abnormality, which may produce a variegated morphological cellular pattern.

When it can be demonstrated that most of the cells of a certain tumour have the same number of

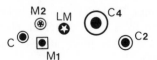

figure 9.9   Tumour cell population of figure 9.8

chromosomes this population is called the 'stemline' population. A tumour cell population can also be referred to as hypoploid, hyperploid, etc. It is not always possible to find the specific stemline because the number of chromosomes per cell can vary considerably (Spriggs, 1974).

Depending upon the circumstances, which can be influenced by such factors as exposure to ionising radiation, chemotherapeutic agents, etc., the population with the most rapid cell division will dominate and will therefore become the monoclonal stemline (figure 9.10). Morphologically a monomorphic pattern develops after cloning.

Invasive growth is often accompanied by loss of chromosomes. The stemline can be diploid or almost diploid but often also hypoploid. This is

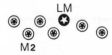

figure 9.10   Monoclonal tumour cell population

called 'ploidy reduction'. In the terminal stage of cervical carcinoma, a clear-cut stemline can no longer be identified; morphologically the pattern is highly polymorphic (Böhm and Sandritter, 1975).

9.4.2 Factors which Increase the Risk of Cancer

For individuals with inherited chromosomal errors, such as Down's syndrome, the risk of developing cancer is enhanced. In a cell population with an abnormal set of genes, it is highly likely that mutants will develop (German, 1972; Hecht *et al.*, 1966). Mutagenic influences from outside (exogenous), such as chemotherapy (Macfarlane, 1974), exposure to ionising radiation (Evans, 1974) and viruses (Harnden, 1974), increase the risk of cancer.

The same applies when no (or defective) 'repair' of somatic mutants occurs. An example of this is in xeroderma pigmentosum, a genetic disease in which DNA in the cells of the skin is destroyed by ultraviolet light and subsequent repair does not occur. The result is a high incidence of skin and other carcinoma (Setlow *et al.*, 1969). In older individuals the number of mutants increases with age, as does the frequency of cancer. For an interesting theoretical explanation of this, see Cairns (1975).

A mechanism which has not been considered here, but which certainly plays a role in the development of cancer, is the immunological defence reaction of the body. However, a discussion of this aspect lies beyond the scope of this book. When this reaction is deficient or has been purposely depressed (for example, for organ transplantation) the chance that a malignant tumour will develop is increased (McKhann, 1969; Prehn, 1969; Good, 1972).

9.5 Cell Morphology

9.5.1 Cell Biology and Morphology

The distribution and staining capacity of the chromatin in the nucleus, the chromatin network, is one of the most important tools for cytodiagnosis when the Papanicolaou stain is used. The chromatin pattern with the nuclear membrane, the nuclear body or nucleolus, and the nuclear sap or karyolymph together form the most important morphological characteristics of the interphase nucleus.

9.5.1.1 Chromatin

Chromatin consists of a DNA protein complex which, because of the affinity of the complex, stains blue in the alkaline stain haematoxylin. The proteins in the DNA protein complex are mainly histones (alkaline proteins) and the so-called 'nonhistone chromosomal' proteins. These proteins are tightly bound to DNA and are considered to be involved in its structure and in the regulation of gene expression in the cell. This regulatory process implies that only certain parts of the genetic code on the DNA are being translated, thus ensuring that cells of different tissues have specific characteristics (Elgin and Weintraub, 1975).

The distribution of the chromatin throughout the nucleus can vary. For instance, in the nuclei of normal intermediate squamous epithelial cells of the ectocervix most of the chromatin is finely granular, dispersed and lightly stained. In several areas, however, the chromatin appears to consist of somewhat larger, darker fragments (chromocentres). In these areas the chromatin is more compact. Biochemical and audioradiographic studies have shown that the noncompact chromatin (euchromatin) is the active part of the chromatin while the compact chromatin (heterochromatin) is less active in protein synthesis (Frenster, 1969).

There is, therefore, a clear relationship between the structure observable with the light microscope and the biochemical function of the nucleus. A good example of this is the nonstimulated small lymphocyte; about 30 per cent of the chromatin in this cell is heterochromatic. By stimulation with a mitogen, a large number of biochemical processes are triggered which are accompanied by an obvious shift in the nucleus from heterochromatin to euchromatin.

In many cases chromosomal duplication with polyploidy of the tumour cells is probably accompanied by elimination of certain genetically active areas on the chromosomes. This is expressed in the interphase nucleus as an increase in the heterochromatin. Cytologically this is manifested as a coarsening of the chromatin pattern.

9.5.1.2 Nucleolus

The nucleolus is the centre of the synthesised ribosomal ribonucleic acid (RNA; see section 1.3.2.2). The nucleolus contains not only RNA but also small quantities of DNA which come from the so-called 'nucleolar organiser' areas found on chromosomes. The protein component of the nucleolus consists of neutral or slightly acidic proteins as well as alkaline proteins and the enzymes necessary for the diverse metabolic processes in the nucleolus. The staining reaction of the nucleolus is often red. The size of the nucleolus in a benign cell depends on protein synthesis. In regenerating tissues, the nucleoli are often enlarged or multiple (Miller and Beatty, 1969).

9.5.1.3 Nuclear Membrane

The nuclear membrane can be observed only with the electron microscope. With the light microscope only the condensation of chromatin along the membrane can be seen. In this text, however, we will refer to what appear to be nuclear membranes under the light microscope (see section 1.2.2.). The degree of condensation (marginal hyperchromasia) depends upon the fixative used and the nature of the cell (Stevens and André, 1969).

Marginal hyperchromasia is slight in benign cells and is often pronounced in malignant and degenerated cells. Even if the nuclear membrane is not electronmicroscopically intact, if may appear so under the light microscope (see section 2.3.1.3).

9.5.1.4 Karyolymph

Karyolymph (also called 'nuclear sap') is a colloidal liquid which contains many types of proteins, including enzymes, as well as RNA molecules and ions in solution, etc. Depending upon the fixative used, some of these proteins will be fixed in the nucleus while the rest will disappear by diffusion.

9.5.2 Nuclear Patterns

The light microscopic pattern of the nucleus (the so-called 'nuclear pattern') obtained by fixation and staining shows the situation in the nucleus at one specific instant. The nuclear pattern is determined by the distribution of the chromatin throughout the nucleus, along the nuclear membrane, and by the presence of nucleoli. Experience in cytology has shown that certain nuclear patterns can be related to malignant and premalignant lesions.

The following descriptions of the various nuclear patterns apply only to cells which have been fixed in fast dehydrating agents. (see (15) below). The morphological picture appears to be very similar to that seen in tissue sections fixed rapidly by freezing (frozen sections) or, for example, in formalin. The appearance of the nuclei in air-dried Giemsa-stained cells is completely different and is not discussed here.

9.5.2.1 Chromatin Pattern of Benign and Malignant Cells

(1) Nucleus with fine chromatin pattern some-times with a few chromocentres. The chromo-centres, which are approximately equal in size, are connected by thin threads of chromatin. In females a Barr body (sex chromatin) may be seen on the edge of the nuclear membrane (see section 5.1). The intact nuclear membrane is visible as a thin taut line. Such a nucleus is found in benign cells.

(2) Large nucleus with large nucleolus (nor-mal nucleolar–nuclear ratio). There are several chromocentres which are larger than those in (1) but are also connected by thin chromatin threads. Lighter areas in the nucleus of about equal size are sometimes mistakenly identified as 'slightly coarsened chromatin pattern'; however, at a higher magnification (1000 x) it can be seen that this effect is caused by larger chromocentres which are round and of the same size. Furthermore, the nuclear membrane is slightly accentuated. Such a nucleus is found in regenerating tissue. Binucleation is common in such cells.

(3) Nucleus with coarse clumps of chromatin which are rounded and of about the same size. This can be a cell in the prophase or the telophase (b), in which case the nuclear membrane is not clearly visible, or a cell of carcinoma *in situ* (a, b and c). In a degenerated malignant cell the clumps lie along the interrupted nuclear membrane (c).

(4) Nucleus with small fragments of chromatin which are sharply angular (rice-flake pattern). The chromatin is more or less evenly distributed over the nucleus. The nuclear membrane seems intact This type of nucleus is found in cells of adeno-carcinoma of the endocervix and small cell carcino-ma *in situ.*

(5) Nucleus with thin threads of chromatin ('wire-netting pattern'). This is seen in dysplastic cells of the metaplastic type and in atypical reserve cells.

(6) Nucleus with marginal hyperchromasia and indistinct chromatin pattern. These nuclei occur frequently in degenerate cells and also in severe inflammation, possibly as a result of degeneration.

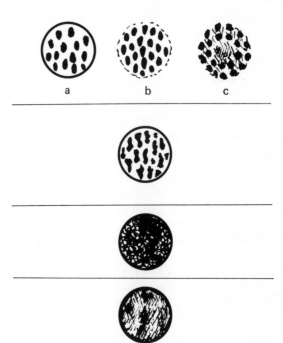

a   b   c

(7) Fairly large nucleus with empty spaces between the threads of chromatin. These spaces are about equal in size. This type is often found in degenerate cells.

(8) Pyknotic nucleus (no visible chromatin pattern). This can be found in a benign cell (a, small round nucleus in abundant cytoplasm) or a malignant cell (b, rather large, often irregularly shaped nucleus in little or no cytoplasm).

(9) Nucleus with several large dark clumps of chromatin which are round and about the same size. Nuclear membrane not always well-defined. This is often seen in degenerate benign cells.

(10) Nucleus with (a) or without (b) well-defined nuclear membrane with dark clumps of chromatin which are angular and of various sizes. These nuclei are often encountered in degenerate malignant cells or highly dysplastic cells.

(11) Nucleus with slightly coarsened chromatin which is evenly distributed. Such nuclei are found in dysplasia of the metaplastic type and in nonkeratinising carcinoma *in situ*.

(12) Nucleus with intact nuclear membrane and coarse clumps of chromatin which are neither round nor equal in size. These nuclei are found in malignant cells and to a lesser extent in markedly dysplastic cells. The clumps are more or less evenly distributed throughout the nucleus in severely dysplastic cells and are irregularly distributed in malignant cells.

(13) Nucleus with irregularly distributed chromatin which can be either markedly coarsened (see (12)) or granular. This is common in malignant cells.

(14) Nulcleus with clear zones in the chromatin. These clear zones are irregularly distributed, vary in size and are often of bizarre shape. This is called 'nuclear clearing'. The chromatin pattern can be either fine or coarse. Such nuclei are found in adenocarcinoma cells (with fine chromatin) and poorly differentiated squamous carcinoma cells (with coarse chromatin).

(15) Nuclei with marginal hyperchromasia and almost no chromatin pattern ('empty' nucleus). This is sometimes seen in cells that have been fixed in 96 per cent ethanol, especially atypical reserve cells.

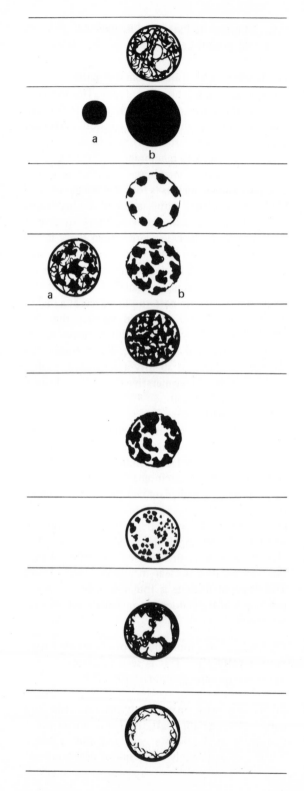

(16) Swollen hypochromatic nucleus with an indistinct chromatin pattern. These nuclei can be encountered in cells which were not fixed quickly enough or in degenerated cells.

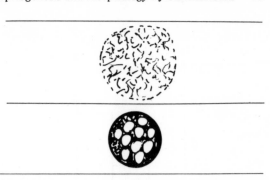

(17) Nucleus with sharply defined vacuoles. This can be either an artefact due to fixation (see section 15.7.(11)) or a change due to degeneration.

It is difficult to distinguish between fixation artefacts and degenerative nuclear abnormalities (see (16) and (17)). Moreover, degeneration phenomana (such as pyknosis and clumping of the chromatin) are found in both benign and malignant cells. The evaluation of an individual cell must be carried out with the aid of the cellular pattern as a whole and the patient's clinical data.

9.5.2.2 The Nucleolus in Benign and Malignant Cells

(1) A nucleolus in benign cells is round or oval. The nucleolar–nuclear ratio (Nc/N ratio) is low. Large nucleoli in large nuclei (normal Nc/N ratio) are found in reparative reactions and inflammation.

(2) Abnormally shaped nucleoli (rods, commas). These are found in inflammation, reparative reactions and in benign cells after exposure to ionising radiation. In these benign cells the Nc/N ratio is always low.

(3) Malignant cells can contain large round nucleoli or irregulat shaped nucleoli – The Nc/N ratio is often high. There can be one large (a) or 3 smaller (b) nucleoli; for the Nc/N ratio the combined area of the nucleoli is compared with that of the nucleus. In undifferentiated carcinoma cells the high Nc/N ratio is sometimes the only available criterion for malignancy.

(4) Perinucleolar halo. This can be found in the malignant cells of a well-differentiated adenocarcinoma. We have also seen such halos in endometrial atypia due to oestrogenic stimulation.

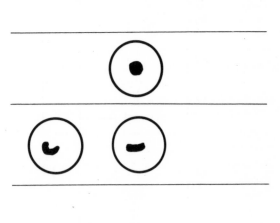

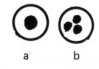

a   b

9.5.2.3 DNA Content and Nuclear Morphology

There is to some degree a relationship between DNA content and nuclear morphology. This may be illustrated in the following.

Characteristic nuclear features as described in section 9.5.2.1 are also found in Feulgen-stained cells (a specific cytochemical DNA staining method). These cells can be identified as benign, dysplastic or malignant, or as atypical reserve cells (see section 10.21.2) just like Papanicolaou-stained cells. Moreover, the DNA content and the nuclear

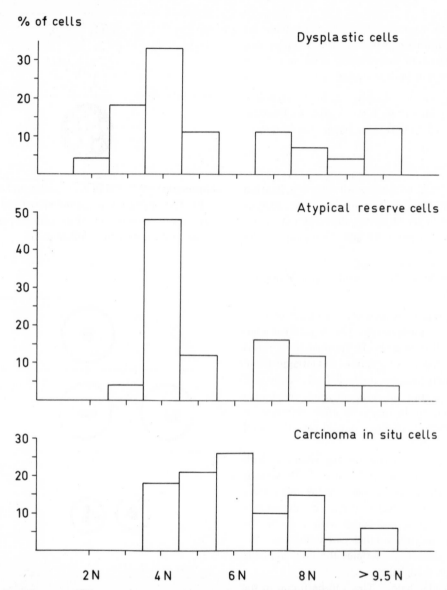

figure 9.11   Histograms of nuclei of dysplastic cells, atypical reserve cells, and carcinoma *in situ* cells. Ninety-two abnormal cells from ten different smears (six smears from cases with atypical reserve cell hyperplasia, dysplasia or both, and four smears from cases with carcinoma *in situ*) were used. For details see figure 9.12

area can be measured. Thus the relationship between nuclear morphology and DNA content can be established. In figure 9.11 histograms of dysplastic cell nuclei, atypical reserve cell nuclei and carcinoma *in situ* nuclei are displayed. All three cell types have elevated DNA values, such as above 5*n*. We did not encounter carcinoma cells

with diploid and near-diploid values (Böhm and Sandritter, 1975) in these samples.

The relationship between nuclear area and DNA content of the three cell types is depicted in the scattergram (figure 9.12). High DNA values, up to 20*n*, are seen in large nuclei with a fine chromatin pattern (for example, atypical reserve cell

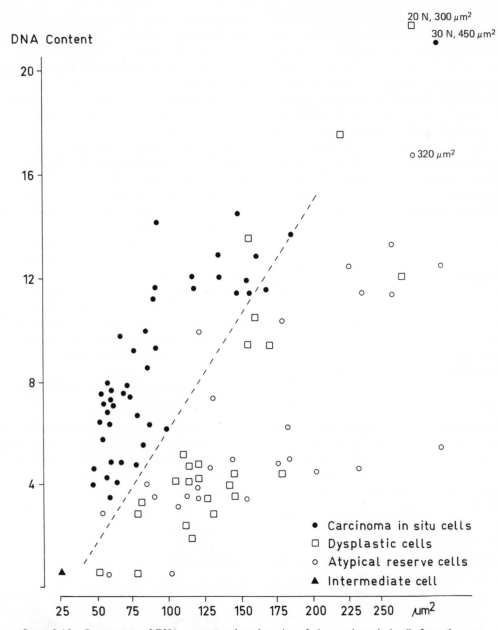

DNA Content

20 N, 300 μm²
30 N, 450 μm²

o 320 μm²

● Carcinoma in situ cells
□ Dysplastic cells
o Atypical reserve cells
▲ Intermediate cell

figure 9.12   Scattergram of DNA content and nuclear size of abnormal cervical cells from the same material as in figure 9.11. Each measured cell was graded cytomorphologically as normal intermediate cell, atypical reserve cell, dysplastic cell or carcinoma cell. The smears were stained Feulgen-Naphthol Yellow-S (Deitch, 1955). The densitometric assessment of DNA content was performed with an MPV II (Leitz), with 564 nm, measuring spot 0.5 μm and stepsize of 0.5 μm. The reliability of the staining results was determined by measuring the Feulgen-DNA levels in leucocytes and normal intermediate cells: no significant differences were found. The mean amount of DNA in normal intermediate cells was taken as the normal diploid nuclear DNA content. The measurements were performed in the Department of Pathology, Leiden, the Netherlands (Dr. C. J. Cornelisse)

nuclei) as well as in relatively small nuclei with marked chromatin clumping (for example, carcinoma *in situ* cells). The difference between dysplastic nuclei and atypical reserve cell nuclei is not significant; the malignant nuclei, however, have significantly higher DNA content per μm^2 ($P = \leqslant 0.001$), thus a high DNA 'packing'. No doubt, malignant nuclei without a high DNA packing can also be found if more samples are examined. However, these results illustrate nicely a rule of thumb in daily routine cervical cytology: the tighter the chromatinic pattern of large nuclei the greater the suspicion of malignancy.

9.5.3 Morphological Diagnosis: Malignant Cell

The morphological diagnosis 'malignant cell' must be based not only on the nuclear and nucleolar patterns but also on the cytoplasm, nuclear shape and size, as well as cellular arrangement and cellular interrelationships.

9.5.3.1 Nuclear Shape and Size

In general malignant cells have larger nuclei than the parent cell (Patten, 1978). In discrete carcinoma cells as well as those arranged in groups, abnormal nuclear shapes (angular, lobular, potato-shaped, etc.) and differences in size can be seen (figure 9.13).

9.5.3.2 Cytoplasm

DNA influences the cytoplasm by means of the arrangement and sequence of the nucleotides of the messenger RNA that is copied from the DNA (see section 1.3.2.2). Protein synthesis, the amount of cytoplasm, secretory products and differentiation products (such as keratin) are thus determined in part by the DNA. When the genetic information changes, as in a malignant cell, not only the nucleus but also the cytoplasm will change with respect to the parent cell. This can be expressed in various ways.

(1) The nucleocytoplasmic ratio (N/C ratio) changes. An abnormal N/C ratio implies a nucleus that is large in relation to the size of the cell. This is frequently encountered in malignant cells. Cells with this feature are frequently immature, undifferentiated or anaplastic.

(2) The differentiation of the cytoplasm is abnormal. There can be a lower degree of differentiation than that of the parent cell, expressed f.e. in a low N/C ratio, or it may show a higher degree of differentiation. An example of the latter is keratinising squamous cell carcinoma of the ectocervix, since ectocervical squamous epithelium does not normally exhibit total keratinisation.

9.5.3.3 Cellular Arrangement and Cellular Interrelationships

Tumour cells can be irregularly arranged; the nuclei can be stacked against each other causing indentations (nuclear moulding, figure 9.14). Nuclear moulding occurs mainly in rapidly growing neoplasms such as small cell anaplastic carcinoma.

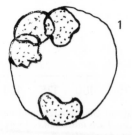

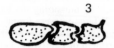

figure 9.14   Irregular arrangement (1) and stacking (2) of nuclei, and nuclear moulding (3)

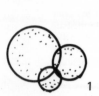
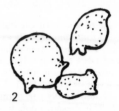

figure 9.13   Differences in nuclear size: anisonucleosis or anisokaryosis (1); and differences in nuclear shape: polymorphism (2)

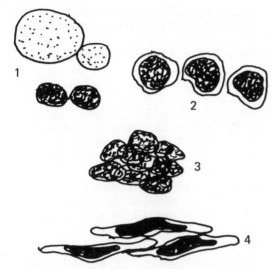

figure 9.15   Cellular interrelationships and cohesiveness. 1. Naked nuclei which just overlap are characteristic of undifferentiated cells. The nuclear pattern may (carcinoma *in situ* cells) or may not (reserve cells) be malignant. 2. Malignant cells lying separately but in a row with a tiny rim of cytoplasm, consistent with moderately differentiated carcinoma *in situ*. The cohesiveness of these cells is slight. 3. Compact group of cells with nuclear stacking, as seen in anaplastic carcinoma *in situ*. The cohesiveness of these cells is pronounced. 4. Ragged groups of cells with cigar-shaped nuclei which lie in parallel as seen in keratinising carcinoma *in situ*

The mutual cohesiveness of neoplastic cells may provide information about the origin and nature of the tumour cells (figure 9.15).

Malignant cells almost never have all the above mentioned characteristics at the same time. On the other hand, some of the characteristics described can also be observed in benign cells – although usually to a lesser degree. It is the combination of several of the morphological features of malignancy which enables one to make the cytological diagnosis of 'malignancy'. It is understandable that for accuracy in this matter considerable experience is needed as well as a thorough knowledge of histology and differential diagnosis.

References

Atkin, N. B., Richards, B. M. and Ross, A. J. (1959). The deoxyribonucleic acid content of carcinoma of the uterus: an assessment of its possible significance in relation to histopathology and clinical course based on data from 165 cases, *Br. J. Cancer*, **13**, 773–87

Baikie, A. G., Court Brown, W. M., Buckton, K. E., Harnden, D. G., Jacobs, P. A. and Tough, I. M. (1960). A possible specific chromosome abnormality in human chronic myeloid leukaemia. *Nature*, **188**, 1165–6

Böhm, N. and Sandritter, W. (1975). DNA in human tumours: A cytophotometric study. In *Current Topics in Pathology*, vol. 60 (eds E. Grundmann and N. H. Kirsten), Springer, New York, pp. 151–213

Brodsky, W. Ya. and Uryvaeva, I. V. (1977). Cell polyploidy: Its relation to tissue growth and function. *Int. Rev. Cytol.*, p. 275

Cairns, J. (1975). Mutation, selection and the natural history of cancer. *Nature*, **225**, p. 197

Comings, D. E. (1972). The structure and function of chromatin. In *Advances in Human Genetics* (eds H. Harris and K. Hirchhorn), Plenum, New York, pp. 137–431

Deitch, S. (1955). Microspectrophotometric study of the binding of the anionic dye Naphthal Yellow-S by tissue sections and purified proteins. *Lab. Invest.*, **4**, 324–51

Elgin, S. C. R. and Weintraub, H. (1975). Chromosomal proteins and chromatin structure. In *Annual Review of Biochemistry*, vol. 44 (eds E. E. Snel *et al.*), Annual Reviews Inc., California, pp. 726–74

Evans, H. J. (1974). Effects of ionizing radiation on mammalian chromosomes. In *Chromosomes and Cancer* (ed. J. German), Wiley, New York, pp. 191–237

Frenster, J. H. (1969). Biochemistry and molecular biophysics of heterochromatin and euchromatin. In *Handbook of Molecular Cytology* (ed. A. Lima-de-Faria), North-Holland, Amsterdam, pp. 251–77

German, J. (1972). Genes which increase chromosal instability in somatic cells and predispose to cancer. *Progr. med. Genet.*, **8**, 61–101

Good, R. A. (1972). Relations between immunity and malignancy. *Proc. natn. Acad. Sci. U.S.A.*, **69**, 1026–32

Harnden, D. G. (1974). Viruses, chromosomes and tumours: the interaction between viruses and chromosomes. In *Chromosomes and Cancer* (ed. J. German), Wiley, New York, pp. 151–91

Harris, H. (1971). Cell fusion and the analysis of Malignancy. *Proc. R. Soc. Lond.*, **179**, 1–20

Hecht, F., Koler, R. D., Rigas, D. A., Dahnke, G. S., Case, M. P., Tisdale, V. and Miller, R. W. (1966). Leukaemia and lymphocytes in ataxia-teleangiectasia *Lancet*, **ii**, 1193

Hirono, I. (1951). Some observations on the mitosis of living malignant tumor cells. *Acta Path. Jap.*, **1**, 40–47

Macfarlane, B. (1974). The biology of cancer. In *Chromosomes and Cancer* (ed. J. German), Wiley, New York, pp. 21–41

McKhann, C. F. (1969). Primary malignancy in patients undergoing immunosuppression for renal transplantation. *Transplantation*, **8**, 209–12

Makino, S. and Kano, K. (1951). Cytological observations on cancer II. Daily observations on the mitotic frequency and the variation of the chromosome number in tumor cells of the Yoshida sarcoma through a transplant generation. *J. Fac. Sci. Hokkaido Univ.*, **10**, 225–42

Miller, O. L. and Beatty, B.R. (1969). Nucleolar structure and function. In *Handbook of Molecular Cytology* (ed. A. Lima-de Faria), North-Holland, Amsterdam, pp. 605–30

Oksala, T. and Therman, E. (1974). Mitotic abnormalities and cancer. In *Chromosomes and Cancer* (ed. J. German), Wiley, New York, pp. 239–67

Patten, S. F. (1978). *Diagnostic Cytology of the Uterine Cervix*, Karger, Basel

Prehn, R. T. (1969). The relationship of immunology to carcinogenesis. *Ann. N.Y. Acad. Sci.*, **164**, 449–57

Reagan, J. W. and Patten, S. F. (1961). Analytic study of cellular changes in carcinoma in situ, squamous cell cancer and adenocarcinoma of uterine cervix. *J. clin. Obstet. Gynec.*, **4**, 1097–127

Scarpelli, D. G. and Haam, E. von. (1957). A study of mitosis in cervical epithelium during experimental inflammation and carcinogenesis. *Cancer Res.*, **17**, 880–4

Setlow, R. B., Reagan, J. D., German, J. and Carrier W. L. (1969). Evidence that xeroderma pigmentosum cells do not perform the first step in the repair of ultraviolet damage to their DNA. *Proc. natn. Acad. Sci. U.S.A.*, **64**, 1035–41

Spriggs, A. I. (1974). Cytogenetics of cancer and precancerous states of the cervix uteri. In *Chromosomes and Cancer* (ed. J. German), Wiley, New York, pp. 432–51

Stadler, L. J. (1931). The experimental modification of heredity in crop plants I. Induced chromosomal irregularities. *Sci. Agric.*, **11**, 557–72

Stevens, B. J. and André, J. (1969). The nuclear envelope. In *Handbook of Molecular Cytology* (ed. A. Lima-de-Faria), North-Holland, Amsterdam, pp. 837–75

Vendrely, R. and Vendrely, C. (1949). La teneur du noyau cellulaire en acide désoxyribonucleique à travers les organes, les individus et les especes animales *Experientia*, **5**, 327–9

Vloten, W. A. van. (1974). *De Betekenis van DNA Cytofotometric voor de vroegtijdige Diagnostiek van Mycosis fungoides. Proefschrift*, Beugelsdijk, Leiden

Wiener, F., Klein, G. and Harris, H. (1971). The analysis of malignancy by cell fusion III. Hybrids between diploid fibroblasts and other tumor cells. *J. Cell Sci.*, **8**, 681–92

Atypical Reserve Cell Hyperplasia, Dysplasia, Carcinoma *in Situ* and Squamous Cell Carcinoma of the Uterine Cervix

10.1 Introduction

In this chapter squamous cell carcinoma of the cervix and its precursors, carcinoma *in situ* dysplasia and atypical reserve cell hyperplasia, will be considered together as a sequence. There are several reasons for this approach. In the first place, a morphological continuity exists between these lesions: for instance, there is a smooth morphological transition between pronounced dysplasia and carcinoma *in situ* (see section 10.2.3.3). Richart and Barron (1969) have coined the term 'cervical intraepithelial neoplasia', which embraces the morphological continuum of these lesions.

Furthermore, the morphogenesis of these different lesions is interrelated: if dysplasia or atypical reserve cell hyperplasia is followed up, progression to carcinoma *in situ* and/or invasive squamous cell carcinoma will be found in a number of cases (see section 10.3).

10.2 Histology, Cytology, Differential Diagnosis and Incidence of the Different Lesions

10.2.1 Atypical Reserve Cell Hyperplasia

10.2.1.1 Histology

The histological pattern of atypical reserve cell hyperplasia is characterised by the presence of several layers of atypical undifferentiated cells beneath the columnar epithelial cells of the endocervical glandular epithelium (Bajardi, 1961). Nuclear polymorphism is not pronounced, being less than that seen in carcinoma *in situ* (Johnson *et al.*, 1964); anisokaryosis can, however, be quite pronounced. Endocervical columnar cells may be absent. The epithelium is then composed of undifferentiated cells throughout its entire thickness. The chromatin pattern is exceedingly important; it is *fine* in atypical reserve cells, in contrast to the coarse chromatin pattern seen in the cells of carcinoma *in situ*. The cytoplasm is hazy (undifferentiated) and ill defined and may vary from very little to abundant.

Atypical reserve cell hyperplasia is always found proximal to the squamocolumnar junction and also always involves the endocervical glands. In regenerating processes (see section 7.5.2) atypical reserve cells can also be encountered.

10.2.1.2 Cytology

The atypical reserve cells display the characteristic exfoliation pattern of normal reserve cells (see sections 2.3.1.2, 7.4.1.2). This includes dense clumps, pairs and rows, often with ramifications. In the clumps and rows nuclear moulding is often present (figure 10.1). Isolated bare nuclei also occur as do cell sheets. The N/C ratio is usually high (see figure 10.5). The shape of the nuclei is usually vesicular; potato-shaped nuclei are also frequently encountered. The nuclei are not as narrow as the nuclei of the (germinal) reserve cells

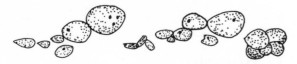

figure 10.1   Atypical reserve cells

in an atrophic smear pattern. The cytoplasm is usually destroyed during the smear procedure (see section 2.3.1.3) or is very hazy with ill-defined borders. The cytoplasm differs greatly in consistency from the dense cytoplasm of dysplastic cells (see section 10.2.2.2). In the scanty cytoplasm vacuolisation may occur, which can make differentiation from an adenocarcinoma difficult. We distinguish two types of atypical reserve cell hyperplasia.

(1) *The anisokaryotic type.* The hypochromatic nuclei vary greatly in size. The chromatin pattern is fine and granular; nuclear clearing also occurs. One or more (large) nucleoli are often seen (nuclear patterns 1, 2, 5, 7, 15, see section 9.5.2.1).

(2) *The monomorphic type.* The nuclei are approximately equal in size; on the average they are slightly smaller than those seen in the anisokaryotic type. Often they lie in sheets; in such cases the cellular margins are easily seen by focussing up and down. There is nuclear moulding but no nuclear overlapping. Mitotic figures are common. The chromatin pattern may be slightly coarse but not as markedly so as in malignant cells. Hyperchromatism may occur.

10.2.1.3 Differential Diagnosis

Atypical reserve cell hyperplasia must be differentiated from the following.

(1) *Endocervical glandular epithelial cells.* Anisokaryotic bare cells may closely resemble endocervical glandular epithelial cells. When the nuclei of endocervical glandular cells lie in a strand of mucus the cells may be incorrectly interpreted as reserve cells.

(2) *Reserve cells.* These cells show neither conspicuous anisokaryosis nor hyperchromatism, and their nuclei are generally narrow and smaller than those of atypical reserve cells.

(3) *Undifferentiated carcinoma cells.* These cells show gross nuclear abnormalities and are often dark.

(4) *Adenocarcinoma cells* (see section 12.2.2.2). This distinction is difficult whenever atypical reserve cells have large nucleoli or their cytoplasm is vacuolated. However, in contrast to cell groups from an adenocarcinoma of the endometrium, groups of atypical reserve cells never have a three-dimensional appearance.

The technical quality of the cytological material must be optimal if differentiation is to be made on basis of chromatin patterns.

10.2.1.4 Incidence of Atypical Reserve Cell Hyperplasia

The mean age of patients with atypical reserve cell hyperplasia is 35.9 years, which is younger than the mean age of patients with carcinoma *in situ* (see table 10.5). The age distribution is shown in figure 10.2. The presence of atypical reserve cells in a high proportion of the smears of patients with carcinoma *in situ* either of the epidermoid type (see section 10.3.1) or adenomatous type (see section 11.2.2) supports the theory that atypical reserve cell hyperplasia is involved directly or indirectly in the development of carcinoma *in situ* (Beyer-Boon and Verdonk, 1978).

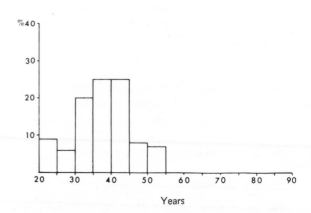

figure 10.2   Age distribution of 70 women with atypical reserve cell hyperplasia (Leiden University and the Leiden Cytology Laboratory, 1970)75

10.2.1.5 Electron Microscopy

In transmission electron microscopy the nucleus has a very irregular shape and the nuclear envelope is intact. A nucleolus is often seen. The outer border of the cytoplasm is often damaged; however, in a few cells mitochondriae can still be discerned.

10.2.2 Dysplasia

Dysplasia is the term used when there is hyperplastic growth of the epithelium characterised by failure of maturation and differentiation combined with abnormally enlarged and hyperchromatic nuclei, short of frankly carcinomatous change.

10.2.2.1 Histology

The hyperplasia of immature cells and the blockage of normal differentiation both result in the

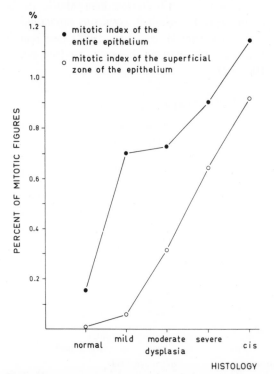

figure 10.3 Graphic representation of the percentage of mitotic figures in normal squamous epithelium, dysplasia and carcinoma *in situ* (cis) of the uterine cervix (courtesy of Dr C. A. Rubio)

presence of relatively immature cells in the higher zones of the epithelium. This is reflected in the morphology of the component cells of the upper layers: low N/C ratio, no glycogen production; and in the biological potentialities: the presence of mitotic figures (figure 10.3) and evidence of DNA synthesis.

The cells generally have abnormal nuclei: (a) the nuclei are larger than normal and anisokaryotic; (b) the shape of the nuclei is irregular (polymorphic); (c) the chromatin pattern of the nuclei is coarse; (d) the nuclei are hyperchromatic, or large and hypochromatic.

Due to anisokaryosis the epithelium has an 'untidy' appearance. Abnormal differentiation in the form of individual cell keratinisation with hyperkeratosis and parakeratosis may occur in keratinising dysplastic lesions (see section 10.2.2.3).

The dysplastic lesions are predominantly in the metaplastic area, and often have deep glandular extensions. Keratinised dysplasia may also occur in the area distal to the squamocolumnar junction, in the area of the native squamous epithelium.

A distinction can be made between mild, moderate and severe dysplasia.

(1) *Mild dysplasia.* If the epithelium is divided into three layers (see section 2.3.1.1) – a deep zone near the stroma, a middle (intermediate) zone and a superficial zone – it may be observed in mild dysplasia that immature cells are present in the deep zone (the nuclei being rounded or elongated with a maximum nuclear diameter perpendicular to the epithelial border). The nuclear density is high in that zone and decreases markedly towards the surface. The cytoplasm of the cells in the intermediate and superficial zones is abundant and dense, suggesting cell maturation (that is, cytoplasmic enlargement as well as decreased cytoplasmic basophilia); the nuclei are enlarged and display some chromatin abnormalities.

(2) *Moderate dysplasia.* Immature cells are present both in the deep zone and in part of or throughout the intermediate zone with a similar nuclear density in both zones. The rest of the epithelium contains cells with nuclear abnormalities and with abundant dense cytoplasm and has a lower nuclear density.

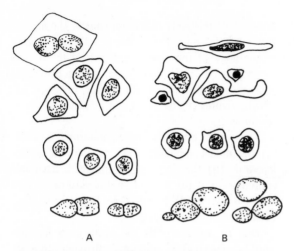

figure 10.4   Cytological pattern of classical dysplasia. A. mild dysplasia and slightly atypical reserve cells; B. severe dysplasia and extremely atypical reserve cells

(3) *Severe dysplasia.*   Immature cells are present in the deep and intermediate zones and in the deeper half of the superficial zone, the nuclear density being similar in these three areas. At the surface, cells with nuclear abnormalities and a moderate amount of cytoplasm occur, resulting in a slightly lower nuclear density. The mitotic indices in the intermediate and superficial layers increase progressively in moderate and severe dysplasia (see figure 10.3).

A special type of epithelial abnormality is that associated with condyloma virus (see section 7.3.5.2). Histologically, the *'condylomatous'* changes include koilocytosis, acanthesis, parakeratosis and multipolar divisions. The warty lesions arise in the native squamous epithelium of the vulva, vagina and cervix; the enodphytic and flat lesions in the metaplstic epithelium. The flat and the papillar lesions are often found in combination (Greene and Peckham, 1954). Especially in condylomatous epithelium of the transformation zone, nuclear enlargement is often pronounced. However, we doubt if the term 'condylomatous *dysplasia*' for these lesions, also used in this book is theoretically correct (see section 10.2.2.2, morphometric data). In our experience condylomatous changes may occur in 10 per cent of cases concurrent with either mild or severe 'classical dysplasia' or with carcinoma *in situ*. Whether these concurrent lesions arise from the same stem cells or are both the result of the same aetiological factors, such as frequent and various venereal contact, remains unclear. Malignant transformation of condylomatous lesions has, however, also been described (Marsh, 1952), resulting in the so-called *'verrucous carcinoma'* of the cervix (Spratt and Lee, 1977) (see section 10.2.4.2). We observed one such case (see section 10.2.4.2).

10.2.2.2 Cytology

The cytological characteristics of *'classical' dysplasia* are as follows (figure 10.4).

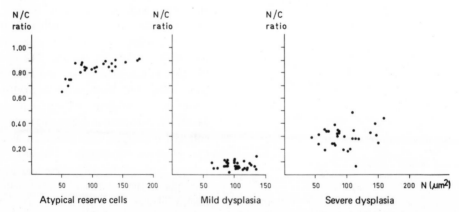

figure 10.5   Scattergram of nuclear area (N) and N/C ratio of cells from a characteristic example of atypical reserve cell hyperplasia, mild dysplasia and severe dysplasia. Extreme values of nuclear area (1000 μm^2) were encountered in other cases of all three conditions

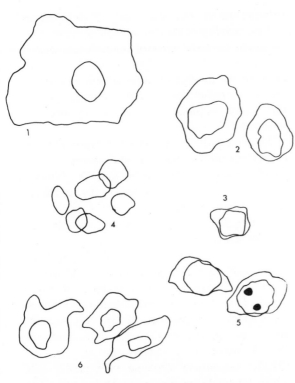

figure 10.6   Dysplastic and malignant cells. Camera lucida drawings. 1. Mildly dysplastic cell; 2. severely dysplastic cells; 3. carcinoma *in situ* cell; 4. malignant cells from a small cell nonkeratinising carcinoma (anaplastic carcinoma); 5. malignant cells from a large cell nonkeratinising carcinoma; 6. malignant cells from a keratinising squamous cell carcinoma

(1) *Disorders of maturation.*   The smear contains many immature cells, such as parabasal epithelial cells, in addition to many epithelial cells which display a failure of maturation, that is, they have the typical shape and cytoplasmic staining reaction of intermediate or superficial epithelial cells, but their nuclei resemble the nuclei of parabasal cells. Another manifestation of failure of differentiation is the fact that the nuclei occupy a relatively large area of the cells (figures 10.5 and 10.6). The N/C ratio of dysplastic cells is, however, not as high as in carcinoma *in situ* cells (see figure 10.13). The cytoplasm of dysplastic cells is always dense (squamous differentiation) and well defined.

(2) *Abnormalities of the nuclei.*   (a) Different sizes (anisokaryosis); (b) irregular shapes (polymorphism); (c) deviations in chromatin pat-

tern, such as coarseness, irregularity of distribution and hyperchromasia (see section 9.5.2.1, nuclear patterns 4, 5, 6, 8, 10, 11, 12); (d) multinucleation.

Usually the dysplastic cells in a smear are isolated; sometimes they lie in sheets in which the cells are regularly arranged. The cytoplasm is dense (squamoid) with distinct cell boundaries, in contrast to the frail and hazy cytoplasm with indistinct cell boundaries in atypical reserve cell hyperplasia. In general, the cell groups are smaller than those encountered in carcinoma *in situ*. The background of the smear is usually 'clean' unless an inflammatory exudate is present due to infection.

The cytological characteristics of *condylomatous dysplasia* as reported by Meisels *et al.* (1977) and Purola and Savia (1977) are (figure 10.7): (1) dysplastic cells with koilocytosis (or koilocytes) (see section 7.3.5.2.); (2) parakeratotic cells with hyperchromatic nuclei, isolated and in sheets; (3) intermediate cells with indistinct cell borders and large pale nuclei with somewhat irregular chromatinic pattern; (4) multinucleated giant (2–25 nuclei) cells with abundant (up to 7000 μm^2) granular cytoplasm. In 84 per cent of the smears of condylomatous lesions these giant cells with a cytoplasmic area over 2000 μm^2 were present (de Graaf Guilloud-Gentenaar and Beyer-Boon, 1977). In a morphometric study of classical dysplastic cells and condylomatous dysplastic cells (or koilocytes) we found that there is a statistically significant difference between these two 'dysplastic' cell types (see table 10.1): in both cell populations there is an increase in nuclear size, however, the

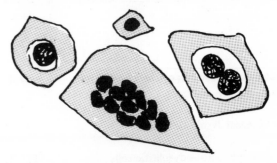

figure 10.7   Cytological pattern of condylomatous dysplasia

koilcytic cells have significantly larger cytoplasmic areas than 'classical' dysplastic cells, and thus also relatively low N/C ratios, and can, therefore, be at the utmost classified as mildly dysplastic (compare with figure 10.5) We interpret these findings as an indication that we deal here with two distinct cell populations (see concurrent lesions, 10.3.2).

10.2.2.3 Classification of Dysplasia

Cytologically also, one can discriminate between mild, moderate and severe dysplasia. The severity of dysplasia is based on the following characteristics.

(1) *Severity of the nuclear abnormalities.* In mild to moderate dysplasia the chromatin pattern is irregular but not coarse. In severe dysplasia hyperchromatism may be pronounced.

(2) *Immaturity of the dysplastic cells.* In mild and moderate dysplasia the dysplastic cells are predominantly of the intermediate type; in severe dysplasia the N/C ratio is increased (see figure 10.5). The amount of cytoplasm, that is, the degree of maturation, can therefore be an important criterion for discrimination. Parabasal cells with slight nuclear abnormalities are, however, classified as mildly dysplastic cells. In severe dysplasia, cells with keratinised cytoplasm and 'immature' relatively large nuclei are sometimes seen (so-called 'keratinising dysplasia').

(3) *Number of abnormal cells in the smear.* According to Patten (1978) there is a relationship between the number of atypical cells in the smear and the severity of the abnormality, assuming that the smear has been obtained correctly (see section 15.3.1). Koss (1968) accepted a clear relationship between the number of atypical cells in a smear and the extent of the lesion. As the lesion spreads, the chance of pronounced cellular abnormalities increases.

In general the morphological features (1) and (2) will decide classification of dysplasia as mild, moderate or severe. Due to the low N/C ratio (see table 10.1) koilocytotic dysplasia cells are always classified as mildly dysplastic.

Dysplasia can also be classified according to *differentiation.*

(1) *Keratinising dysplasia.* Dysplastic polygonal cells with strongly orangeophilic cytoplasm, parakeratotic cells and cells with abnormal shapes (spool, fibre, club or tadpole-shaped cells). Sometimes anucleated squamous cells are also encountered. The majority of the cells are isolated and there is often extensive nuclear pyknosis.

(2) *Nonkeratinising dysplasia.* Dysplastic cells which resemble mature metaplastic cells. The majority of the dysplastic cells are isolated (mature cells), and the cells are predominantly polygonal.

(3) *Metaplastic dysplasia.* Dysplastic cells which resemble immature metaplastic cells. Again the majority of the cells are isolated; however, cell aggregates are also found. The cell shape is oval or rounded, like immature metaplastic cells. The cytoplasm is dense (squamoid).

table 10.1   Mean cell dimensions of 1000 dysplastic cells measured in ten different slides from ten different patients

	Nuclear area		Cytoplasmic area		N/C Ratio	
	μm^2	s.d.	μm^2	s.d.		s.d.
Normal squamous epithelial cells from negative controls	47.21	20.60	2105.20	824.14	0.038	0.018
Classical dysplastic cells	92.34	80.86	279.30	232.96	0.358	1.275
Condylomatous dysplastic cells (koilocytes)	115.23	134.76	1752.06	1410.9	0.0940	0.503

A combination of these specific types of dysplasia may occur, and of classical and koilocytotic or condylomatous dysplasia. Also a combination with atypical reserve cells is frequently encountered. The reader should realise that in the smear only the cells from the upper layers of the epithelium are found. In histological diagnosis the morphology of the upper layers plays a decisive role. Therefore a high degree of correlation is obtainable between histological and cytological diagnosis.

10.2.2.4 Differential Diagnosis

Dysplasia must be differentiated from the following.

(1) Changes due to inflammation. To distinguish between dysplasia and an inflammatory reaction, for instance as a result of trichomoniasis (see section 7.3.3.1), a second smear should be taken after the inflammation has been treated.

(2) Tissue repair (see section 7.5.2).

(3) Folic acid deficiency (see section 14.5).

(4) Changes due to irradiation (see section 14.5).

(5) Decidual cells (see section 3.3.3).

(6) Carcinoma *in situ* (see section 10.2.3).

(7) Invasive squamous cell carcinoma. Cytologically it is not always possible to discriminate keratinising dysplasia from keratinising invasive quamous cell carcinoma. Biopsy is then indicated.

(8) Effect of chemotherapeutic drugs (see section 14.7).

10.2.2.5 Incidence of Dysplasia

The average age of patients with mild 'classical' dysplasia in our series was 30.8 years; the average age of patients with severe 'classical' dysplasia was 38.6 years. The average age of patients with condylomatous dysplasia in our material was 29.8 years, thus almost ten years younger than patients with severe 'classical' dysplasia. The age distribution of both 'classical' and condylomatous dysplasia is depicted in figure 10.8. The occurrence of dysplasia appears to remain more or less constant when the same group of women is examined several years in succession (table 10.1).

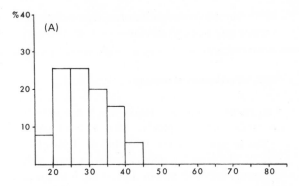

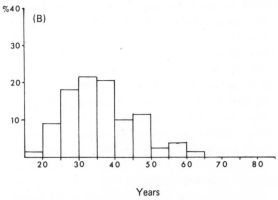

Years

figure 10.8 Age distribution of 51 women with a condylomatous dysplasia (A) and 234 women with a 'classical' severe dysplasia (B). (Leiden University and the Leiden Cytology Laboratory, 1974–5)

10.2.2.6 Electron Microscopy

At the SEM level an epithelial surface covered by microridges was found not only in normal squamous epithelium but also in dysplastic epithelium. In cases with dysplasia, however, only fragments of microridges were observed, intermingled with microvilli-like formations (Rubio and Kranz,

table 10.2 Frequency of dysplasia found in a population screening programme in Louisville, Kentucky (Christopherson and Parker, 1964b)

First screening	4.8/1000
Second screening	5.6/1000
Third screening	5.5/1000
Fourth screening	5.8/1000
Fifth screening	4.8/1000

1976). In transmission electron microscopy the nucleus may be partly absent.

10.2.3 Carcinoma *In Situ*

Carcinoma *in situ* is a lesion which can only be recognised microscopically. After a latent period it can progress to invasive carcinoma (Koss *et al.*, 1963). The term 'carcinoma *in situ*' is used when immature cells and mitotic figures are found in all layers of the epithelium ('full thickness' lesion), and the architecture of the epithelium is totally disrupted. In contrast to dysplasia, there are no features of cytoplasmic maturation (for example, clear cell boundaries and abundance of cytoplasm) in the superficial layers of the epithelium. Mitoses are present at all levels of the epithelium (see figure 10.3). Carcinoma *in situ* is a type of cancer which displays *no* signs of invasion of the underlying stroma (Koss, 1968). In 1961, the international Committee on Histological Terminology gave the following definition:

> Only those cases should be classified as carcinoma *in situ* which, in the absence of invasion, show a surface epithelium in which no differentiation takes place throughout the whole thickness. The process may involve the lining of the cervical glands without thereby creating a new group. It is recognised that cells of the uppermost layers may show some flattening. The very rare case of an otherwise characteristic carcinoma *in situ* which shows a greater degree of differentiation belongs to the exception for which no classification can provide.

This definition is restricted since there is no reference to the fact that the cells which make up this epithelium should show nuclear abnormalities (especially in the chromatin pattern). The presence of nuclear abnormalities is, however, considered by some authors, such as Govan *et al.*(1966), a prerequisite for the histological diagnosis of carcinoma *in situ*. In the 1950s the following criteria were established for a carcinoma *in situ*.

(1) *Cellular abnormalities.* (a) Anaplasia — variation in cell form, increased N/C ratio, basophilic cytoplasm, lack of glycogen. (b) Abnormal nuclei — multiple or multilobed nuclei. (c) Abnormalities of proliferation — frequent or abnormal (multipolar) mitotic figures, mitotic figures in epithelial cells near the surface.

(2) *Structural abnormalities.* (a) A sharp boundary between normal and pathological epithelium. (b) Disorder of epithelial structure (loss of normal stratification and polarity).

Carcinoma *in situ* occurs mainly in the metaplastic area, proximal to the squamocolumnar junction. In the majority of cases the underlying glands are also involved. The distribution of carcinoma *in situ* is comparable to that observed for reserve cell hyperplasia and squamous metaplasia (Patten, 1978). Dysplastic changes are found in general distal to the carcinoma *in situ* (Reagan and Patten, 1962), thus on the ectocervical side. In a large number of cases the two processes may be encountered in combination. Carcinoma *in situ* is often *multifocal*; in a later stage the lesions may merge together. It is usually diagnosed by chance during a routine examination. Sometimes the clinician will see an erosion or leucoplakia. When carcinoma *in situ* is established cytologically a histological examination (biopsy) must always follow to exclude invasive carcinoma.

10.2.3.1 Histology

Histologically three types of carcinoma *in situ* can be recognised (Reagan and Hamonic, 1956). The various types may be present in one patient.

(1) *Keratinising carcinoma in situ.* The surface of the epithelium is keratinised, thus the uppermost epithelial layers consist of cells with hyperchromatic fusiform nuclei which lie with their axes parallel to the surface (figure 10.9). Often many parakeratotic cells with relative large pycnotic nuclei are present.

It appears that this type in particular is the precursor of an invasive carcinoma with metastases to the lymph nodes. Some pathologists may classify these lesions as keratinising or pleomorphic dysplasia (Patten, 1978). However, we contend that, from a biological point of view, these lesions may antedate the development of keratinising squamous cell carcinoma.

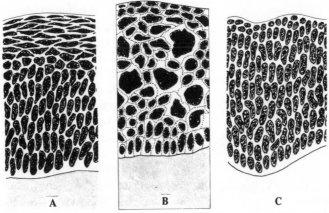

Figure 10.9 Histological pattern of carcinoma *in situ*. A. Keratinising carcinoma *in situ*; B. moderately differentiated carcinoma *in situ*; C. anaplastic carcinoma *in situ*

(2) *'Moderately differentiated' large cell carcinoma in situ.* The entire epithelium consists of malignant cells with large, often bizarre nuclei. The nuclear density is high in all zones. The cytoplasm is dense (squamoid differentiation) as in squamous metaplasia, and intracellular bridges may be observed (figure 10.9).

(3) *Anaplastic carcinoma in situ.* The epithelium displays little or no maturation. The nuclei are fusiform and polychromatic (figure 10.9). The cytoplasm is hazy and ill defined. No intercellular bridges are observed. It is possible to distinguish between a type with very small nuclei (small cell anaplastic carcinoma *in situ*) and a type with fairly large nuclei (large cell anaplastic carcinoma *in situ*).

10.2.3.2 Cytology

In the smear, the cells of carcinoma *in situ* (especially the small cell anaplastic type) show pronounced cohesion with respect to one another: most of these cells form groups in the smear. The malignant epithelium is easily detached from the underlying stroma. This explains why malignant cell groups can be found in the smear even when the lesion is very small. These 'microbiopsies' of malignant epithelium may be flat on one side (the surface) and undulating on the other (the rete pegs).

The cells from carcinoma *in situ* often lie in cell groupings with ill-defined cellular margins. On the other hand dysplastic epithelial cells are found mainly in sheets with clearly defined cell borders. The malignant cell groups appear ragged and the cells are irregularly arranged, thus enabling them to be distinguished from a group of endocervical glandular cells. In addition to malignant cells, the smear often also contains dysplastic cells and atypical reserve cells (table 10.3).

The background of the smear is usually clean unless there is an inflammatory reaction. A true tumour diathesis is seldom seen. A high K.I. is often encountered (Rubio, 1973) in fertile women as well as in postmenopausal women and also in patients using oral contraceptives. Fraser *et al.* (1967) established that patients with carcinoma *in situ* have elevated levels of curculatory oestrogen; this may explain the cytohormonal finding.

Cytologically three types of carcinoma *in situ* can usually be distinguished, but often components of all three types will be found in one smear.

(1) *Keratinising carcinoma in situ.* In the smear the keratinised cells (fibre cells, parakeratotic cells) predominate. The nuclei of these fibre cells are equal in shape and lie in parallel to each other (figure 10.10). In addition, round or oval malignant cells with acidophilic or cyanophilic cytoplasm also occur. The nuclei are hyperchromatic and/or pycnotic. The nuclear structure is irregular

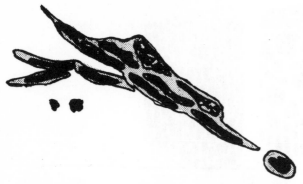

figure 10.10   Cytological pattern of keratinising carcinoma *in situ*

(nuclear patterns 8, 12, 14, section 9.5.2.1). The nuclei are not as bizarre as those seen in invasive squamous cell carcinoma (see section 10.2.4.2).

(2) *'Moderately differentiated' large cell carcinoma in situ.*   The smear contains mainly moderately differentiated malignant cells with centrally located nuclei and acidophilic or cyanophilic cytoplasm. There is little variation in nuclear size. The N/C ratio is higher than in dysplastic cells (compare figures 10.11 and 10.5 and 10.6). The nuclear pattern is coarse and irregular (nuclear patterns 10, 11, 12, 13, 14 section 9.5.2.1). Sometimes the cells are star-shaped like metaplastic cells. The carcinoma cells tend to lie separately; occasionally they appear in rows (figure 10.12).

(3) *Anaplastic carcinoma in situ.*   The smear consists of ragged or compact groups of malignant cells which are either irregularly arranged or neatly stacked. The nuclei can be indented so that moulding occurs (figure 10.13). Mitotic figures are seen in the groups. In the small cell type there is little variation in cell size; in the large cell type anisokaryosis becomes more prominent. In general the cells consist of naked nuclei; the cytoplasm, when present, is sparse and poorly defined (see section 10.2.1.2). The nuclei are round to oval or potato-shaped with a slightly wrinkled or lobed nuclear membrane (Graham, 1972). The chromatin pattern is irregular; granular chromatin as well as nuclear clearing can be seen. In contrast to atypical reserve cells, anaplastic carcinoma *in situ* cells *always* have an abnormal chromatin pattern (nuclear patterns 3, 4, 5; 11, 12, 13, 14, section 9.5.2.1).

10.2.3.3 Differential Diagnosis

Morphologically there is a gradual transition between severe dysplasia or atypical reserve cell hyperplasia and a carcinoma *in situ*. In a number of cases the cytological report will not be sufficient to establish a definite diagnosis and a biopsy will be necessary. In addition, cytological differentiation between carcinoma *in situ* and invasive squamous cell carcinoma can also be difficult. In general carcinoma *in situ* is characterised by a 'clean' background to the smear (figure 10.14), or a diathesis consisting only of protein (smooth even pink material) and leucocytes. The carcinoma *in situ* cells are relatively monomorphic.

table 10.3   The simultaneous occurrence of dysplastic cells, atypical reserve cells and carcinoma cells in smears of 96 women with a histological diagnosis of carcinoma *in situ* **(90) or possible microinvasive carcinoma (6) (Leiden, Cytological Laboratory 1976)**

	Number of smears	Percentage
Dysplastic cells	31	32
Atypical reserve cells	10	10
Both	51	53
Neither	4	4
Total	96	99

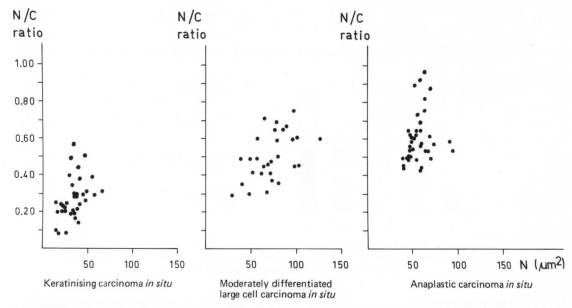

figure 10.11 Scattergram of nuclear area and N/C ratio of cells from typical examples of a keratinising carcinoma *in situ*, a moderately differentiated carcinoma *in situ* and an anaplastic carcinoma *in situ*. Extreme values of 1000 μm^2 for nuclear areas were encountered in other cases

Atrophic patterns can be difficult to evaluate. To establish the correct diagnosis, the clinician can be asked to treat the patient with an oestrogen preparation (locally or orally) for several days: the smear is then repeated a few days later. Under the influence of the oestrogen the epithelium will show maturation. Malignant cells, however, are not affected by the oestrogen (Keebler and Wied, 1974).

Keratinising carcinoma *in situ* must be differentiated from:

(1) keratinising dysplasia;
(2) parabasal cells in an atrophic smear;
(3) keratinising squamous cell carcinoma.

Large cell moderately differentiated carcinoma *in situ* must be differentiated from:

(1) dysplasia with naked nuclei as a result of cytolysis;
(2) tissue repair;
(3) 'blue blobs' in atrophic smear patterns (Ziabkowski and Naylor, 1976);
(4) severe dysplasia of the metaplastic type;
(5) microinvasive carcinoma.

Anaplastic carcinoma *in situ* must be differentiated from:

(1) overstained endocervical glandular cells (especially in older women);
(2) degenerated endocervical glandular cells;

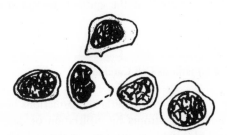

figure 10.12 Cytological pattern of moderately differentiated large cell carcinoma *in situ*

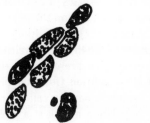
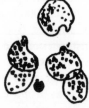

figure 10.13 Cytological pattern of anaplastic carcinoma *in situ*

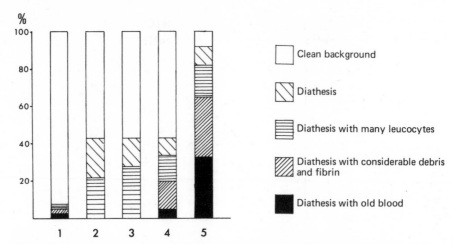

figure 10.14   **The occurrence of diathesis in positive and negative smears (Leiden University, 1975). 1. Negative smears (not atrophic); 2. negative smears (atrophic); 3. carcinoma *in situ*; 4. microinvasion; 5. invasive squamous cell carcinoma**

(3) clusters of histiocytes;

(4) reserve cell hyperplasia;

(5) chronic lymphocytic cervicitis;

(6) endometrial cells;

(7) adenocarcinoma of the endometrium or the endocervix;

(8) degenerated parabasal cells;

(9) undifferentiated carcinoma.

10.2.3.4 Incidence of Carcinoma *in situ*

The average age of women with carcinoma *in situ* is between 40 and 50 years. In Patten's study the youngest woman with carcinoma *in situ* was 22 years old, the oldest woman was 91 years old; the average age was 42.3 (Patten, 1978). The age distribution in our series is illustrated in figure 10.15. The average age of the women with carcinoma *in situ* was 43.5 years. The first screening of a population group may yield 3—4 cases of carcinoma *in situ* per 1000 women, depending on the population screened (see section 10.4). In a study by Christopherson and Parker (1964b) the prevalence was 3.7 per 1000 women. The *prevalence* is the number of cases of the condition (for example, carcinoma *in situ* or invasive squamous cell carcinoma) present in the population at risk at a given time. The *incidence* is the number of new cases occurring in a period of one year in a well-defined

population of known size and age distribution. The incidence for carcinoma *in situ* appears to be relatively constant: 0.6 and 0.5 per 1000 women for the second and third annual screening, respectively (Christopherson and Parker, 1964b).

10.2.3.5 Electron Microscopy

In transmission electron microscopy the nucleus of a carcinoma *in situ* cell may be large, with an irregular contour, and highly electron dense. In many cells the nuclear envelope is partly absent. The cytoplasm may be similar to that of a normal intermediate cell or it may resemble that of reserve cells.

At the SEM level carcinoma *in situ* is characterised by the presence of altered microvilli formations in cobblestone-like epithelial structures. This indicates that the malignant cells have reached the exfoliating surface of the epithelium (Rubio and Kranz, 1976).

10.2.4 Squamous Cell Carcinoma

'Any lesion in which epithelial formations invade the underlying stroma by infiltration or destruction is classified as invasive carcinoma' (International Committee on Histological Terminology,

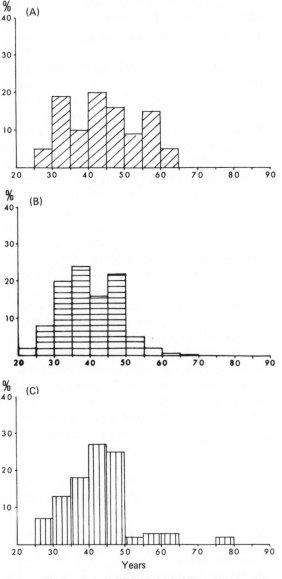

figure 10.15   Age distribution of 361 women with carcinoma *in situ*. A. Population screening programme 1974, 1975 (*n* = 77); B. smears from general practitioners 1974, 1975 (*n* = 218); C. smears from the Department of Gynaecology and Obstetrics 1970–75 (*n* = 66) (A, B, Leiden Cytology Laboratory; C, Leiden University)

Vienna, 1961). The term *microinvasive* is used when the tumour has not penetrated deeper than 5 mm into the stroma. The distinction between microinvasive growth and deep infiltration is important in view of the therapeutic considera-

tions. The question has been raised as to whether the 5-mm limit is the correct one, since lymph-nodal metastasis has been found in a few such cases (Boronow, 1977). Therefore, the International Federation of Gynaecology and Obstetrics (FIGO) has recently subclassified microinvasive carcinoma into cases with *early stromal invasion* and cases with *occult cancer* but with frankly invasive histological patterns (see section 10.5.3.1) (Boronow, 1977).

10.2.4.1 Microinvasive Squamous Cell Carcinoma

(1) *Histology.*   Microinvasion is more frequently encountered in cases with extensive carcinoma *in situ*. One of the first signs of early stromal invasion in histological sections is the formation of buds in areas of carcinoma *in situ* (Rubio *et al.*, 1974) and loss of palisade arrangement of the cells near the

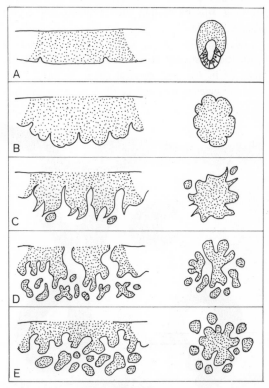

figure 10.16   Various infiltration patterns. Left, the squamous epithelium; right, a glandular duct. A. Carcinoma *in situ*; B. bulging carcinoma *in situ*; C. thorny infiltrating growth; D. extensive net-like infiltrating growth; E. extensive club-shaped infiltrating growth

stroma. In the majority of cases the epithelium at the site of invasion may show some squamous differentiation, in the remaining cases the micro-invasive foci are composed of small undifferentiated cells (Rubio *et al.*, 1974). These more mature cells often have an irregular chromatin pattern and a macronucleolus. Where the basement membrane is damaged, carcinoma cells invade the stroma (figure 10.16). Lymphocytes and plasma cells are often found around the clusters of carcinoma cells. Sometimes the nests of carcinoma cells degenerate and evoke a granulomatous reaction (Christopherson and Parker, 1964a). Oedema-like halo formations around invading foci are frequently encountered (Rubio *et al.*, 1974). Microinvasion may be accompanied by tissue destruction, although to a lesser degree than is seen with a deeply infiltrating carcinoma. It may be very difficult to distinguish histologically between microinvasion and carcinoma *in situ* extending into endocervical crypts (figure 10.17).

Microinvasion is in the majority of cases a multifocal process. It is found in the metaplastic area or in the endocervical canal; in only 2 per cent of cases is it found in the squamous epithel-

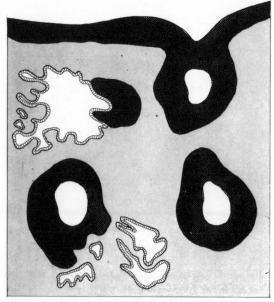

figure 10.17   Growth of carcinoma *in situ* along glandular crypts

ium. It can arise in an area with carcinoma *in situ* (68.2 per cent), at the junction of carcinoma *in situ* and dysplasia (13.6 per cent), in a dysplastic area (4.6 per cent), or even in morphologically benign epithelium (1.5 per cent) (Ng and Reagan, 1969).

(2) *Cytology*.   When a carcinoma begins to infiltrate, its cellular pattern may change qualitatively as well as quantitatively. Smears from patients with microinvasion contain a large number of malignant cells compared with carcinoma *in situ* This is mainly attributable to the large extent of the carcinomatous epithelium (see (1) above).

The nuclei may contain *macronucleoli* (Ng *et al.*, 1972), especially the nuclei of anaplastic carcinoma cells. *Nuclear clearing* is more pronounced than in carcinoma *in situ*. Patten (1978) considers the occurrence of nucleoli and nuclear clearing as signs of increased metabolic activity heralding infiltrative capacities of the cells. Often there are many bizarre malignant cells corresponding with the differentiation at the site of infiltration (see (1)). However, cells from microinvasive carcinoma cannot be distinguished from carcinoma *in situ* cells on morphometrical parameters such as nuclear size and N/C ratio (Rubio, 1974). The background is usually clean as in carcinoma *in situ* (see figure 10.14); however, a background with detritus, fibrin and old blood is more frequently encountered than in the latter case.

As infiltration proceeds the pattern will differ less from that of a deeply infiltrating carcinoma. Of the seventeen histologically confirmed micro-invasive carcinomas in our series, nine were cytologically recognised as invasive and eight were classified as carcinoma *in situ*.

(3) *Occurrence of microinvasive carcinoma*.   The average age in our series of women with micro-invasion is 45 years (figure 10.18). Like carcinoma *in situ*, microinvasive carcinoma is usually diagnosed during a routine examination of the cervix.

10.2.4.2 Invasive Squamous Cell Carcinoma

(1) *Histology*.   There are various histological classifications of epidermoid carcinoma of the cervix (Broders, 1926; Warren, 1931). The clas-

sification according to Wentz and Reagan (1959) is used here: (a) *keratinising* squamous cell carcinoma; (b) *large cell nonkeratinising* squamous cell carcinoma; (c) *small cell nonkeratinising* carcinoma. This classification has clinical significance in

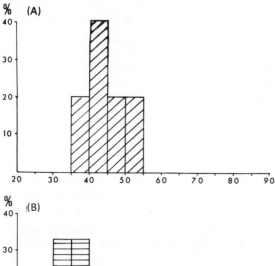

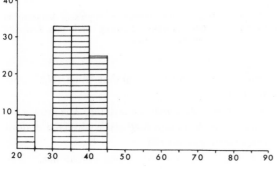

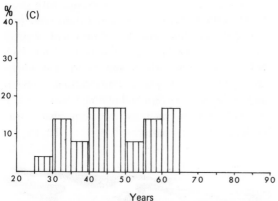

figure 10.18 **Age distribution of 40 women with a microinvasive carcinoma. I, Population screening programme 1974, 1975 (*n* = 5); II, smears from general practitioners 1974, 1975 (*n* = 12); III, smears from the Department of Gynaecology and Obstetrics 1970–75 (*n* = 23) (I, II, Leiden Cytology Laboratory; III, Leiden University)**

that prognosis and therapy depend in part on the category.

(a) *Keratinising squamous cell carcinoma.* The pattern is characterised by cells with fairly abundant keratinising cytoplasm and highly polymorphic nuclei. Many nuclei are hyperchromatic. In histological sections epithelial pearls and isolated cell keratinisation are seen. Sometimes the surface of the neoplasm is covered with squames; this keratinisation is a form of abnormal differentiation. The mitotic index, that is, the number of normal and abnormal mitotic figures per microscopic field, is low.

(b) *Large cell nonkeratinising squamous cell carcinoma.* The pattern is characterised by cells with large pale nuclei, macronucleoli and relatively little cytoplasm. Isolated areas of cell keratinisation may be found. Epithelial pearls and squames are not seen. There is a moderately high mitotic index.

(c) *Small cell nonkeratinising carcinoma.* The pattern is characterised by cells with uniform small nuclei and hazy, ill-defined cytoplasm. Individual cell keratinisation is not seen. The mitotic index is high.

A special type of cervical cancer is the uncommon *verrucous carcinoma* of the cervix, presumably arising from condylomata acuminata (Spratt and Lee, 1977). Verrucous carcinomas are insidious and slow growing, and lack distant metastasis (Jennings and Barclay, 1972).

(2) *Cytology.* The smear may contain numerous malignant cells. Many cells have bizarre shapes; the nuclear abnormalities are more pronounced than in carcinoma *in situ*. Mitotic figures are found mainly in cell groups and seldom in isolated cells. Usually there is a background with considerable debris and fibrin (tiny pinkish-orange threads or fragments) or old blood (smooth, even, orange-pink material) (see figure 10.14). When such a 'tumour diathesis' is present it may be difficult or even impossible to find malignant cells, especially in the case of an ulcerating carcinoma. Tumour diathesis may be absent in the case of an exophytic growth pattern.

(a) *Keratinising squamous cell carcinoma.* The smear may contain many parakeratotic cells with

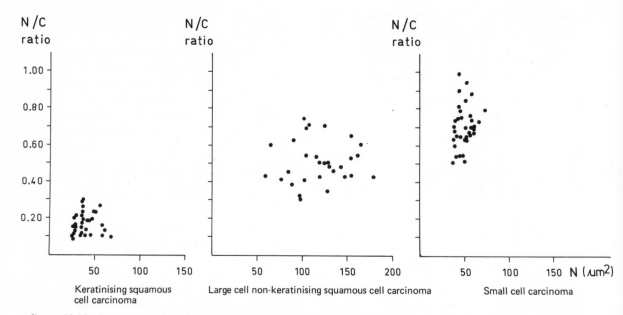

figure 10.19 Scattergram of nuclear area (N) and N/C ratio of malignant cells from typical examples of keratinising squamous carcinoma, large cell nonkeratinising squamous carcinoma and small cell nonkeratinising carcinoma. Extreme values of 1200 μm² for nuclear areas were encountered in other cases

relatively large nuclei, next to bizarre cells (tadpole and fibre cells) and malignant epithelial pearls. Also abnormal cells with cytoplasmic granulae may be observed. The nuclei are hyperchromatic with a coarse chromatinic pattern (see nuclear patterns 8, 10, 12, 13, section 9.5.2.1). The cytoplasm is still fairly plentiful and is keratinised (N/C ratio low, figures 10.19 and 10.6). Sometimes *only* abnormally shaped squames (figure 10.20) will be seen in the smear, especially when the lesion is lightly scraped. In general the cells of a keratinising squamous cell carcinoma are more polymorphic and show more marked nuclear abnormalities than the cells of a keratinising carcinoma *in situ*.

(b) *Large cell nonkeratinising squamous cell carcinoma.* In the smear are many malignant cells which vary markedly in size. Nuclear shapes are often very abnormal (potatoes, etc.). The nuclei display a coarse chromatin pattern (see nuclear patterns 11, 12, 13, 14, section 9.5.2.1), and often possess macronucleoli (figure 10.21). The nucleolar/nuclear ratio (Nc/N ratio) may be high. Pyknotic nuclei are seldom present. The cytoplasm is

scarce and ill-defined or absent (high (N/C ratio, figure 10.22).

Nuclear moulding may be striking. The groups are always flat. A tumour diathesis is observed in most cases (see figure 10.14).

(c) *Small cell nonkeratinising carcinoma.* The pattern is characterised by cell groups with small nuclei with a coarse chromatin pattern and pronounced polychromasia, sometimes with a small rim of cytoplasm but predominantly bare (high N/C ratio, figures 10.19 and 10.6). The nuclei are abnormal in shape (indentations, bulges) and are sometimes thin and oblong (figure 10.22). Nucleoli can be seen in the somewhat larger nuclei (see nuclear patterns, 3, 4, 8, 11, 12, 13, 14,

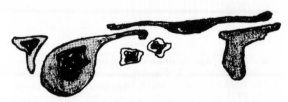

figure 10.20 Cytological pattern of a keratinising squamous cell carcinoma

figure 10.21 Cytological pattern of a large cell non-keratinising squamous cell carcinoma

section 9.5.2.1). The Nc/N ratio may be high. In groups, cells of small cell carcinoma will contain many mitotic figures. The nuclei may be very tiny, which makes differentiation from groups of endometrial cells difficult.

We have seen only one case of verrucous carcinoma of the cervix. The diagnosis of malignancy was not rendered cytologically, as in the smear only morphologically benign parakeratotic and koilocytotic cells were found. In biopsy material the true nature of the process with its infiltrating capacity can only be appreciated in the deeper parts of the lesion.

(3) *Differential diagnosis.* Sometimes one of the following can be used to discriminate between carcinoma *in situ* and invasive squamous cell carcinoma.

In squamous cell carcinoma:

(a) there is often a tumour diathesis, frequently containing old blood and fibrin (see figure 10.14);

(b) there may be numerous malignant cells in the smear;

(c) the cells and the nuclei are markedly polymorphic

(d) macronucleoli are often present;

(e) the undifferentiated malignant cells in particular are characterised by a high Nc/N ratio.

Keratinising squamous cell carcinoma must be differentiated from:

(a) keratinising carcinoma *in situ*;

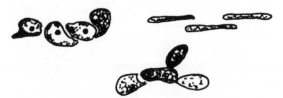

figure 10.22 Cytological pattern of a small cell non-keratinising (anaplastic) carcinoma

(b) keratinising dysplasia.

Although the cell pattern for keratinising dysplasia is also highly varied (tadpole and fibre cells), the background is generally clean and the nuclear

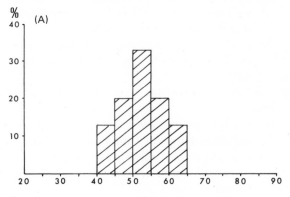
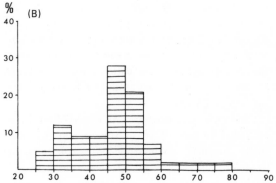
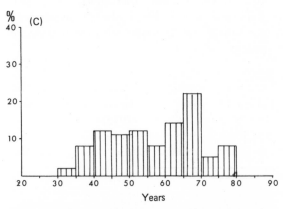

figure 10.23 Age distribution of 106 women with invasive squamous cell carcinoma. I. Population screening programme 1974, 1975 (*n* = 15); II. smears from general practitioners 1974, 1975 (*n* = 42); III. smears from the Department of Gynaecology and Obstetrics 1970–75 (*n* = 49) (I, II, Leiden Cytology Laboratory; III, Leiden University)

abnormalities are slight. Biopsy may be needed to settle the matter.

Nonkeratinising squamous cell carcinoma must be differentiated from:

(a) repair cells (never isolated, but always in aggregates; low Nc/N ratio; no irregularly shaped nuclei; no tumour diathesis);

(b) poorly differentiated adenocarcinoma (lopsided cytoplasm and spherical groupings) (see section 12.2.2.2).

Small cell carcinoma must be differentiated from:

(a) small cell carcinoma *in situ* (no macronucleoli, coarse but more evenly distributed chromatin);

(b) endometrial cells (spherical cell groupings);

(c) overstained reserve cells (no abnormal nuclear shapes).

(4) *Occurrence of infiltrating squamous cell carcinoma.*   On the average women with invasive squamous cell carcinoma are about 10 years older than women with carcinoma *in situ*. In our series the average age of these patients was 55.9 years (figure 10.23); in Patten's study (1978) the average age was 51.7 years.

(5) *Electron microscopy.*   At the SEM level the epithelial surface of an invasive carcinoma may show irregular cobblestone-like structures or irregular formations in between mosaics and cobblestones. Cellular overlapping is present (Rubio and Einhorn, 1977). Also bizarre deformity of microvilli was associated with the presence of invasive carcinoma.

10.3 The Relationship between Atypical Reserve Cell Hyperplasia, Dysplasia, Carcinoma *in situ* and Squamous Cell Carcinoma

10.3.1 The Relationship between Atypical Reserve Cell Hyperplasia, Carcinoma *in situ* and Squamous Cell Carcinoma

There is a variety of reasons for assuming that carcinoma *in situ* develops as a malignant change in reserve cell hyperplasia.

(1) The carcinoma *in situ* is often located in an area of atypical reserve cell hyperplasia. This was demonstrated by Johnson *et al.* (1964) in 34 of 47 cone biopsies taken from patients with carcinoma *in situ*.

(2) In our series it appeared that as the severity of the lesions increased, the likelihood of finding atypical reserve cells in the smear increased (table 10.3). Ten per cent of the smears with carcinoma *in situ* contained atypical reserve cells in addition to the malignant cells, but no dysplastic cells (see table 10.3 and section 10.3.2).

(3) In our series the average age of the patients with atypical reserve cell hyperplasia was 35.9 years, considerably less than the average age of patients with carcinoma *in situ* (table 10.5)

(4) The natural history of atypical reserve cell hyperplasia.

Morphologically, atypical reserve cell hyperplasia is highly similar to 'alpha carcinoma *in situ*' described by Old *et al.* (1965) as a lethargic type

table 10.4   Occurrence of atypical reserve cells in normal and abnormal smears (Leiden University and Leiden Cytological Laboratory, 1975)

Number of cases	Diagnosis	% Smears with atypical reserve cells
30 000	Normal smear	0.5
170	Mild dysplasia	4.8
90	Severe dysplasia	42.2
90	Carcinoma *in situ*	63.0
90	Squamous cell carcinoma	66.0

table 10.5 Average age of women with atypical reserve cell hyperplasia, dysplasia or carcinoma *in situ*

	Patten (1978)	Christopherson and Parker (1964b)	Our material
Atypical reserve cell hyperplasia	—	—	35.9 years
Dysplasia	34.7 years	35.0 years	38.6 years
Carcinoma *in situ*	42.3 years	39.6 years	43.5 years

of carcinoma *in situ*. As far as biological behaviour is concerned, they ranked it with dysplasia. This agrees with our own findings: cytological follow-up of patients with atypical reserve cell hyperplasia indicates that in a number of cases carcinoma *in situ* will develop (table 10.6)

The possible genesis of a carcinoma *in situ* via an atypical reserve cell hyperplasia can be illustrated schematically, as shown in figure 10.24.

This type of carcinoma develops in the region originally covered with columnar epithelium, that is in the metaplastic area proximal to the squamo-columnar junction (Burghardt, 1970). The biological behaviour of the atypical reserve cell hyperplasia cannot be predicted on the morphology alone. Therefore clinical and cytological follow-up is advisable (section 10.5.3).

10.3.2 The Relationship between Dysplasia, Carcinoma *in situ* and Squamous Cell Carcinoma

There is also a variety of reasons for assuming that there is a relationship between dysplasia, carcinoma *in situ* and squamous cell carcinoma.

(1) In 1962 Reagan *et al.* described the surgical specimens of 189 patients with invasive squamous cell carcinoma. In 128 cases carcinoma *in situ* was also found; in 61 cases there was also dysplasia. In a high percentage (80 per cent) of patients with carcinoma *in situ* severe dysplasia was also discovered (Reagan and Hicks, 1953). The dysplasia is always distal to the carcinoma *in situ*.

(2) The occurrence of dysplastic cells and of carcinoma *in situ* cells in the same smear. In 85 per cent of the smears of patients with carcinoma *in situ*, dysplastic cells are also seen (see table 10.3).

(3) On average, women with dysplasia are younger than those with carcinoma *in situ* (table 10.5); patients with invasive squamous cell carcinoma are the oldest (figure 10.23). This agrees with the theory that in a few cases mild dysplasia can progress to severe dysplasis, then to carcinoma *in situ* and ultimately to invasive squamous cell carcinoma. The biological behaviour of a given

table 10.6 Follow-up of 41 women with atypical reserve cell hyperplasia (Leiden University and Leiden Cytology Laboratory, 1975)

Number of patients	Cytological diagnosis after a follow-up of at least one year
12	Negative
8	Atypical reserve cell hyperplasia
4	Dysplasia
17	Carcinoma *in situ* (histologically confirmed)

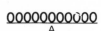 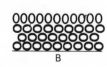 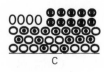 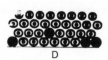 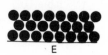

A   B   C   D   E

O Endocervical glandular epithelial cell

◯ Reserve cell

◉ Atypical reserve cell

● Anaplastic carcinoma *in situ* cell

figure 10.24   The genesis of cervical squamous carcinoma *in situ* via atypical reserve cell hyperplasia (after Patten, 1978). A. Endocervical columnar epithelium; B. proliferation of reserve cells, leading to reserve cell hyperplasia; C. atypical reserve cell hyperplasia; D. severe atypical reserve cell hyperplasia; E. small cell anaplastic carcinoma *in situ*

dysplasia cannot be predicted on the morphology alone. So it is advisable to survey these patients both clinically and cytologically (section 10.5.3). Clarke and Anderson (1979), consider in a retrospective study the 'Pap smear an effective screening procedure helping to control the development of cervical cancer.

Bangle *et al.* (1963) described several rare cases in which dysplasia developed directly into an invasive carcinoma. Assuming that this can happen, then the following schematic representation results (Langley and Crompton, 1973):

1. Normal epithelium —————————→ invasive squamous
2. Dysplasia ⟶ carcinoma *in situ* ⟶ cell carcinoma
3. Dysplasia —————————→

Ashley (1966) considered the possibility of two types of squamous cell carcinoma. One type would develop explosively (pathway 1) and a second

type, which is more susceptible to therapy, would grow more slowly and develop along pathway 2 or 3. With respect to pathway 1, it should be noted that the duration of the *in situ* stage may be so short that it is not observed. In our material of over 450 000 cases, we encountered 5 cases in which clinically detected invasive cervical carcinoma was preceded by a completely negative smear (qualitatively excellent) taken within 1.5 years prior to the diagnosis of cancer. Therefore a negative smear *never* offers a 100 per cent certainty that an 'explosive' cancer may not develop within a short period of time.

(4) The natural history of dysplasia. Follow-up studies have shown that many patients with dysplasia will develop at some time (varying between one and ten years) carcinoma *in situ* or invasive squamous cell carcinoma (Koss *et al.*, 1963). According to Richart and Barron (1969) 80 per cent of all dysplasias progress within ten years

table 10.7   Average age of patients with dysplasia, carcinoma *in situ* or invasive squamous cell carcinoma

	Patten (1978)	Beyer-Boon (1976)*
Mild 'classical' dysplasia	32.0 years	30.8 years
Moderate dysplasia	35.7 years	—
Severe 'classical' dysplasia	38.4 years	38.6 years
'Condylomatous' dysplasia	—	29.8 years
Carcinoma *in situ*	42.3 years	43.5 years
Invasive squamous cell carcinoma	51.7 years	55.9 years

* Unpublished data

to carcinoma *in situ*. The chance that carcinoma *in situ* will develop is 1600 times greater for a woman with dysplasia than for a woman without abnormalities of the portio (Stern and Neely, 1964). Studies in the United States (Koss, 1968; Patten, 1975) showed that severe dysplasia in particular may progress to carcinoma *in situ*. Women with a mild dysplasia of the uterine cervix have 5—10 times more chance of developing carcinoma *in situ* (Melamed and Flehinger, 1976).

In our series we found progession to carcinoma in 66 of 2615 cases of mild to moderate dysplasia cases after a follow-up period of one year (table 10.8). The severe dysplasia ('classical' type) showed progression to carcinoma (*in situ*) in 196 out of 642 cases (table 10.7). So far no data have been published concerning the natural history of condylomatous dysplasia. In our experience, it is largely dependent on the concurrent 'classical' dysplasia which is illustrated in our follow-up study of 50 patients with classical severe dysplasia and 50 patients with classical severe dysplasia *and* koilocytosis. This study failed to show that patients with both severe dysplasia and condyloma were at higher risk of developing a progressive lesion than patients with dysplasia alone. However, an invasive verrucous carcinoma may develop in condylomatous epithelium (see section 10.2.4.2).

Dysplasia diagnosed during pregnancy deserves special attention because its natural history differs from dysplasia diagnosed in nonpregnant women. According to Reagan *et al.* (1961) dysplasia occurs in pregnant women more frequently than in nonpregnant women. However, when the nonpregnant women with severe dysplasia were re-examined six months after the first examination, the dysplasia persisted in 84 per cent of cases. In contrast, when pregnant women with pronounced dysplasia were re-examined six months later, after delivery, only 10 per cent of these women still had severe dysplasia. During pregnancy the dysplastic reaction may mature, for example, the dysplastic cells in the first trimester have relatively large nuclei in relatively small cells, whereas in the last trimester this is reversed (Patten 1978). Persistence of immature abnormal cells through the last months of pregnancy is a reason for great concern (Patten, 1978).

table 10.7   Natural history of 4054 cases of mild to moderate dysplasia and 781 cases of severe dysplayia, diagnosed in a routine cervical material of 245 686 smears (Leiden Cytology Laboratory, 1974—1978). In the table are the diagnoses after a follow-up period of one year (Beyer-Boon, 1977)

Cytological diagnosis	Number of smears	Repeat smear unknown, histology unknown	Follow-up							
			Negative	Mild/moderate dysplasia	Arch. severe dysplasia	Carcinoma *in situ*	Adeno-carcinoma *in situ*	Squamous cell carcinoma	Adeno-carcinoma	
Mild/mod. dysplasia	4054 16.5‰	1439 5.65‰	1707 (+ 27) 1734 6.81‰	684 (+ 13) 697 2.74‰	102 (+ 16) 118 0.4‰	53 (+ 8) 61 0.24‰	—	2 (+ 3) 5 0.02‰	—	
Severe dysplasia	781 3.2‰	139 0.55‰	122 (+ 11) 133 0.52‰	120 (+ 9) 129 0.51‰	160 (+ 24) 184 0.72‰	104 (+ 77) 181 0.71‰	2 0.01‰	3 (+ 10) 13 0.05‰	—	

(+ . . .) histology

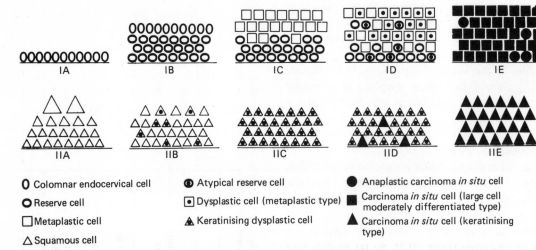

O Colomnar endocervical cell   ● Atypical reserve cell   ● Anaplastic carcinoma *in situ* cell

O Reserve cell   ▣ Dysplastic cell (metaplastic type)   ■ Carcinoma *in situ* cell (large cell moderately differentiated type)

□ Metaplastic cell   ▲ Keratinising dysplastic cell   ▲ Carcinoma *in situ* cell (keratinising type)

△ Squamous cell

figure 10.25 Morphogenesis of carcinoma *in situ* via dysplasia. IA. endocervical columnar epithelium; IB. reserve cell hyperplasia, IC. metaplasia; ID. dysplasia (metaplastic type); IE. 'moderately differentiated' large cell carcinoma *in situ*. IIA. stratified squamous epithelium; IIB. mild dysplasia (keratinising type); IIC. moderate dysplasia (keratinising type); IID. severe dysplasia (keratinising type); IIE. keratinising carcinoma *in situ*

Patients who are treated with chemotherapeutic or immunosuppressive drugs are subject to a high risk of developing dysplasia (Rilke, 1976; Coleman, 1976); the same is true for patients undergoing radiotherapy. These iatrogenic types of dysplasia are discussed in chapter 14.

Not every dysplasia will lead to carcinoma. In some patients the dysplasia may disappear spontaneously, although the possibility of a recurrence some time later must be considered. Traumata (obstetric delivery, cervical biopsy) may cause dysplasia to disappear. Local application of tetracycline may cause the epithelium to shed (Koss *et al.*, 1963).

The morphogenesis of carcinoma *in situ* from dysplasia is influenced by the following. The ectocervix is partly covered with 'native' squamous epithelium, partly with metaplastic epithelium and columnar epithelium. Various types of dysplasia or carcinoma *in situ* can develop from these epithelia (figure 10.25). The keratinising dysplasia or carcinoma *in situ* is usually located in the distal part of the ectocervix, the area of the native squamous epithelium. The nonkeratinising and

table 10.9 Occurrence of columnar endocervical cells, reserve cells and metaplastic cells in the smears from 87 women with mild dysplasia of the uterine cervix with a follow-up period of more than 5 years

	42 Cases mild dysplasia regression to normal		45 Cases mild dysplasia progression to malignancy		17 Cases persistent mild dysplasia		13 000 Cases (control group) normal cytology
Columnar endocervical cells	26	61.9%	30	66.7%	12	70.6%	63%
Reserve cells	2	4.8%	14	31.1%	5	29.4%	0.5%
Metaplastic cells	11	26.2%	26	57.8%	14	82.4%	38%

metaplastic dysplasia and the moderately differentiated carcinoma *in situ* can lie in the metaplastic area (native columnar area) as well as (less frequently) in the 'native' squamous area (Burghardt, 1970). The undifferentiated small cell carcinoma *in situ* is located in the area of the 'native' columnar epithelium. More than 70 per cent of carcinomata *in situ* are located in the area of the glandular ducts, that is, the metaplastic and endocervical area (Burghardt, 1970).

In a follow-up study, over a period of 5 or more years, of 87 women with a mild dysplasia of the cervix, we registered the presence of columnar endocervical cells, metaplastic cells and reserve cells (table 10.9). Reserve cells and metaplastic cells were found much more frequently in the lesions progressing into malignancy than in the disappearing lesions, and much more frequently than in the normal smears. This underlines the importance of an exposed immature epithelium (either immature metaplasia or reserve cell hyperplasia) in the development of cervical cancer (see also section 7.4.2.3).

10.3.3 Summary

The morphogenesis of carcinoma *in situ* from atypical reserve cell hyperplasia or from dysplasia

has been described above. In practice it appears that all of these processes occur in close proximity and in close association with each other so that the various types of carcinoma *in situ* or dysplasia can occur together in the same patient. Moreover, areas with carcinoma *in situ* can be found adjacent to, for instance, dysplastic epithelium.

The smears of patients with carcinoma *in situ* often contain not only malignant cells but also atypical reserve cells and dysplastic cells (see table 10.2). The cancer cells are seldom of one type; usually various types are found together. Patten (1975) summarised the theories about the development of carcinoma *in situ* and squamous cell carcinoma (Reagan *et al.*, 1962; Johnson *et al.*, 1964; von Haam and Old, 1964) as shown in figure 10.26.

10.3.4 The Biological Behaviour of Carcinoma *in situ*

Carcinoma *in situ* can in the long run progress to invasive carcinoma. In general there is a large variation in the duration of the *in situ* stage. On average it will last about ten years, several years longer in young women (Kashgarian and Dunn, 1970). In some patients, however, the *in situ* stage is very short. As yet, little is known about the spontaneous behaviour of carcinoma *in situ* since the diagnosis usually leads to surgical intervention and the lesion is removed in its entirety. On the basis of the morphological pattern we cannot predict whether a particular example of carcinoma *in situ* will be aggressive or not. Large-scale population screening programmes have shown that progression of carcinoma *in situ* to invasive carcinoma does not occur in all patients. Various percentages are given in the literature, for example, Fidler and Boyes (1959), 43 per cent, and Stern and Neely (1964), 50 per cent. The values are calculated from the difference between the incidence of invasive squamous cell carcinoma and the incidence of carcinoma *in situ*. Less than 50 per cent of cases with carcinoma *in situ* eventually progress to invasive cancer when followed for prolonged periods (Murphy and Coleman, 1976).

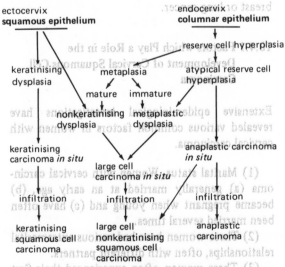

figure 10.26 Morphogenesis of cervical carcinoma (modified from Patten, 1978)

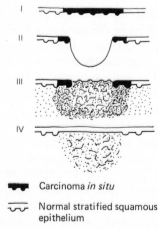

Carcinoma *in situ*

Normal stratified squamous epithelium

figure 10.27   Schematic diagram of the disappearance of carcinoma *in situ* after a biopsy (based on Koss *et al.*, 1963). I. before biopsy; II. biopsy is taken; III. formation of granulation tissue, inflammation; IV. state after re-epitheliasation

Carcinoma *in situ* is a fragile lesion which can disappear easily as a result of a trauma (delivery, biopsy, coitus, surgical intervention) or spontaneously for no known reason. When the superficial layers of the epithelium have disappeared this may lead to a false-negative diagnosis cytologically. Histologically the correct diagnosis can be made on the carcinomatous changes in the endocervical glands. It is obvious that the extent of the lesion is important as well as the location. A small lesion will disappear sooner than an extensive one; when the carcinoma *in situ* is localised in the endocervix it is not easily removed.

As a result of biopsy a focus of carcinoma *in situ* can be removed partly or entirely (figure 10.27). During the healing process fragments of the carcinoma *in situ* may be shed so that ultimately healthy tissue is formed at the site of the biopsy. A new carcinoma *in situ* may develop at another site. When a smear is taken immediately after a biopsy it will be found that the number of carcinoma cells has decreased markedly (Koss *et al.*, 1963). Usually cells from the deeper layers of squamous epithelium and many repair cells are found. The same occurs after local application of tetracycline. These drugs cause extensive shedding of the abnormal epithelium. The smear contains sheets of squamous epithelial cells with a charac-

teristic yellowish cytoplasm. The background of the smear is strikingly clean due to the absence of the normal bacterial flora (Koss *et al.*, 1963).

The occurrence of negative smears after biopsy or after administration of drugs can provide incorrect information about the lesion. A report that the 'carcinoma *in situ* has disappeared' must be interpreted with the greatest care.

10.4 Epidemiology of Cervical Squamous Cell Carcinoma

The occurrence of cervical carcinoma varies from country to country and from district to district. In South America and Africa it is very common and accounts for 40 per cent of carcinomas in women; in the United States the figure is 11 per cent. Particularly when a country has just been exposed to western culture the number of cervical carcinomas increases markedly. In Israel cervical carcinoma is relatively rare; possibly circumcision and the strict Niddah ritual play a role here. The average annual incidence per 100 000 women is: Columbia 148.8; Israel 11.4; the Netherlands 24.2; United Kingdom 34.2 (Waterhouse *et al.*, 1976). In the Netherlands about 450 women die each year of cervical carcinoma. The number of deaths is fairly low in comparison with those due to breast or lung cancer.

10.4.1 Factors which Play a Role in the Development of Cervical Squamous Cell Carcinoma

Extensive epidemiological investigations have revealed various common factors in women with cervical carcinoma.

(1) Marital status. Women with cervical carcinoma (a) generally married at an early age, (b) became pregnant when young and (c) have often been married several times.

(2) These women have had various extramarital relationships, often with different partners.

(3) These women often experienced their first coitus at an early age.

(4) Cervical carcinoma occurs frequently in prostitutes and rarely in virgins such as nuns.

(5) The sexual partners of women with cervical carcinoma have often had numerous other sexual partners themselves.

(6) Women with cervical carcinoma have often had syphilis or gonorrhoea.

(7) Cervical carcinoma occurs most frequently among women of low socioeconomic status.

(8) Cervical carcinoma is more common in cities (especially sea ports) than in the rural areas. Incidence of cervical carcinoma *in situ* in rural areas in the Netherlands is 1.8 per 1000, in cities ±5.5 per 1000 (Collette, 1976). In some seaside resorts (Katwijk, Noordwijk, Zandvoort) cervical carcinoma also appears to be relatively frequent (Collette, 1976).

(9) Women who marry a man whose former wife died of cervical cancer have an increased risk of contracting the same disease (Kessler 1977).

On the basis of the above mentioned data two theories have been developed concerning the aetiology of cervical carcinoma.

(1) The cervical epithelium in young females is susceptible to carcinogens. The age at which the first coitus and the first pregnancy occur is, therefore, of essential importance. The relevant carcinogens include: cervical infections, smegma, DNA from spermatozoa, DNA from bacteria, trauma and the influence of hormones.

(2) The number of sexual partners is very important, not only of the woman herself but also of her partners. One could say that cervical carcinoma behaves like a 'venereal disease' whereby the aetiological factor is transmitted during coitus by a 'high-risk male'.

What is the role of cervical infections, such as for instance trichomoniasis, herpes infection, condyloma, in the development of carcinoma *in situ*? A causative relationship between trichomoniasis and carcinoma *in situ* has not been demonstrated (Koss and Wolinska, 1959). The cellular atypia caused by trichomoniasis is in general less marked than that seen in carcinoma *in situ* (Christopherson and Parker, 1965). It is, however, true that trichomoniasis and cervical carcinoma occur predominantly in women of the same socioeconomic environment (Collette, 1976). The same applies for infections such as syphilis, gonorrhoea and condylomata. During World War II the incidence of gonorrhoea and syphilis in England was very high among women; in 1972 the incidence of cervical carcinoma in the same group of women was also very high (Beral, 1974). Beral's study showed that, in comparison with the total female population, women with venereal diseases live mainly in cities, come from low socioeconomic classes and also have sexual relationships with more than one partner. A similar epidemiological pattern is shown by the genital warts or condylomata acuminata occurring on the vulva, vagina, uterine cervix and penis. Virus particles were demonstrated in the nuclei of metaplastic koilocytotic cells by electron microscopy (Laverty *et al.*, 1978). These genital warts seem to be transmitted by sexual contact. The incidence is high among populations of high sexual promiscuity (Stormby, 1974; Zur Hausen, 1976). Progressions of these lesions to malignancy has been described (Bauer and Friedrich, 1965; Domaniewski and Gustowski, 1968; Kerl and Pickel, 1971). In the majority of cases, however, the condylomatous lesion is probably concomitant with a true premalignant lesion (see section 10.3.2). The herpes simplex virus type II (HSV) is considered an oncogenic virus. Carcinoma of the uterine cervix often occurs in combination with a herpes type II infection (Rawls *et al.*, 1969).

A real causative relationship has not (yet) been established. The effect of all these carcinogenic factors on the exposed immature epithelium (immature metaplasia and reserve cells) needs further research.

10.4.2 Some Results from a Routine Laboratory

In a cytology laboratory the chance of detecting carcinoma *in situ*, microinvasion and invasive squamous carcinoma is partly dependent on the patient population being screened. For example, the occurrence of the different lesions is related to the age of the women being screened (see figures

table 10.10 Occurrence of carcinoma *in situ*, microinvasion and invasive squamous carcinoma of the uterine cervix in various patient material

Age (years)	Number of smears			Occurrence of carcinoma *in situ* (‰)			Occurrence of microinvasion (‰)			Occurrence of invasive squamous cell carcinoma (‰)		
	I	II	III	I	II	III	I	II	III	I	II	III
15–19	0	301	1332	–	1.2	0.0	–	0.0	0.0	–	0.0	0.0
20–24	0	3870	6018	–	1.2	0.0	–	0.2	0.0	–	0.0	0.0
25–29	8129	12230	7910	0.4	1.4	0.6	0.0	0.0	0.2	0.0	0.1	0.0
30–34	8096	15573	5005	1.7	2.8	0.6	0.0	0.3	0.6	0.0	0.3	0.2
35–39	7342	14349	3816	1.8	3.6	3.1	0.1	0.2	0.5	0.0	0.3	1.3
40–44	7028	11962	2904	2.1	2.8	6.1	0.1	0.3	1.4	0.2	0.3	2.1
45–49	5931	9201	2762	2.1	5.1	6.1	0.1	0.0	1.5	0.5	1.3	1.8
50–54	5629	6391	1784	1.2	1.5	0.6	0.7	0.0	1.1	0.8	1.4	3.4
55–59	3822	2510	983	3.1	1.9	2.0	0.0	0.0	3.0	0.7	1.1	4.1
60–64	2793	1244	631	1.4	0.8	3.1	0.7	0.0	7.9	1.1	0.8	9.5
65–69	0	688	525	–	2.9	0.0	–	0.0	0.0	–	1.4	19.0
70–74	0	218	1089	–	0.4	0.1	–	0.0	0.0	–	4.5	2.8
>75	0	0	384	–	–	0.0	–	0.0	0.0	–	–	10.4
Total	48110	78687	35143	1.6	2.1	1.8	0.1	0.2	0.7	0.3	0.5	1.4

I, Population screening programme, 1974, 1975; II, Smears from general practitioners, 1974, 1975; III, Smears from the Department for gynaecology and obstetrics, 1970–75 (I, II, Leiden Cytology Laboratory; III, Leiden University)

10.2, 10.8, 10.15, 10.18). Material from screening programmes may offer fewer abnormalities than material from a clinic for gynaecology and obstetrics (table 10.10). The histological diagnoses for the positive smears are given in table 10.11.

10.5 Clinical Aspects of Cervical Squamous Cell Carcinoma

10.5.1 Symptoms

Carcinoma *in situ* is often discovered by chance in the smear of a woman who claims to be free of gynaecological complaints. However, if the family doctor then asks specific questions, one or more of the following complaints will often be found: postcoital bleeding, bloody vaginal discharge or vague complaints such as a heavy feeling in the lower abdomen (possibly attributable to an accompanying cervicitis) and dryness of the vagina (Kern, 1964). In the literature, therefore, discussions of the symptoms vary widely, depending upon whether an extensive history was taken or a questionnaire was used which the woman had to fill in herself.

In our series about 80 per cent of the patients with carcinoma *in situ* reported no complaints to the general practitioner (table 10.12).

An invasive cervical carcinoma will in general lead to obvious complaints. When the carcinoma infiltrates and tissue destruction begins, the following complaints can be expected: yellowish discharge, foul-smelling discharge, severe postcoital bleeding and intermenstrual or postmenopausal vaginal bleeding. According to Kuipers (1972) vaginal bleeding will often be the first symptom, followed by postcoital bleeding, vaginal discharge, and, in a small number of cases, pain. When the carcinoma invades the bladder and ureters, recurrent infections of the urinary tract may develop; extension to the rectum may lead to proctitis. Should pronounced tissue destruction take place, fistulas may develop between the vagina and the bladder, between the vagina and rectum or both, resulting in incontinence of urine or faeces or both. Neoplastic growth may obstruct one or both ureters leading to hydronephrosis, renal malfunction and possibly death.

Pain is usually a late symptom which develops

table 10.11   Histological diagnoses of the cases in table 10.10

	Population screening material (*n* = 97)	Smears from general practitioners (*n* = 272)	Smears from Department of Gynaecology and Obstetrics (*n* = 138)
No known histology	4%	15%	4%
Negative	2%	6%	2%
Dysplasia	8%	10%	6%
Carcinoma *in situ*	68% (4%)*	55% (10%)*	42% (5%)*
Microinvasion	5%	2% (1%)*	21% (1%)*
Invasive squamous cell carcinoma	14% (2%)*	11% (1%)*	34% (1%)**
	101% (6%)***	99% (12%)***	99% (7%)***

* Cytological diagnosis: dysplasia or atypical reserve cell hyperplasia
** Cytological diagnosis: carcinoma *in situ* or invasive squamous cell carcinoma
***Cytological under-diagnosis

only when metastatic neoplasm in the lymph nodes exerts pressure on nerve bundles or when the carcinoma invades the sheath of a nerve. Metastasis to the regional lymph nodes can also cause impairment of the venous blood flow. Haematogenous dissemination of carcinoma, which tends to occur later, may cause metastasis to the lungs and liver (table 10.13). Generally, anaemia, loss of appetite and loss of weight do not develop until the disease is advanced.

table 10.12   Symptoms of 348 women with carcinoma *in situ*

	I		II	
	n	%	*n*	%
No complaints	69	76	201	78
Menorrhagia or metrorrhagia	–	–	5	2
Postmenopausal bleeding	7	8	22	9
Postcoital bleeding	13	14	12	5
Vague complaints in lower abdomen	1	1	5	2
Combination of complaints	–	–	13	5
Total	90	99	258	101

Data from Leiden Cytology Laboratory, 1975/1976
I, population screening, programme (*n* = 90);
II, family doctor's practice (*n* = 258)

10.5.2 Macroscopic and Microscopic Examination of the Portio

Carcinoma *in situ* may lead to macroscopically visible changes in the portio: leucoplakia or the more common 'suspicious' erosion. The latter can appear as a bright red polypous portio, a readily bleeding portio (the superficial epithelium sheds easily) or a flat 'blushing' portio due to the granulated surface of the endocervical epithelium being replaced by immature metaplastic epithelium (van den Bosch, 1968). In our series 10 per cent of the

table 10.13   Spread by contiguity or metastasis of cervical carcinoma in 100 patients as established at necropsy (Kuipers, 1972)

To the bladder	28%
To the rectum	15%
In pelvic region ('frozen pelvis')	23%
Stenosis of the ureters	67%
Metastasis to lymph nodes	26%
Mestastasis to peritoneum	17%
Metastasis to lungs	9%
metastasis to liver	32%

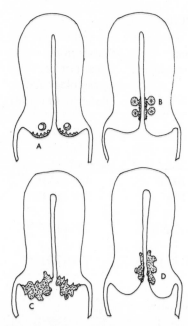

figure 10.28   Possible localisation of carcinoma *in situ* and squamous cell carcinoma. A. Ectocervical carcinoma *in situ* growing into the endocervical glandular crypts; B. endocervical carcinoma *in situ* with extensive growth into the endocervical glandular crypts; C. exophytic invasive squamous cell carcinoma; D. endophytic invasive squamous cell carcinoma

women with carcinoma *in situ* were found to have a suspicious erosion. For more precise evaluation the clinician should use colposcopy or the Schiller test, or both. Invasive carcinomas are often visible macroscopically. The exophytic ectocervical tumour is seen as a bulging friable mass; the endophytic tumour appears as an ulcer covered with fibrin and cellular and necrotic cellular debris (figure 10.28). The uncommon endophytic endocervically located carcinomas cannot be seen macroscopically.

10.5.2.1 The Schiller Test

The Schiller test makes use of the fact that, in contrast to normal squamous epithelial cells, cancer cells contain little or no glycogen. It is carried out as follows: the portio is painted with a watery solution of one part iodine (which has a marked affinity for glycogen) and two parts potassium iodide (Lugol's solution). Within several minutes the normal glycogen-rich squamous epithelium will turn dark brown; endocervical epithelial cells remain unstained. Abnormal squamous epithelial cells will in general take on a light colour or none at all. Thus the stain forms a map which can be used as a guide for biopsy or to determine the outer margin of a cone biopsy (the site of the incision must always pass through the dark brown area).

10.5.2.2 Colposcopy

An important aid for the clinician is the colposcope, a stereoscopic microscope with which the surface of the portio can be studied at a magnification of 6–20. The portio is first painted with 2 per cent acetic acid so that the mucus will be white and opaque. Vascular changes are best seen with a green filter. The endocervical glandular epithelium is slightly eversed by speculum examination and the whole metaplastic zone can usually be studied (Coppleson *et al.*, 1976). By colposcopic examination the following morphological features can be assessed: the extent and relationship of native squamous epithelium, metaplastic epithelium and glandular epithelium; the colour of the ectocervix, modified by epithelial height, cell density, keratin production; the surface configuration; the vascular pattern (punctate pattern, ground structure, mosaic structure, dotting (figure 10.29), etc.); and the degree of atypia (Coppleson *et al.*, 1976). In general the colposcope is used for patients with a macroscopically abnormal portio or abnormal cytological findings. As with the Schiller test, the colposcope can be used as a guide for biopsy of an abnormal area. It is important to establish a definite histological diagnosis as treatment depends on it.

10.5.3 Diagnosis

Correct diagnosis requires good cooperation between the clinician and the cytopathologist. Our diagnostic routine is as follows. After the clinical history has been taken, the patient undergoes physical examination. A cellular sample is prepared from the portio and sent to the cytopathology laboratory. When mild dysplasia or atypical reserve cell hyperplasia is diagnosed

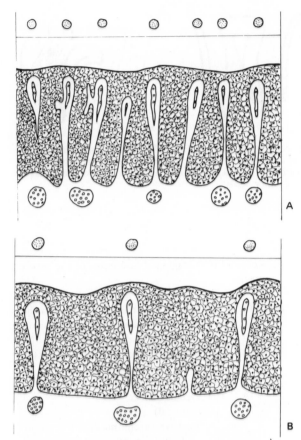

figure 10.29 Vascular bed and thickness of the epithelium determine the colposcopic pattern. A. Papillae with blood vessels close together; colposcopic pattern: crowded dots; B. the papillae are further apart: dots not as crowded.

If the cytological findings indicate carcinoma *in situ* or invasive carcinoma, the examination is supplemented with colposcopy and biopsy, sometimes preceded by the Schiller test for guidance. Naked-eye abnormalities of the portio may also be a sufficient reason to perform a biopsy. If there are no indications of an invasive carcinoma (infiltrating deeper than 5 mm) conisation or cryosurgery is performed. Cytological and colposcopic follow-up is recommended. If there are clinical indications of invasive neoplasm, or the histological examination leads to such a conclusion, then the patient must be admitted to the hospital for more extensive studies and for treatment.

10.5.3.1 Staging of Cervical Carcinoma

In order to determine whether a cervical carcinoma has extended to the bladder or the rectum the gynaecological examination must be supplemented with cystoscopy and proctoscopy. X-ray films of the lungs are prepared, to ascertain whether there is pulmonary metastasis, and of the kidneys, to ascertain whether there is hydronephrosis as a result of neoplastic obstruction of the ureters. Lymphography is carried out to ascertain whether there is metastasis to pelvic lymph nodes. Since the 1920s the following system of clinical staging of cervical cancer has been used internationally (figure 10.30).

Stage 0	Intraepithelial carcinoma (carcinoma *in situ*)
Stage I	Carcinoma is limited to the cervix
IA	Microinvasive carcinoma
IB	Invasive carcinoma
Stage II	Extension beyond the cervix, but not as far as the walls of the pelvis
IIA	Extension of the carcinoma within the cervix and in the upper two-thirds of the vagina
IIB	Extension of the carcinoma within the cervix and to the parametrium
Stage IIIA	The carcinoma extends to the lower third of the vagina
IIIB	The carcinoma extends to the wall of the pelvis
Stage IV	Invasion by carcinoma of bladder or rectum; distant metastasis

cytologically, the patient is then followed clinically and cytologically at 6-monthly intervals (see chapter 16). When severe dysplasia or atypical reserve cell hyperplasia is diagnosed the intervals should be shortened to 3 months. In cases of doubt (for instance, few abnormal cells but with outstanding pleomorphism, or a great number of abnormal cells) a biopsy is advised. Also persistence of severe dysplasia beyond 1 year is an indication for histological evaluation (Villasanta and Durkan, 1966). If there is evidence of extensive involvement (many dysplastic cells) some prefer cryosurgery (freezing) (Townsend, 1975) or laser surgery. Colposcopy can also play a crucial role in the management of dysplasia patients (Coppleson *et al.*, 1976).

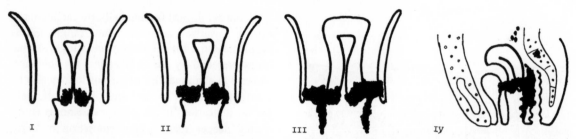

I   II   III   IY

figure 10.30   Clinical stages of cervical carcinoma (drawing according to Pschyrembel, 1966). I. Carcinoma restricted to cervix; II. spread of carcinoma into parametrium and upper two-thirds of the vagina; III. extension of carcinoma in parametrium to the walls of the pelvis and/or lower third of the vagina; IV. invasion of bladder and/or rectum, or metastasis of carcinoma beyond minor pelvis

In 1974 and 1977 modifications of stages IA and IB were published.

(1) 1974 modification of FIGO staging of carcinoma of the cervix uteri		(2) Recent FIGO staging of carcinoma of the cervix uteri	
*Stage I	Carcinoma strictly confined to the cervix (extension to the corpus should be disregarded)	Stage I	Carcinoma strictly confined to the cervix (extension to the corpus should be disregarded)
IA	Microinvasive carcinoma (early stromal invasion)	IA	The cancer cannot be diagnosed by clinical examination
IB	All other cases of Stage I: occult cancer should be marked 'occ'	IA	(1) Early stromal invasion
		IA	(2) Occult cancer
		IA	(postsurgical)
			Invasive carcinoma (a microscopic focus found on histological examination of the removed uterus)
		IB	All other cases of Stage I

*Notes to the staging. Stage IA (microinvasive carcinoma) represents those cases of epithelial abnormalities in which histological evidence of early stromal invasion is unambiguous. The diagnosis is based on microscopic examination of the tissue removed by biopsy, conisation, or portio amputation of the removed uterus. Cases of early stromal invasion should thus be allotted to Stage IA. The remainder of Stage I cases should be allotted to Stage IB. As a rule, these cases can be diagnosed by routine clinical examination. Occult cancers are evidently invasive cancers that cannot be diagnosed by routine clinical examination. They are as a rule diagnosed by a cone or on the amputated portio. They should be included in Stage IB and should be marked 'Stage Ib—occ.'. Stage I cases can thus be indicated in the following ways.

Stage IA	Carcinoma *in situ* with early stromal invasion diagnosed on tissue removed by biopsy, conisation, or portio amputation or on the removed uterus
IB	Clinically invasive carcinoma confined to the cervix
IB—occ	Histological invasive carcinoma of the cervix that could not be detected at a routine clinical examination but was diagnosed on a large biopsy, a cone, or the amputated portio

In the old system in ±10 per cent of stage IA cases positive lymph nodes were found, which influences prognosis in a negative sense. In the newest staging system lymph node metastases are found exclusively in the 'occult' stages, that is, IA (2 and postsurgical) and IB (Boronow, 1977).

As the neoplasm continues to spread, the prognosis of the patient worsens. At more advanced stages (II–IV) metastasis to the lymph nodes can occur more frequently. The presence of metastasis also influences the prognosis in a negative sense.

The cell type and the degree of differentiation of the neoplasm also appear to be important for prognosis and therapy. Wentz and Reagan (1959) divided cervical carcinomas into keratinising and nonkeratinising types, with the nonkeratinising type having a more favourable prognosis; in addition, it responds to radiotherapy. Keratinising squamous cell carcinoma has an unfavourable prognosis and does not respond as well to radiotherapy. Anaplastic carcinoma has the worst prognosis. A small cell carcinoma of the uterine cervix is probably a highly aggressive tumour and behaves quite differently from other types of squamous cell carcinoma of the cervix (van Nagel *et al.*, 1977).

10.5.4 Treatment of Cervical Carcinoma

10.5.4.1 Treatment of Carcinoma *in situ* (Stage 0)

Cervical carcinoma *in situ* can frequently be treated adequately by surgery alone. It is generally sufficient to use conisation, which serves the dual purpose of diagnosis and therapy. Using the Schiller test as a guide, a cone-shaped biopsy with the cervical canal as the axis is removed from the cervix (figure 10.31) taking care to remove tissue well up in the endocervix. The cone biopsy is then examined histologically. The data of Rubio *et al.* (1978) indicate that the frequency of lesions incompletely removed at conisation increase with decreasing size (that is, length and volume) of the specimen. When cancerous epithelium is found at the margins of the cone or if local microinvasion is established, further therapy is indicated. After

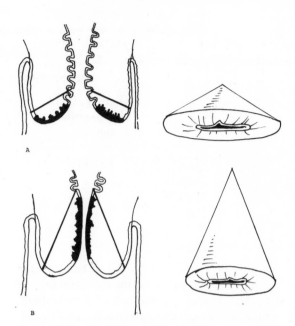

figure 10.31 Cervical cone biopsy. The shape of the cone depends partly on the location of the transition zone (schematic drawing according to Kern, 1964). A. Sexually mature female: blunt cone; B. elderly female: sharply pointed cone

conisation, periodic cytological follow-up for life is desirable. According to the literature, 0.5–2 per cent of patients treated in this way will show recurrence of the carcinoma within one year. The five-year survival after therapy of carcinoma *in situ* is 100 per cent. In the near future carcinoma *in situ* will probably be treated more frequently with cryotherapy or laser surgery, procedures which can be carried out in the outpatient clinic. However, histological examination of excised tissue is then not possible.

10.5.4.2 Treatment of an Invasive Carcinoma

There are various methods for treating a patient with invasive carcinoma: (1) radiotherapy; (2) surgery; (3) a combination of 1 and 2.

(1) *Radiotherapy.* Radiotherapy usually consists of the local application of radium to treat the primary neoplasm, followed by treatment of any lymph-nodal metastasis by irradiation of the entire pelvis using telecobalt. Radiotherapy can be used in all stages with good results (table 10.14;

table 10.14   Five-year survival from cervical squamous carcinoma (Ketting, 1976; Kok, 1976; Kuipers, 1972)

	after combined therapy		after irradiation	
	(Ketting, 1976) with negative lymph nodes	with positive lymph nodes	Kok, 1976	Kuipers, 1972
Stage I	89–90%	50%	88.5%	71%
Stage II	–	50–60%	72 %	62%
Stage III	–	25–30%	52.6%	44%
Stage IV	–	0%	9 %	20%

Kuipers, 1972; Kok, 1976). The success of radiotherapy depends partly on the radiosensitivity of the carcinoma and on the lack of complications, such as infection of the intestine and bladder which could lead to ulcerative proctitis, ulcerative cystitis, even rectovaginal or vesicovaginal fistula formation or both.

(2) *Surgery.* Microinvasive carcinoma can be treated by conisation or hysterectomy. The treatment of invasive carcinoma consists of a radical hysterectomy. This operation was first developed in Vienna by Schauta and later by his student Wertheim, among others. It consists of the removal of the uterus, adnexa, part of the vagina and the parametrium as far as possible. Schauta approached the uterus from the vagina; Wertheim used the abdominal approach and performed a lymphadenectomy at the same time.

In general, surgery is used for Stages I–IIA (growth into the upper two-thirds of the vagina); more advanced stages are usually considered inoperable. Surgical complications include urinary symptoms, fistular formation and proctitis, apart from the general risks of surgery such as venous thrombosis.

In Stages III and IV or when neoplasm persists following therapy, pelvic exenteration may be necessary. This is a very major operation (associated with the name Brunschwig) whereby the minor pelvis is 'emptied': depending upon the severity of the neoplasm, the rectum, sigmoid, bladder, distal part of the ureters, internal iliac blood vessels, internal genitalia, lymph nodes and pelvic floor are removed. If metastasis has already occurred outside the minor pelvis this operation serves no purpose. The surgical risk involved in such an operation is obviously very high.

(3) *Combined therapy.* This is used for Stages I and II, sometimes also Stage III. Preoperative application of radium to the cervix is common, in addition, most operations are followed by irradiation (Ketting, 1976). In a number of cases the carcinoma is clinically recurrent, often within two years of treatment. Such a neoplasm is presumed to have been not completely eradicated, that is, it is a *persistent* neoplasm. Late recurrences (after an interval of at least five years) occur in 5–10 per cent of cases (Noordijk, 1976). Survival from recurrent carcinoma is very poor: 97 per cent die within five years (Truelsen, 1949). Treatment of persistent or recurrent carcinoma is usually accompanied by numerous complications. In a few cases chemotherapy is also used for palliation.

References

Ashley, D. J. B. (1966). The biological status of carcinoma in situ of uterine cervix. *J. Obstet. Gynaec. Br. Commonw.*, 73, 373–81

Bajardi, F. (1961). Histomorphology of reserve cell hyperplasia, basal cell hyperplasia and dysplasia. *Acta Cytol.*, 5, 133–42

Bangle, R., Berger, M. and Levin, M. (1963). Variations in morphogenesis of squamous cell carcinoma of the cervix. *Cancer,* **16**, 1151–9

Bauer, K. M. and Friederich, H. C. (1965). Peniscarcinom auf dem Boden vor-behandelter Condylomata acuminata. *Z. Haut-Geschlechtskrankh.,* **39**, 150–3

Beral, V. (1974). Cancer of the cervix: a sexually transmitted infection? *Lancet,* 1037–40

Beyer-Boon, M. E. (1977). *Year report of the Leiden Cytology Laboratory,* Leiden.

Beyer-Boon, M. E. and Verdonk, G. W. (1978). The identification of atypical reserve cells in smears of patients with premalignant and malignant changes in the squamous and glandular epithelium of the uterine cervix. *Acta Cytol.,* **22**, 305–11

Boronow, R. C. (1977). Stage I cervix cancer and pelvic node metastasis. *Am. J. Obstet. Gynec.,* **127**, 135–8

Bosch, J. Th. M. van den. (1968). *De Waarde van de Cytologische Controle bij de Behandeling van het Carcinoma in situ van de Cervix Uteri,* Bronder, Rotterdam

Broders, A. C. (1926). Carcinoma: grading and practical application. *Arch. Path. Lab. Med.,* **2**, 376–81

Burghardt, E. (1970). Latest aspects of precancerous lesions in squamous and columnar epithelium of the cervix. *Int. J. Gynec. Obstet.,* **8**, 573–80

Chi, C. H., Rubio, C. A. and Lagerlöf, B., (1977). The frequency and distribution of mitotic figures in dysplasia and carcinoma in situ. *Cancer,* **39**, 1218–23

Christopherson, W. M. and Parker, J. E. (1964a). Microinvasive carcinoma of the uterine cervix. *Cancer,* **17**, 1123–31

Christopherson, W. M. and Parker, J. E. (1964b). *Dysplasia, Carcinoma in situ and Microinvasive Carcinoma of the Cervix Uteri* (ed. L. A. Gray), Thomas, Springfield

Christopherson, W. M. and Parker, J. E. (1965). Relation of cervical cancer to early marriage and childbearing. *New Engl. J. Med.,* **273**, 235–9

Clarke, E. A. and Anderson, T. W. (1979). Does screening by 'Pap' smears help prevent cervical cancer? *Lancet,* **ii**, 1419–22

Coleman, D. V. (1976). *Cell changes due to therapeutic measures – their clinical significance and cytological recognition,* 6th European Congress of Cytology, Weimar

Collette, H. J. A. (1976). *De Epidemiologische Aspecten van het Cervix Carcinoom,* Boeijinga, Apeldoorn

Coppleson, M., Pixley, E. and Reid, B. (1976). *Colposcopy: a Scientific and Practical Approach to the Cervix in Health and Disease,* Thomas, Springfield

Domaniewski, J. and Gustowski, A. (1968). Planoepithelial, spinocellular cancer of the vulva, originating from condylomata acuminata. *Ginekol. Pol.,* **39**, 239–43

Fidler, H. K. and Boyes, D. A. (1959). Patterns of early invasion from intraepithelial carcinoma of the cervix. *Cancer,* **12**, 673–80

Fraser, R. C., Cudmore, D. C., Melanson, J. and Morse, W. I. (1967). The metabolism and production rate of estradiol-17 in pre-menopausal women with cervical carcinoma. *Am. J. Obstet. Gynec.,* **98**, 509–15

Govan, A. D. T., Haines, R. M., Langley, F. A., Taylor, C. W. and Woodcock, A. S. (1966). Changes in the epithelium of the cervix uteri. *J. Obstet. Gynaec. Br. Commonw.,* **73**, 883–96

Graaf Guilloud-Gentenaar, J. C. de and Beyer-Boon, M. E. (1977). Cytologic and histologic differences between 'classical' and condylomatous dysplasia, Abstract. *7th European Congress of Cytology, Luik*

Graham, R. M. (1972). *The Cytologic Diagnosis of Cancer,* Saunders, Philadelphia and London

Greene, R. R. and Peckham, B. M. (1954). Squamous papilloma of the cervix. *Am. J. Obstet. Gynec.,* **67**, 883–98

Haam, E. von and Old, J. W. (1964). Reserve cell hyperplasia, squamous metaplasia and epidermidization. In: *Dysplasia, Carcinoma in situ and Micro-invasive Carcinoma of the Cervix Uteri* (ed. L. A. Gray), Thomas, Springfield, pp. 41–82

Jennings, R. H. and Barclay, D. L. (1972). Verrucous carcinoma of the cervix. *Cancer,* **30**, 431–4

Johnson, L. D., Easterday, C. L., Gore, H. and Hertig, A. T. (1964). The histogenesis of carcinoma in situ of the uterine cervix. A preliminary report of the origin of carcinoma in situ in subcylindrical cell anaplasia. *Cancer,* **17**, 213–29

Kashgarian, M. and Dunn, J. E. (1970). The duration of intraepithelial and pre-clinical squamous cell carcinoma of the uterine cervix. *Am. J. Epidem.,* **92**, 211–22

Keebler, C. M. and Wied, G. L. (1974). The estrogen test: an aid in differential cytodiagnosis. *Acta. Cytol.,* **18**, 482–92

Kerl, H. and Pickel, H. (1971). Maligne Umwandlung von Condylomata Acuminata der Vulva. *Z. Haut-Geschlechtskrankh,* **46**, 155–62

Kern, G. (1964). *Carcinoma in situ,* Springer, Berlin

Kessler, I. I. (1976). Human cervical cancer as venereal disease. *Cancer Res.,* **36**, 783

Ketting, B. W. (1976). *De Chirurgische Therapie,* Boerhaave cursus, Leiden

Kirk, M. E. (1974). Progress in human pathology, gynecology. *Hum. Path.,* **5**, 253–64

Kok, G. (1976). *De Radiologische Therapie,* Boerhaave cursus, Leiden

Koss, L. G. (1968). *Diagnostic Cytology and its Histopathologic Bases,* Lippincott, Philadelphia

Koss, L. G. Stewart, F. W., Foote, F. W., Jordan, M. J., Bader, G. M. and Day, E. (1963). Some histological aspects of behaviour of epidermoid carcinoma in situ and related lesions of the uterine cervix. *Cancer,* **9**, 1160–211

Koss, L. G. and Wolinska, W. H. (1959). Trichomonas vaginalis cervicitis and its relationship to cervical cancer; a histocytological study. *Cancer,* **12**, 1171–93

Kuipers, T. (1972). Carcinoma of the uterine cervix. *Acta Radiol,* Stockholm

Langley, F. A. and Crompton, A. C. (1973). *Epithelial Abnormalities of the Cervix Uteri,* Springer, Berlin

Laverty, C. R., Russell, P., Hills, E. and Booth, N. (1978). The significance of noncondylomatous wart virus infection of the cervical transformation zone. A review with discussion of two illustrative cases. *Acta Cytol.,* **22**, 195–201

Marsh, M. (1952). Papilloma of the cervix. *Am. J. Obstet. Gynec.,* **64**, 281–91

Meisels, P. A., Fortin, R. and Roy, M. (1977). Condylomatous lesions of the cervix II. *Acta Cytol.,* **21**, 379–90

Melamed, M. R. and Flehinger, B. J. (1976). Non-diagnostic squamous atypia in cervico-vaginal cytology as a risk factor for early neoplasia. *Acta Cytol.,* **20**, 108–10

Murphy, W. M. and Coleman, S. A. (1976). The long-term course of carcinoma in situ of the uterine cervix. *Cancer,* **38**, 957–63

Nagel, J. R. van, Donaldson, E. S., Wood, E. G., Maruyama, Y. and Utley, J. (1977). Small cell cancer of the uterine cervix. *Cancer,* **40**, 2243–9

Ng, A. B. P. and Reagan, J. W. (1969). Microinvasive carcinoma of the uterine cervix, *Am. J. clin. Path.,* **52**, 511–29

Ng, A. B. P., Reagan, J. W. and Lindner, E. A. (1972). The cellular manifestations of microinvasive squamous cell carcinoma of the uterine cervix. *Acta Cytol.,* **16**, 5–13

Noordijk, E. M. (1976). *De Therapie van het Recidiverende Cervix Carcinoom,* Boerhaave cursus, Leiden

Old, J. W., Wielenga, G. and Haam, E. von (1965). Squamous carcinoma in situ of the uterine cervix I. Classification and histogenesis. *Cancer,* **18**, 1598–611

Patten, S. F. (1975). Morphologic subclassification of preinvasive cervical neoplasia. In: *Compendium on Diagnostic Cytology* (eds. G. L. Wied, L. G. Koss and J. W. Reagan), Tutorials of Cytology, Chicago, pp. 121–33

Patten, S. F. (1978). *Diagnostic Cytopathology of the Uterine Cervix,* Karger, New York

Pschyrembel, W. (1966). *Praktische Gynäkologie für Studierende und Ärzte,* de Gruyter, Berlin

Purola, E. and Savia, E. (1977). Cytology of gynecologic Condyloma acuminatum. *Acta Cytol.,* **21**, 26–32

Rawls, W. E., Tompkins, W. A. F. and Melnick, J. L. (1969). The association of herpesvirus type 2 and carcinoma of the uterine cervix. *Am. J. Epidemiol.,* **89**, 547–54

Reagan, J. W., Bell, B. A., Neuman, J. L., Scott, R. B. and Patten, S. F. (1961). Dysplasia in the uterine cervix during pregnancy: an analytical study of the cells. *Acta Cytol.,* **5**, 17–30

Reagan, J. W. and Hamonic, M. J. (1956). The cellular pathology in carcinoma in situ: a cytohistopathological correlation. *Cancer,* **9**, 385–402

Reagan, J. W. and Hicks, D. J. (1953). A study of in situ and squamous cell cancer of the uterine cervix. *Cancer,* **6**, 1200–14

Reagan, J. W. and Patten, S. F. (1962). Dysplasia: a basic reaction to injury in the uterine cervix. *Ann. N. Y. Acad. Sci.,* **97**, 662–82

Reagan, J. W., Seidemann, I. B. and Patten, S. F. (1962). Developmental stages of in situ carcinoma in uterine cervix: an analytical study of the cells. *Acta. Cytol.*, **6**, 538–46

Richart, R. M. and Barron, B. A. (1969). A follow-up study of patients with cervical dysplasia. *Am. J. Obstet. Gynec.*, **105**, 386–93

Rilke, F. (1976). Prevalence of malignant tumors in immunosuppressed patients and their cytologic presentation, *Abstract. 6th European Congress of Cytology, Weimar*

Rubio, C. A. (1973). Estrogenic effect in vaginal smears in cases of carcinoma in situ and microinvasive carcinoma of the uterine cervix. *Acta Cytol.*, **17**, 361–5

Rubio, C. A. (1974). Cytologic studies in cases with carcinoma in situ and microinvasive carcinoma of the uterine cervix. *Acta Path. Microb. Scand.*, Section A, **82**, 161–8

Rubio, C. A. and Einhorn, N. (1977). The exfoliating epithelial surface of the uterine cervix IV: Scanning electron microscopical study in invasive squamous carcinoma of human subjects. *Beitr. Path.*, **161**, 72–81

Rubio, C. A. and Kranz, I. (1976). The exfoliating cervical epithelial surface in dysplasia, carcinoma in situ and invasive squamous carcinoma I. Scanning electron microscopic study. *Acta Cytol.*, **20**, 144–50

Rubio, C. A., Söderberg, G. and Einhorn, N. (1974). Histological and follow-up studies in cases of microinvasive carcinoma of the uterine cervix. *Acta Path. Microb. Scand.*, Section A, **82**, 397–410

Rubio, C. A., Thomassen, P., Söderberg, G. and Kock, Y. (1978). Big cones and little cones. *Histopathology*, **2**, 133–43

Spratt, D. W. and Lee, S. C. (1977). Verrucous carcinoma of the cervix. *Am. J. Obstet. Gynec.*, **129**, 699–700

Stern, E. and Neely, P. M. (1964). Dysplasia of the uterine cervix: incidence of regression, recurrence and cancer. *Cancer*, **17**, 508–12

Stormby, N. (1974). Morphology of virus induced changes, *Abstract. 4th European Congress of Cytology, Ljubljana*

Townsend, D. E. (1975). Cryosurgery in gynecology. In: *Progress in Gynecology 6* (ed. Taymor and Green), Grune & Stratton, New York, pp. 583–95

Truelsen, F. (1949). *Cancer of the Uterine Cervix*, Thesis. Rosenhild 109 Bagger, Copenhagen

Villasanta, V. and Durkan, J. P. (1966). Indications and complications of cold conization of the cervix; observations of 200 consecutive cases. *Obstet. Gynec.*, **27**, 717–23

Warren, S. (1931). The grading of carcinoma of the cervix uteri as checked at autopsy. *Arch. Path.*, **12**, 783–6

Waterhouse, J., Muir C., Correa, P. and Powell, J. (eds.) (1976). *Cancer Incidence in Five Continents*, Vol II. International Agency for Research on Cancer, Lyon

Wentz, W. B. and Reagan, J. W. (1959). Survival in cervical cancer with respect to cell type. *Cancer*, **12**, 384–8

Ziabkowski, T. A. and Naylor, B. (1976). Cyanophilic bodies in cervicovaginal smears. *Acta Cytol.*, **20**, 340–3

Zur Hausen, H. (1976). Condylomata acuminata of the cervix. *Am. J. Obstet. Gynec.*, **75**, 1354–62

Adenocarcinoma of the Cervix

11.1 Introduction

This chapter contains a discussion of gland cell atypia, adenocarcinoma *in situ*, and invasive adenocarcinoma of the endocervix (with or without a squamous component). As in squamous epithelium morphological transitions are fluid and the different lesions are often found together in the same surgical specimen (Friedell and McKay, 1953). Cases have also been published of an initial diagnosis of atypia of the endocervical epithelium which later became an infiltrating adenocarcinoma (Novak and Woodruff, 1974).

11.2 Histology, Cytology and Differential Diagnosis of Lesions of Endocervical Glandular Epithelium

11.2.1 Atypia of the Endocervical Glandular Epithelium

11.2.1.1 Histology

The nuclei of the endocervical glandular epithelium may be somewhat anisokaryotic and hyperchromatic with prominent nucleoli. These changes in the cells often occur in patients with chronic inflammation, but can also be seen when there are no signs of inflammation.

11.2.1.2 Cytology

The smear will contain endocervical gland cells with changes in the nuclei similar to those seen in the histological sections. Within the groups of cells, the arrangement of the nuclei may be highly irregular. Anisokaryosis and prominent nucleoli may be quite striking. Atypical endocervical gland cells should be differentiated from immature metaplastic cells, a distinction which is not always possible. In general, the latter lie in clusters with a greater nuclear density and their nuclei are also somewhat smaller. They must also be distinguished from endometrial cells with slightly swollen nuclei. The nuclei of the latter are much smaller than those of the endocervical cells and their groupings appear more three-dimensional.

11.2.2 Adenocarcinoma of the Endocervix

11.2.2.1 Histology

Adenocarcinoma arising in endocervical epithelium is characterised by the presence of an acinar or 'grape-like' histological pattern of the glandular ducts, as well as by morphological changes in the epithelial cells. Cellular atypia may vary from slight to marked. The precursor of infiltrating adenocarcinoma is adenocarcinoma *in situ* (Friedell and McKay, 1953). In adenocarcinoma *in situ* the preexisting glands are lined by cells with nuclear enlargement, coarse chromatin, reduced N/C ratio and many mitoses. This abnormal epithelium may display pseudostratification and papillary intraluminal budding (Qizilbash, 1975). In the well-differentiated adenocarcinoma the structure of the glandular ducts is still largely intact; in contrast, it is rare or absent in the poorly differentiated carci-nomas (Broders, 1925). The mucus-producing type of adenocarcinoma of the endocervix (mucoid carcinoma) is relatively rare (Novak and Woodruff, 1974). A special type of adenocarcinoma of the cervix, clear cell carcinoma, is found in young girls whose mothers took large doses of diethylstil-boestrol during pregnancy. There are 170 cases of clear cell carcinoma with such an aetiological background registered with the Registry of Clear Cell Adenocarcinomas of the Genital Tract in Young Females; of these, 100 arose in the vagina and 70 in the cervix (Herbst *et al.*, 1975) (see section 13.4.1).

11.2.2.2 Cytology

The smear will contain a large number of malignant cells, discrete and in groups (Wied *et al.*, 1974). In contrast, a smear from a patient with endometrial adenocarcinoma usually contains only a small number of carcinoma cells (Koss, 1968). The cyto-logical pattern is determined to a large extent by the degree of differentiation.

(1) A *well-differentiated* endocervical adeno-carcinoma *without* evidence of pronounced mucus formation is characterised by more or less flat cell groups with nuclear stacking; moreover, it may be perceived that these cells form glandular arrange-ments in which the cells in a group lie in a rosette pattern with a central 'lumen' (figure 11.1). An arrangement of the nuclei in palisades is common. Mitotic figures occur in approximately one-third of the cases. The cells are often clearly columnar with basal nuclei which are oval and hyperchromatic with a characteristic coarsening of the chromatin ('rice chromatin', nuclear patterns 3, 4, 14, section 9.5.2.1). Nucleoli may be prominent; perinuclear halos may be seen.

(2) A *well-differentiated mucus-secreting* adeno-carcinoma exfoliates cells which are a caricature of normal endocervical cells. The cells may lie in papillary groups and they may be arranged in a somewhat disorganised honeycomb with vacuoles of unequal size. The nuclei are hyper chromatic and anisokaryotic. Large mucous vacuoles may flatten the nucleus.

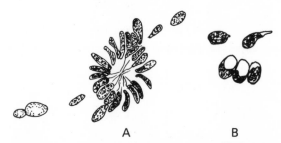

figure 11.1   Cytological pattern of an endocervical adeno-carcinoma. A, rosette pattern in a will-differentiated adenocarcinoma; B, cells from a nucus-secreting adeno-carcinoma

(3) A *poorly differentiated* adenocarcinoma is characterised by vesicular 'three-dimensional' (less pronounced than in an endometrial carcinoma) cells which are irregularly arranged and show marked nuclear atypia. The cells of a poorly differentiated adenocarcinoma are rounded with round hyper-chromatic nuclei (nuclear pattern 14, section 9.5.2.1) and several nucleoli, which are often abnormally shaped. With decreasing differentiation the mean nuclear area increases (figure 11.2). Cyto-plasmic vacuolisation is absent or inconspicuous. The cytoplasm has a granular appearance. Leuco-phagocytosis may occur, but is seen less frequently in comparison with endometrial adenocarcinoma. In a smear there are often poorly differentiated cells as well as cell groups showing better differen-tiation (figure 11.3).

A background diathesis is almost always seen with an infiltrative lesion (figure 11.4). However, the smears of six patients with adenocarcinoma *in situ* showed no signs of a diathesis.

11.2.2.3 Atypical Reserve Cells and Squamous Cell Components in Endocervical Adenocarcinoma

Adenocarcinoma of the endocervix is frequently associated with a (pre)malignant squamous com-ponent (Reagan and Ng, 1973). This also applies to adenocarcinoma *in situ* (Melnick *et al.*, 1957; Lauchlan and Penner, 1967). In our 20 cases of early adenocarcinoma (14 *in situ*, 2 microinvasive and 4 invasive carcinomas) 13 of the smears con-tained malignant squamous cells, 9 dysplastic cells

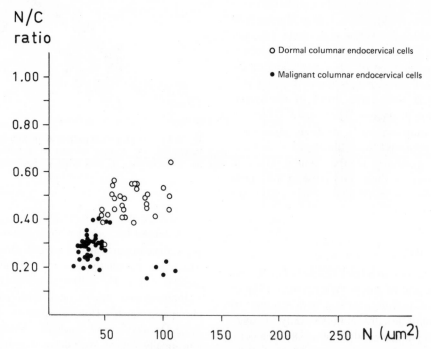

figure 11.2   Scattergram of N/C ratio and nuclear area (N) of adenocarcinoma cells of the endocervix compared with normal columnar cells

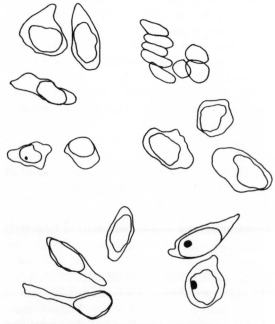

figure 11.3   Camera lucida drawings. Several examples of malignant endocervical adenocarcinoma cells

and 13 atypical reserve cells (table 11.1) (Kirk and Beyer-Boon, in preparation). The presence of atypical reserve cells in association with malignant squamous and glandular epithelial cells supports the theories of previous workers (Johnson *et al.*, 1964; Burghardt, 1970) that the reserve cell has a potential to differentiate to either squamous carcinoma cell or an adenocarcinoma cell (Beyer-Boon and Verdonk, 1978). This process is illustrated in figure 11.5. Squamous cell carcinomas occur frequently without an associate adenocarcinoma, and Qizilbash (1975) reported an incidence of adenocarcinoma *in situ* in association with squamous carcinoma *in situ* of 2.5 per cent. The disparity in incidence of squamous cell carcinoma and adenocarcinoma could perhaps be due to an innate tendency of reserve cells to develop into squamous epithelium. Another possibility is the fact that carcinomatous change of the columnar epithelium is frequently overlooked in cases of

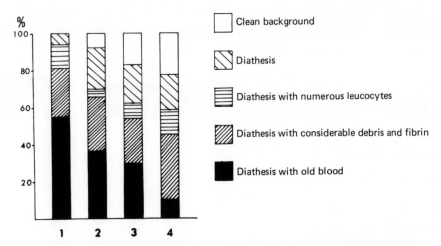

figure 11.4 Frequency of diathesis in smears from 79 females with adenocarcinoma (University of Leiden, 1975). 1. Endocervical carcinomas (15); 2. endometrial carcinomas (42); 3. ovarian carcinomas (13); 4. metastasis of adenocarcinoma (9)

squamous carcinoma *in situ*, cytologically and histologically (Lauchlan and Penner, 1967; Weisbrot *et al.*, 1972). When there are two malignant components, one component may be infiltrating whilst the other is still in an *in situ* phase.

11.2.2.4 Differential Diagnosis

Endocervical adenocarcinoma must be distinguished from:
(1) endometrial adenocarcinoma (only possible if the tumour is well-differentiated (Nuovo, 1960));
(2) anaplastic carcinoma *in situ*;
(3) anaplastic carcinoma;
(4) tissue repair;
(5) endocervicitis.
It may be very difficult to discriminate cytologically between endocervicitis and well-differentiated endocervical adenocarcinoma. The following points are important in this respect.
(1) *Shape of the nuclei.* In endocervicitis the nuclei are round to oval (egg-shaped); in endocervical adenocarcinoma they are elongated (cigar-shaped).
(2) *Chromatin pattern.* In endocervicitis there

Table 11.1 Number of cases with different cell types in cervical smears from twenty cases of early adenocarcinoma diagnosed in a health screening programme

Histological classification	Malignant columnar cells	Atypical reserve cells	Dysplastic squamous cells	Malignant squamous cells
Adenocarcinoma *in situ*	13/14	9/14	6/14	9/14
Microinvasive adenocarcinoma	2/2	1/2	1/2	0/2
Invasive adenocarcinoma	4/4	3/4	2/4	4/4
Total	19/20	13/20	9/20	13/20

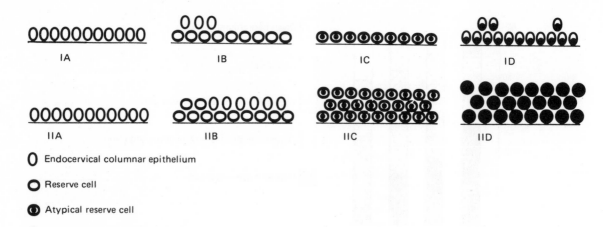

O Endocervical columnar epithelium

O Reserve cell

Ⓞ Atypical reserve cell

◖ Adenocarcinoma cell

● Malignant cell from anaplastic carcinoma *in situ*

figure 11.5   Morphogenesis of adenocarcinoma *in situ* and squamous carcinoma *in situ* of the endocervix. IA. Endocervical glandular epithelium; IB. reserve cells; IC. atypical reserve cells; ID. adenocarcinoma *in situ*; IIA. endocervical glandular epithelium; IIB. reserve cells; IIC. atypical reserve cell hyperplasia; IID. anaplastic carcinoma *in situ*

is at most a slight coarsening of the chromatin pattern. Well-differentiated endocervical carcinoma cells may show a characteristic coarsening of the chromatin ('rice' chromatin) (see nuclear pattern 4, section 9.5.2.1).

(3) *Arrangement of the cells.* In endocervicitis the groups of cells resemble a regular honeycomb; in endocervical carcinoma they form an irregular honeycomb or the nuclei lie in a typical palisade arrangement. Sometimes there will be as many as 12 nuclei lying in a row. The palisade pattern can sometimes be observed along the edge of a large group of cells.

(4) *Number of mitotic figures.* Although occasional mitotic figures may be seen in a smear manifesting endocervicitis, they may be strikingly numerous in endocervical carcinoma; thus a large number of mitotic figures increases the likelihood of the lesion being carcinoma.

(5) In endocervicitis the cell groups almost never lie in a rosette pattern.

11.2.2.5 Incidence of Endocervical
        Adenocarcinoma

The age of patients may vary from about 25 to 85 years (Hertig and Gore, 1960). The average age of

patients with adenocarcinoma *in situ* is 38.4 years (Qizilbash, 1975). In our series the peak age for adenocarcinoma *in situ* was in the 30–40 age group, whereas for evident clinical invasive adeno-carcinoma it was 55–64 (figure 11.6).

11.3 Clinical Aspects of Endocervical Adenocarcinoma

In our 14 *in situ* cases only one patient complained or irregular bleeding. All our patients with frankly invasive adenocarcinoma of the endocervix had clinical complaints, of which vaginal bleeding was the most common.

Endocervical carcinoma metastasises early via lymphatic channels (Butenberg and Stoll, 1960). The prognosis after treatment is not as good as that for cervical squamous cell carcinoma. The 5-year survival rate at the Free Hospital for Women in Boston was 17.8 per cent, whereas in the same hospital the survival rate for all cervical carcinomas was 43.7 per cent (Hertig and Gore, 1960). A biological difference in endocervical adenocarci-

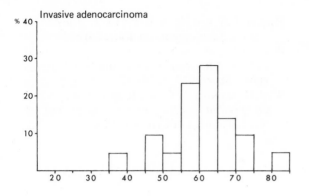

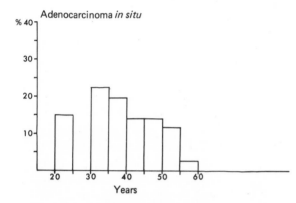

figure 11.6　Age distribution of 47 women with endo-cervical adenocarcinoma (Leiden University, 1970–5) and of 14 women with adenocarcinoma *in situ* (Leiden Cytology Laboratory, 1976–9).

nomas developing before and after menopause may exist. The latter display a particularly malignant behaviour (Kjörstad, 1977). The overall prognosis has improved over the last 20 years. The most important factor in this improvement is a change in attitude towards more radical surgery. Yet these patients are still more at risk than patients with squamous cell carcinoma (Kjörstad, 1977). Poor survival rates are found also in cases of mixed adenosquamous carcinomas (Julian *et al.*, 1977).

The diagnosis of cervical adenocarcinoma can often be made on a cervical smear taken with a modified Ayre spatula; in some cases from an endocervical swab (see sections 15.3.1 and 15.3.2).

References

Beyer-Boon, M. E. and Verdonk, G. W. (1978). The identification of atypical reserve cells in smears of patients with premalignant and malignant changes in the squamous and glandular epithelium of the uterine cervix. *Acta Cytol.*, **22**, 305–11

Broders, A. C. (1925). The grading of carcinoma. *Minn. Med.*, **8**, 726

Burghardt, E. (1970). Latest aspects of precancerous lesions in squamous and columnar epithelium of the cervix. *Int. J. Gynec. Obstet.*, **8**, 573–80

Butenberg, D. and Stoll, P. (1960). Incidence and clinical course of endocervical adenocarcinoma. *Acta Cytol.*, **4**, 341–3

Friedell, G. H. and McKay, D. G. (1953). Adenocarcinoma in situ of the endocervix. *Cancer*, **6**, 887–97

Herbst. A. L., Scully, R. E. and Robboy, S. J. (1975). Significance of adenosis and clear cell adenocarcinoma of the genital tract in young females. *J. reprod. Med.*, **15**, 5–11

Hertig, A. T. and Gore, H. (1960). *Tumours of the Female Sex Organs*, Armed Forces Institute of Pathology, Washington

Johnson, L. D., Easterday, C. L., Gore, H. and Hertig, A. T. (1964). The histogenesis of carcinoma in situ of the uterine cervix: a preliminary report of the origin of carcinoma in situ in subcylindrical cell anaplasia. *Cancer*, **17**, 213–29

Julian, C. G., Daikoku, N. H. and Gillespie, A. (1977). Adenoepidermoid and adenosquamous carcinoma of the uterus. *Am. J. Obstet. Gynec.*, **128**, 106–16

Kjörstad, K. E. (1977). Adenocarcinoma of the uterine cervix. *Gynec. Oncol.*, **5**, 219–23

Koss, L. G. (1968). *Diagnostic Cytology and its Histopathologic Bases*, 2nd edn, Lippincott, Philadelphia

Lauchlan, S. C. and Penner, D. W. (1967). Simultaneous adenocarcinoma in situ and epidermoid carcinoma in situ. Report of two cases. *Cancer*, **20**, 2250–4

Melnick, P. J., Lee, L. E. and Walsh, H. M. (1957). Endocervical and cervical neoplasms adjacent to carcinoma in situ. *Am. J. Clin. Path.*, **28**, 354–76

Novak, E. R. and Woodruff, J. D. (1974). *Gynaeco-*

logic and Obstetric Pathology, 7th edn, Saunders, Philadelphia and London

Nuovo, V. M. (1960). Can one distinguish by means of cytology the endocervical and endometrial adenocarcinoma? *Acta Cytol.,* **4,** (1960)

Qizilbash, A. H. (1975). In situ and microinvasive adenocarcinoma of the uterine cervix. A clinical, cytological and histological study of 14 cases. *Am. J. clin. Path.,* **64,** 155–70

Reagan, J. W. and Ng, A. B. P. (1973). *The Cells of Uterine Adenocarcinoma,* Karger, Basel

Weisbrot, I. M., Stabinsky, C. and Davis, A. M. (1972). Adenocarcinoma in situ of the uterine cervix. *Cancer,* **29,** 1179–92

Wied, G. L., Koss, L. G. and Reagan, J. W. (1974). *Compendium on Diagnostic Cytology,* Vol. III, No. 1, Tutorials of Cytology, Chicago

Adenocarcinoma of the Endometrium

12.1 Introduction

Endometrial hyperplasia and adenocarcinoma of the endometrium are discussed together in this chapter because, once again, there are morphological transitions between the two (Novak and Yui, 1936). Adenocarcinoma of the endometrium develops mainly in postmenopausal women. Risk factors include obesity, hypertension, diabetes mellitus, delayed menopause, a history of anovulatory menstrual cycles (as in the Stein—Leventhal syndrome (Andrews and Andrews, 1960)), low fertility and high oestrogen levels as a result, for instance, of an oestrogen-producing ovarian neoplasm (Novak and Woodruff, 1974). In general, women with endometrial hyperplasia are younger than women with endometrial adenocarcinoma, unless the hyperplasia is associated with hormonal therapy in postmenopausal women.

12.2 Histology, Cytology and Differential Diagnosis of Endometrial Lesions

12.2.1 Endometrial Hyperplasia

12.2.1.1 Histology

There are various forms of endometrial hyperplasia (Ng *et al.*, 1973a) with frequent transitions.
(1) *Cystic glandular hyperplasia.* This is characterised by increased formation of stroma as well as glandular ducts. The diameter of some glandular ducts is considerably increased, whereas others show a small diameter; this causes the 'Swiss cheese' appearance (figure 12.1). The glandular ducts are lined by columnar epithelium which appears at the most to be slightly atypical. Proliferation of the glandular ducts may be greater than that of the stroma, so that the ducts end up lying very close together.
(2) *Adenomatous hyperplasia.* There is a marked increase in the number of glandular ducts; cellular atypia is slight or negligible.
(3) *Atypical hyperplasia.* In addition to a pronounced increase in the formation of glandular ducts and the appearance of multiple layers of epithelium, there is also cellular atypia (figure 12.1).

12.2.1.2 Cytology

The smear may unexpectedly contain endometrial epithelial cells; unexpectedly because the patient is postmenopausal or in the second half of the menstrual cycle. Depending upon the oestrogen level, the K.I. varies from very high (75 or over) to very low or even zero when there will be only intermediate squamous epithelial cells present. Cells from glandular cystic hyperplasia do not differ much from normal endometrial cells. Cells from adenomatous and atypical hyperplasia, on the other hand, are slightly larger (figures 12.2 and 12.3) and have a slightly irregular chromatinic pattern; in a cell group several, but not all, of the nuclei will have an obvious nucleolus (Ng *et*

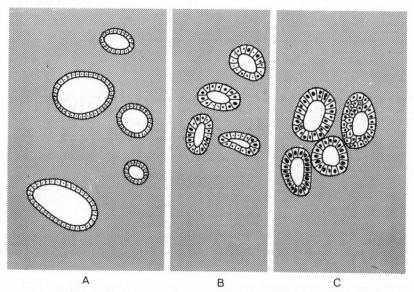

figure 12.1   Histology of endometrial epithelium. A. Cystic glandular hyperplasia (area of glandular ducts with increased diameter); B. atypical hyperplasia; C. adenocarcinoma of the endometrium

al., 1973a). The cellular changes of atypical hyperplasia may be more pronounced than those of adenomatous hyperplasia; also the abnormal cells are more numerous.

12.2.1.3 Differential Diagnosis

Cells from endometrial hyperplasia may often be distinguished from normal endometrial cells. Normal endometrial cells are usually smaller (figure 12.2) and generally have no visible nucleoli. On the other hand, cells derived from hyperplastic endometrium must also be distinguished from a well-differentiated endometrial adenocarcinoma. The carcinoma cells almost always possess fairly small nucleoli and their chromatin pattern is more 'open' than in the cells derived from hyperplastic endometrium. Atypical endometrial cells may resemble reserve cells. Endometrial cells, however, never display the characteristic exfoliation pattern of reserve cells.

12.2.1.4 Incidence of Endometrial Hyperplasia

Women with endometrial hyperplasia are on average younger than women with endometrial carcinoma.

Hyperplasia of the endometrium is often seen (1) during the climacteric as a result of enhanced oestrogen production which is not followed by subsequent progesterone activity, such as in the presence of a persistent ovarian follicle; (2) during oestrogen therapy for menopausal complaints; and (3) in the presence of an oestrogen-producing ovarian neoplasm.

12.2.2 Adenocarcinoma of the Endometrium

12.2.2.1 Histology

The growth of endometrial carcinoma may be diffuse, polypoid or focal. Carcinoma rarely occurs in an endometrial polyp (Novak and Woodruff, 1974). Adenocarcinomas of the endometrium can be classified according to their differentiation or to the extent of invasion of the myometrium. Broders (1925) classified carcinomas according to their degree of differentiation: grade I (well differentiated) to grade IV (poorly differentiated). The degree of differentiation and the extent of invasion play an important role in the prognosis

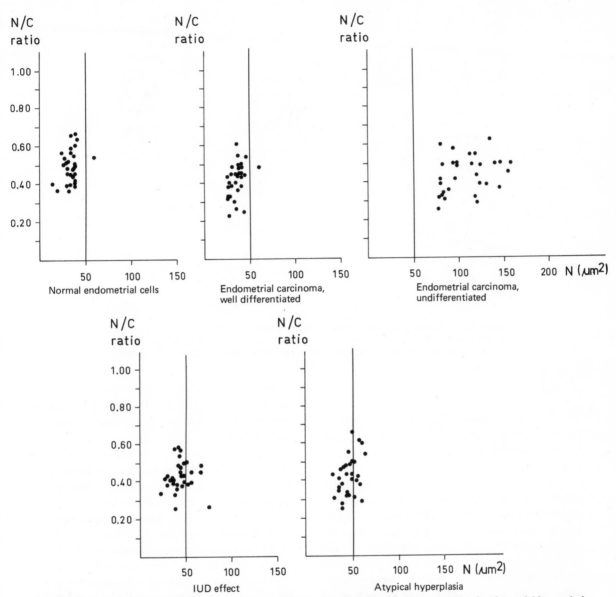

figure 12.2   Scattergram of N/C ratio and nuclear area (N) of endometrial cells in an example of endometrial hyperplasia; the effect of an IUD; well-differentiated adenocarcinoma cells, undifferentiated adenocarcinoma cells and normal endometrial cells. There are no great differences in nuclear size of normal endometrial cells, cells from well-differentiated endometrial carcinoma, from patients with an IUD and from atypical hyperplasia (the latter being larger than the well-differentiated adenocarcinoma cells). Also in histological sections, the nuclear areas of these cell types show a considerable overlap. Yet, considering the means, the normal nuclei are the largest, whereas the nuclei of the well-differentiated carcinoma cells show an intermediate value (Baak and Diegenbach, 1977).

of endometrial adenocarcinoma (see section 12.3). Opinions differ as to whether the *in situ* stage can be diagnosed histologically: Reagan and Ng (1973) believed they could diagnose this form, whereas

Novak and Woodruff (1974) repudiated this diagnosis because it is so vaguely defined. A clear cell carcinoma is seldom encountered (see section 13.4.2.3) in the endometrium.

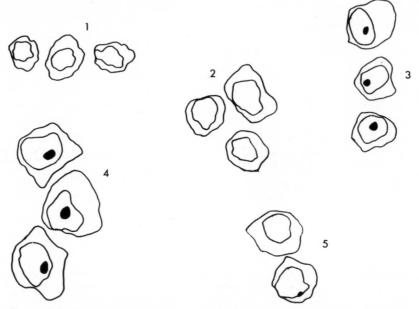

figure 12.3   Endometrial cells. Camera lucida drawings. 1. Normal endometrial cells;
2. endometrial cells with IUD effect; 3. endometrial cells in atypical hyperplasia; 4. poorly
differentiated endometrial carcinoma cells; 5. well-differentiated endometrial carcinoma
cells

12.2.2.2 Cytology

The cytological pattern of adenocarcinoma of the
endometrium is determined to a large extent by its
degree of differentiation (Broder's grades I, II, III,
IV).

The nuclei of well-differentiated adenocarcinoma cells are slightly larger than the nuclei of
intermediate squamous epithelial cells (figure 12.4),
hardly larger than normal endometrial cells, but
have a lower mean N/C ratio. Cells from atypical
hyperplasia have a larger mean nuclear area (figure
12.2). The nuclei are relatively monomorphic.
Most of the nuclei contain one micronucleolus
(Reagan and Ng, 1973). The Nc/N ratio may be
increased. This is a particularly important criterion
of malignancy when the nuclei are small. As the
degree of differentiation of the neoplasm decreases,
the size of the nuclei (Reagan and Ng, 1973) as
well as of the nucleoli increases (see figures 12.2
and 12.3).

In poorly differentiated adenocarcinoma cells
there are almost always multiple irregularly shaped
macronucleoli (Symposium, 1958). Anisokaryosis

is very prominent (figure 12.4). The groups are not
as three-dimensional as in a well-differentiated
endometrial carcinoma. Psammoma bodies (see
section 13.1.1.2) are very rarely seen in the papillary groups. There are fewer morphologically
malignant cells in the smears than in smears from
patients with endocervical carcinoma. The number
of cells increases as the differentiation of the carcinoma decreases. The number of malignant cells
depends also on the degree of necrosis, the presence
of inflammation (favouring desquamation) and the
extent of infiltration (Reagan and Ng, 1973).
Adenocarcinoma cells from the endometrium may
be solitary or in groups (Wied *et al.*, 1974). The
groups are often three-dimensional (in contrast to
the cell groups in an endocervical carcinoma). The
nuclei are irregularly arranged and may overlap.
There is no palisade arrangement of the nuclei.
The shape of the nucleus is predominantly oval to
round but it may be irregular (indentations, lobulated nuclei, wrinkled nuclear membrane, sharp
points on the nuclei, etc.). The chromatin pattern
is generally fine, but the distribution is irregular
(Graham, 1972). Between the threads of chromatin

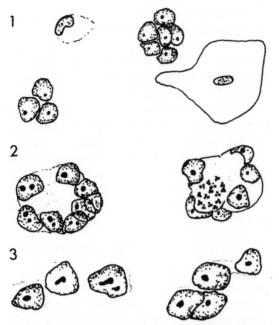

figure 12.4 Cytological pattern of endometrial carcinoma. 1. Adenocarcinoma grade I, well-differentiated; 2. adenocarcinoma grade II, III, moderately differentiated; 3. adenocarcinoma grade IV, poorly differentiated

there are often 'empty spaces' (nuclear clearing) which cause the nuclei to appear markedly *hypochromatic.* Some hyperchromatism along the margins is found in most adenocarcinoma cells (Reagan and Ng, 1973). Almost always nucleoli are seen; there is often a halo around the nucleolus (perinucleolar halo).

Screening with low power magnification may reveal striking cells with enormous vacuoles full of leucocytes while the background of the smear is sparsely cellular (Koss, 1968). When this type of leucophagocytosis is encountered the possibility of endometrial adenocarcinoma must be considered and, therefore, the nuclei should be scrutinised under high power. Leucophagocytosis is seen mainly in spontaneously exfoliated cells. When the cytoplasm is coarsely vacuolated the malignant nucleus will generally lie at the periphery of the cell. In general, however, cytoplasm is sparse and poorly defined.

Diathesis is not encountered as frequently as in endocervical adenocarcinoma (see figure 11.4).

Histiocytes are often seen. A large variation in the K.I. is possible (Liu, 1970) (figure 12.5).

12.2.2.3 Squamous Cell Component and Squamous Cell Carcinomas

Areas of squamous epithelium may occur in an endometrial adenocarcinoma (Baggish and Woodruff, 1967). When this squamous epithelium appears benign, the term *'adenoacanthoma'* is used. The squamous component can either be well differentiated or it may resemble immature squamous metaplasia. The origin of this squamous metaplasia is not known, nor whether it develops simultaneously with the adenocarcinoma or antedates it, which is most likely in pure squamous cell carcinoma (White *et al.*, 1973). Immature metaplasia may be found in endometrium without squamous neoplastic changes (Silverberg *et al.*, 1972) especially in connection with oestrogen deficiency. If the area of squamous epithelium appears to be malignant then the term *'adenosquamous carcinoma'* (or mixed carcinoma) is used. In the adenosquamous carcinoma the glandular component is poorly differentiated, in contrast to adenoacanthomas with their well-differentiated glandular component (Ng *et al.*, 1973b). Because of the prognostic differences associated with these neoplasms it is important to determine whether an adenocarcinoma is accompanied by a morphologically benign or malignant squamous cell component (Ng, 1968; Silverberg *et al.*, 1972). Adenoacanthoma can be definitely diagnosed only when benign squamous cells are

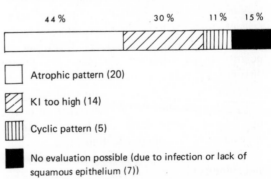

Atrophic pattern (20)

KI too high (14)

Cyclic pattern (5)

No evaluation possible (due to infection or lack of squamous epithelium (7))

figure 12.5 The hormonal patterns in the smears taken from 46 patients with endometrial carcinoma (University of Leiden, 1970–74)

juxtaposed with adenocarcinoma cells. This is seldom the case, however. The smear from a patient with an adenosquamous carcinoma usually contains both squamous carcinoma cells and adenocarcinoma cells.

Pure squamous cell carcinomas of the endometrium are very rare (White *et al.*, 1973). In our case (see the atlas section) we found it in combination with benign squamous epithelium of the tumour-free endometrium.

12.2.2.4 Differential Diagnosis

Adenocarcinoma cells from the endometrium must be distinguished from the following.

(1) Benign endometrial cells, which lie in more compact groups. Furthermore their nuclei are more polymorphic and darker, and nucleoli are not visible. Compared with undifferentiated carcinoma cells the nuclei are smaller (see figure 12.2).

(2) Atypical endometrial cells from hyperplasia due, for instance, to oestrogen therapy. These cells have large rounded nuclei which are sometimes hyperchromatic; nucleoli may be present but are not present in most nuclei (Ng *et al.*, 1973a). We have examined cytological specimens from five such patients. The exfoliated endometrial cells showed such a marked atypia that they could not be distinguished morphologically from adenocarcinoma cells. These patients were all postmenopausal and had been treated with oestrogens. When therapy was discontinued the atypia disappeared.

(3) The pattern of tissue repair can resemble that of an adenocarcinoma because of the cytoplasmic vacuolisation and leucophagocytosis which may be present in the reparative epithelial cells. The cells of tissue repair are, however, arranged in flat ragged groups with abundant cytoplasm; nuclear polarity is not disturbed; chromatin is regularly distributed (Geirrson *et al.*, 1977).

(4) Epithelium showing the effect of irradiation. The pattern resembles that of tissue repair, although the cellular abnormalities may impart a bizarre appearance to the cells (see section 14.5).

(5) Immature metaplasia with leucophagocytosis and cytoplasmic vacuolisation.

(6) After endometrial curettage endometrial cells with atypia may be encountered in a cervical smear.

(7) Adenocarcinoma cells which do not originate in the endometrium. It is often possible to discriminate between endocervical and endometrial adenocarcinoma cells by means of the difference in the shape and arrangement of the nuclei (see also section 11.2). However, in the case of undifferentiated adenocarcinomas it may well be difficult or impossible to determine their origin.

(8) Anaplastic cervical carcinoma.

(9) Histiocytic cells with nucleoli and vacuoles as a result of chronic inflammation or an intrauterine contraceptive device (IUD).

(10) Slightly atypical endometrial cells due to an IUD.

12.2.2.5 Incidence of Endometrial Carcinoma

It has been found that recently the number of patients with endometrial adenocarcinoma has increased, whereas the number of cases of cervical squamous cell carcinoma has decreased. This increase can be attributed mainly to the larger number of patients with an adenosquamous carcinoma (Ng, 1968). It is also influenced by the increase in the average age of the population. The average age of women with endometrial adenocarcinoma is greater than that of women with cervical squamous cell carcinoma. Endometrial adenocarcinoma develops generally in postmenopausal women; however, it is also possible for it to occur in younger women (figure 12.6). In our series the youngest patient with endometrial adenocarcinoma was 36 years old.

12.3 Clinical Aspects of Endometrial Carcinoma

In postmenopausal women the presenting symptom is usually vaginal bleeding and in premenopausal women menometrorrhagia. Endometrial carcinoma may metastasise via the lymphatics, the bloodstream, and, possibly, the fallopian tubes (to the peritoneum). Metastasis of the ovary is common. The prognosis for endometrial adenocarcinoma is better than for cervical squamous cell carcinoma. The 5-year survival rate is 75 per cent (Novak and Woodruff, 1974). The factors which influence the prognosis are as follows.

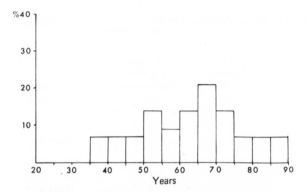

figure 12.6 **Age distribution of 153 women with an adenocarcinoma of the endometrium. The series is drawn from three hospitals in Leiden (1969–75). Cytology had been carried out in 50 of these patients: 19 patients (38%): cytology negative, histology positive; 5 patients (10%): cytology atypia, histological examination indicated (positive); 26 patients (52%): cytology positive, histology positive**

(1) *Extent of the carcinoma.* The extent of an endometrial carcinoma may be classified as follows.

Stage 0 Carcinoma *in situ.*

Stage I Carcinoma confined to corpus.

> IA the length of the uterine cavity is 8 cm of less.

> IB the length of the uterine cavity is greater than 8 cm.

Stage II The carcinoma has involved the corpus and cervix.

Stage III The carcinoma has extended outside the uterus but not outside the true pelvis.

Stage IV The carcinoma has extended outside the true pelvis or has obviously involved the mucosa of the bladder or rectum.

(FIGO staging carcinoma corpus uteri, January 1971).

(2) *Degree of differentiation of the carcinoma.* The stage I cases should be subgrouped with regard to the histological type of the adenocarcinoma as follows: highly differentiated adenomatous carcinomas (G1, corresponding to Broders' grade I); differentiated adenomatous carcinomas with partly solid areas (G2, corresponding to Broders' grade II); and predominantly solid or entirely undifferentiated carcinomas (G3, corresponding to Broders' grades III and IV) (FIGO staging, 1971). In stage IA disease, the 5-year and 10-year overall survival decreases from 88 and 77 per cent with

G1 lesions to 65 and 57 per cent with G3 lesions. For stage IB the 5-year and 10-year overall survival decreases from 98 and 93 per cent to 38 and 38 per cent as the grade progresses from G1 to G3 disease (Malkasian, 1978).

Well-differentiated adenocarcinomas have a better prognosis than poorly differentiated ones.

(3) *Presence of squamous epithelium.* Not only the degree of differentiation but also the presence of squamous epithelium is important for the prognosis. Adenoacanthomas have the best prognosis followed by adenocarcinomas. Adenosquamous carcinomas have the poorest prognosis with a 5-year survival rate of 19.2 per cent (Ng, 1968).

12.3.1 Diagnosis of Endometrial Carcinoma

Cervical carcinomas are readily detectable cytologically at an early stage; however, the detection of endometrial carcinoma has not been the subject of mass screening programmes. From the literature it appears that two-thirds to three-quarters of all known endometrial carcinomas were not discovered by means of routine cervical cytology. In our series only one endometrial adenocarcinoma was diagnosed in an asymptomatic patient by a routine cervical smear. The success of cytological detection of endometrial adenocarcinoma depends on the method used to obtain the cellular sample (table 12.1). Various methods have been described, such as endometrial aspiration and endometrial washings (see section 15.3.3). In practice, it appears that the direct techniques give the best results.

At present endometrial cancer is a histological diagnosis for all practical purposes and neither clinicians nor the public should expect cervical cancer screening to detect a major portion of endometrial cancers by cervical smears.

References

Andrews, W. C. and Andrews, M. C. (1960). Stein-Leventhal syndrome with associated adenocarcinoma of the endometrium. *Am. J. Obstet. Gynec.*, **80**, 632–6

Baak, J. P. A. and Diegenbach, P. C. (1977). Quantitative nuclear image analysis: differentiation between normal, hyperplastic and malignant appearing uterine glands in a parafin section. I.

table 12.1 Comparison of the various methods used to obtain material for detection of endometrial carcinoma (from Wyss et al., 1975)

Author	Total number endometrial carcinomas	Correct diagnosis: smear from posterior fornix	Correct diagnosis: cervical smear	Correct diagnosis: endometrial smear	Intrauterine method
Hecht (1956)	52	–	–	92.3%	aspiration
Boschann (1958)	96	–	–	86.0%	aspiration
Graham (1953)	218	77.0%	–	–	
Graham (1958)	49	92.0%	–	–	
Jordan (1956)	25	76.0%	–	84.0%	smear with cannula
Jordan (1956)		–	–	92.0%	combined with endometrial biopsy
Wied (1958)	12	41.5%	67.0%	80.3%	–
Reagan (1965)	225	41.5%	67.0%	80.3%	aspiration
Jameson (1961)	51	–	55.0%	–	–
Jameson (1961)	29	–	–	83.0%	aspiration
Jameson (1961)	7	–	–	57.0%	brush

Elementary features for differentiation. *Eur. J. Obstet. Gynec. reprod. Biol.*, 7, 33–42

Baggish, M. A. and Woodruff, J. D. (1967). The occurrence of squamous epithelium in the endometrium. *Obstet. Gynec. Survey*, 22, 69–115

Broders, A. C. (1925). The grading of carcinoma. *Minn. Med.*, 8, 726

Geirrson, G., Woodworth, F. E., Patten, S. F. Jr and Bonfiglio, T. A. (1977). Epithelial repair and regeneration in the uterine cervix I. An analysis of the cells. *Acta Cytol.*, 21, 371–8

Graham, R. M. (1972). *The Cytologic Diagnosis of Cancer*, 3rd edn, Saunders, Philadelphia and London

Koss, L. G. (1968). *Diagnostic cytology and its histopathologic bases*, Lippincott, Philadelphia

Liu, W. (1970). Hypoestrogenism and endometrial carcinoma. *Acta Cytol.*, 14, 583–6

Malkasian, G. D. (1978). Carcinoma of the endometrium: effect of stage and grade on survival. *Cancer*, 41, 996–1001

Ng, A. B. P. (1968). Mixed carcinoma of the endometrium. *Am. J. Obstet.*, 102, 506–15

Ng, A. B. P., Reagan, J. W. and Ceckner, R. L. (1973a). The endometrial cancer: a study of their cellular manifestations. *Acta Cytol.*, 17, 439–48

Ng, A. B. P., Reagan, J. W., Storaasli, J. P. and Wentz, W. B. (1973b). Mixed adenosquamous carcinoma of the endometrium. *Am. J. clin. Path.*, 59, 765–81

Novak, E. R. and Woodruff, J. D. (1974). *Gynecologic and Obstetric Pathology*, Saunders, Philadelphia and London

Novak, E. R. and Yui, E. (1936). Relation of endometrial hyperplasia to adenocarcinoma of uterus. *Am. J. Obstet. Gynec.*, 32, 674

Reagan, J. W. and Ng, A. B. P. (1973). *The Cells of Uterine Adenocarcinoma*, Karger, Basel

Silverberg, S. G., Bolin, M. G. and De Giorgi, L. S. (1972). Adenoacanthoma and mixed adenosquamous carcinoma of the endometrium. A clinico-pathologic study. *Cancer*, 30, 1307–14

Symposium on endometrial cytology (1958). *Acta Cytol.*, 2, 481–635

White, A. J., Buchsbaum, H. J. and Macasaet, M. A. (1973). Primary squamous cell carcinoma of the endometrium. *Obstet. Gynec.*, 41, 912–19

Wied, G. L., Koss, L. G. and Reagan, J. W. (1974). *Compendium on Diagnostic Cytology*, Vol. III, No. 1, Tutorials of Chicago

Wyss, R., Vassilakos, P. and Riotton, G. (1975). *Verschiedene Methoden der Früherfassung endometrialer Veranderungen*, J. Jenny, Zurich

Other Malignant Tumours and Related Lesions of the Genital Tract

13.1 Ovarian Tumours

Because the ovary is made up of several different elements, the structure of ovarian tumours varies considerably and is sometimes quite complex. A classification based on these various elements has become generally accepted; when reduced to its simplest form, the following categories are found.

(1) tumours originating in the germinal epithelium.

(2) tumours originating in the sex cells.

(3) tumours originating in the stroma.

(4) metastatic neoplasms (primary tumour elsewhere in the body).

(5) rare tumours of uncertain origin.

Stroma cell tumours are significant because they frequently give rise to hormonal activity which can affect the epithelium of the uterus and the vagina. Granulosa-thecacell tumours usually produce oestrogen; Sertoli–Leydig cell tumours, also called arrhenoblastomas, sometimes secrete androgen. Occasionally tumours originating in the superficial epithelium may secrete oestrogen.

13.1.1 Tumours of the Superficial Epithelium

13.1.1.1 Histology

The superficial epithelium of the ovary is related to the coelomic epithelium that gave rise to the müllerian ducts. This relationship becomes apparent in the histological pattern of its tumours.

Thus the epithelium of serous papillary cystadenocarcinoma shows some resemblance to tubal epithelium; the epithelium of an endometrioid adenocarcinoma is similar to endometrial epithelium; and the epithelium of a mucinous cystadenocarcinoma resembles columnar epithelium.

13.1.1.2 Cytology

(1) *Serous papillary adenocarcinoma.* The cells of a serous papillary adenocarcinoma lie in papillary clusters, often with several 'offshoots' which are clearly visible at low magnification (figure 13.1). The cells of these groups are arranged in acini (rosettes). The adenocarcinoma cells can be very small (figure 13.2); they then resemble endometrial cells with pleomorphic nuclei.

Some of the serous papillary adenocarcinomas will contain so-called 'psammoma bodies' (calcospherites): these are calcified spheroids which contain concentric lamellae (at least two), probably a consequence of dystrophic calcification associated with cellular degeneration (Ferenczy *et al.*, 1977).

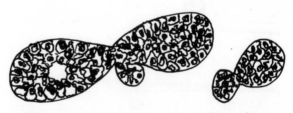

figure 13.1   Cytological pattern of an ovarian carcinoma. Papillary groups with offshoots (low magnification)

Usually they lie within the cellular clusters but they can also appear as solitary bodies in the smear. With the Papanicolaou stain psammoma bodies will take on a light blue to dark purple colour; they may vary greatly in size. If a smear contains psammoma bodies *and* adenocarcinoma cells, then an ovarian carcinoma must be strongly suspected. The occurrence of this combination has been described in detail in the literature (Graham and van Niekerk, 1962; Differding, 1967; Koss, 1968; Dance and Fullmer, 1970; Beyer-Boon, 1974); we have 6 such cases in our material. In one patient, psammoma bodies and adenocarcinoma cells were found in a preclinical stage of the disease. We also have one case of endometrial carcinoma with psammoma bodies.

Sometimes numerous psammoma bodies are found in a smear although neoplastic cells cannot be found. Highman (1971), for example, observed them in smears from patients wearing an intra-uterine contraceptive (IUD). The histological sections of endometrial curettings as well as the material scraped from an IUD which had been removed contained many structures resembling psammoma bodies. Another possible source of confusion is the presence of prostatic calculi which can enter the vagina during coitus (Meisels and Ayotte, 1976).

(2) *Mucinous cystadenocarcinoma.* Mucinous cystadenocarcinoma of the ovary can be of the large cell variety (figure 13.2). In the smear three-dimensional groups of cells and vesicular vacuolised cytoplasm can be found or 'flat' clusters. The nuclei may have very large nucleoli and thus a high Nc/N ratio; it is then difficult to distinguish between such cells and the cells of tissue repair (figure 13.3) or endocervical cells with prominent nucleoli.

(3) *Endometrioid adenocarcinoma.* The cytological pattern of this tumour cannot be distinguished from that of adenocarcinoma of the endometrium (figure 13.3). There may also be either a benign or a malignant squamous cell component.

13.1.2 Ovarian Tumours which Produce Sex Hormones

When an ovarian tumour secretes sex hormones, it may be evident in the cytological pattern. Thus an oestrogen-producing tumour in a woman in the menopausal phase will cause high oestrogen levels

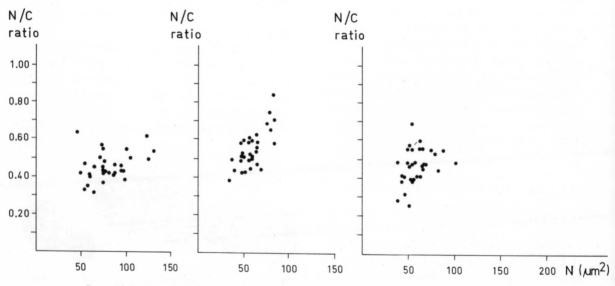

figure 13.2   Scattergrams of N/C ratio and nuclear area (N) of three examples of ovarian carcinoma

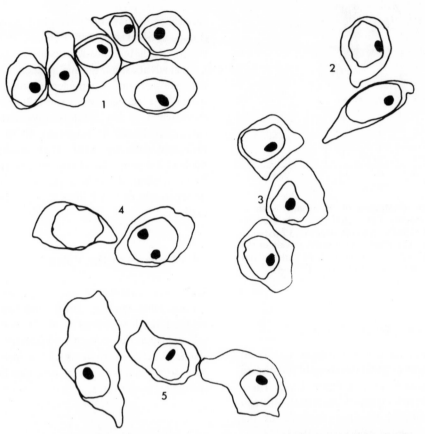

figure 13.3 **Differential diagnosis of ovarian carcinoma cells. Camera lucida drawings.**
1. Ovarian carcinoma cells; 2. endocervical adenocarcinoma cells; 3. endometrial adenocarcinoma cells; 4. squamous cervical carcinoma cells; 5. repair cells

which cannot be explained physiologically. In the smear this is indicated by the extremely high K.I. and, in some cases, the presence of endometrial cells.

The rare tumour which produces male hormones (arrhenoblastoma) can develop in the sexually mature female; it is characterised cytologically by the presence of numerous parabasal cells with a rectangular outline. Such cells are almost never seen in a smear; nearly all of these tumours are benign.

13.1.3 Clinical Aspects of Ovarian Tumours

Ovarian carcinoma develops mainly in women between 50 and 80 years of age (figure 13.4).

Sixty per cent of malignant ovarian tumours are serous papillary cystadenocarcinomas, 5–10 per cent are mucinous cystadenocarcinomas. Malignant tumours which originate in the sex cells, as well as stroma cell tumours, occur mainly in children and young women.

Malignant ovarian tumours do not cause symtoms until the disease is in an advanced stage; for this reason they are frequently called 'silent killers'. These patients often present with symptoms due to the bulk of the neoplasm: increasing abdominal girth, a heavy feeling in the pelvis, difficulty of urination and defaecation, and abdominal pain. Abdominal swelling due to ascites caused by metastasis to the peritoneum may be the first symptom.

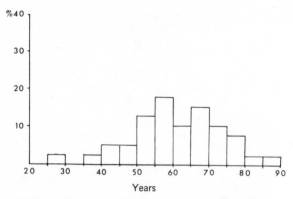

figure 13.4   Age distribution of 38 women with an ovarian adenocarcinoma. Cytological data were available for 20 women: 3 patients: cytology negative, 17 patients: cytology positive. The number of positive smears in this series is relatively high because most of the patients were terminal cases (Leiden University, 1970–4)

13.1.3.1 Diagnosis of Ovarian Tumours

The cells of a malignant ovarian tumour usually do not appear in cervicovaginal smears until the disease is in an advanced stage (see figure 13.4). These cells may reach the vagina by metastasis through the fallopian tube or by direct invasion of the uterus or vagina (Umiker and Skeen, 1953).

When an ovarian carcinoma grows through the ovarian capsule, neoplastic cells may be found in the pouch of Douglas. By means of aspiration (culdocentesis) material can be collected for examination (Graham and Graham, 1967). However, the surface of the ovary may be covered with benign papillary structures containing psammoma bodies; when such material is obtained by culdocentesis, these bodies and their surrounding cells must not be confused with adenocarcinoma (Kern, 1969; Picoff and Meeker, 1970). Ovarian carcinomas can also be diagnosed by aspiration biopsy with or without the aid of the laporoscope (Geier *et al.*, 1974; Wagman and Brower, 1974).

13.2 Tubal Carcinoma

Malignant tumours of the fallopian tubes are exceedingly rare. Several cases with a positive

cervical smear have been described in the literature (Song, 1955; Dance and Fullmer, 1970). In our experience it is impossible to distinguish between a tubal adenocarcinoma and an adenocarcinoma of the endometrium. When adenocarcinoma cells are found in a cervicovaginal smear but endometrial curettage does not yield positive material, tubal carcinoma should be suspected. In the smear the malignant cells are small. Their nuclei are oval; nucleoli are seen. The chromatin pattern is coarse. The cytoplasm shows little vacuolisation. The cells lie separately or in papillary groups, and there is a diathesis.

13.3 Diseases of the Vulva

The vulva consists of the mons veneris, labia majora, labia minora, clitoris and vestibule. The external urethral orifice is in the vestibule. The subcutaneous fat contains sebaceous and sweat glands as well as remnants of the wolffian ducts. Accessory mammary tissue may also be found in the region of the vulva.

13.3.1 Benign Abnormalities

13.3.1.1 Papilloma

This is a solitary benign tumour composed predominantly of stratified squamous epithelium. Cytologically papilloma cells cannot be differentiated from normal squamous epithelial cells.

13.3.1.2 Condylomata Acuminata

These lesions of viral origin appear in and around the vulva as white warty growths. Histological examination reveals pronounced hyperplasia of the epithelium as well as hyperkeratosis, parakeratosis and koilocytosis (see section 7.3.5.2). The smears contain parakeratotic cells and anucleate squames; if cells from the deeper layers of the lesion are present, then koilocytosis, multinucleation and granular cytoplasm will be seen. There is suggestive evidence that some of these lesions could progress into verrucous carcinoma (Boxer and Skinner,

1977). Vulvar condylomata are often accompanied by similar lesions in the vagina and flat lesions in the cervix (see section 7.3.5.2.), which points to a multifocal involvement of the genital epithelium. Cytology is not a good method of diagnosing verrucous carcinoma: the malignant cells are not reached by scraping (see section 10.2.4.2).

13.3.1.3 Hyperplasia and Hyperkeratosis of the Stratified Squamous Epithelium

The squamous epithelium of the vulva may (in older women) be characterised by hyperplasia and hyperkeratosis, sometimes accompanied by nuclear atypia and elongation of rete pegs. Macroscopically these lesions appear as white patches (leucoplakia). In other cases the epithelium may be very thin (lichen sclerosis). Most of these lesions are accompanied by changes in the underlying connective tissue (collagenisation). Manifestations of the accompanying disturbed maturation include an increase in thickness of the basal and parabasal cell layers, parakeratosis, dyskeratosis (individual cell keratinisation) and irregular maturation of the epithelium.

Depending upon the histological pattern, cytological examination will reveal parakeratosis and, in the event of atypia, nuclear changes such as hyperchromasia and slight clumping of the chromatin. The nuclear changes are not as pronounced as in squamous cell carcinoma, nor does the smear contain irregularly shaped anucleate squames.

13.3.2 Malignant Tumours of the Vulva

13.3.2.1 Squamous Cell Carcinoma *in situ*

Squamous cell carcinoma *in situ* of the vulva often develops in combination with carcinoma *in situ* of the perineum, the vagina and/or the cervix. In the vulva, as elsewhere, carcinoma *in situ* may be multifocal. The histological pattern often closely resembles that of carcinoma *in situ* of the skin (Bowen's disease) with acanthosis, hyperkeratosis, parakeratosis, keratinisation of individual cells and marked nuclear atypia. In addition, patterns may be seen which resemble the typical cervical squamous carcinoma *in situ*, with its lack of maturation and of keratin production. These two types of carcinoma *in situ* often occur together. Depending upon the type, the cytological pattern will resemble that of Bowen's disease of the skin (with pronounced nuclear polymorphism, anisokaryosis and anucleate squames) or that of a carcinoma *in situ* of the cervix (primarily with large malignant nuclei of equal size).

13.3.2.2 Squamous Cell Carcinoma

Women with vulval carcinoma will often have a history of leucoplakia or a granulomatous inflammation of the vulva (Novak and Woodruff, 1974). Macroscopically, vulval carcinoma in the early stage resembles a small white nodule; later these nodules may ulcerate.

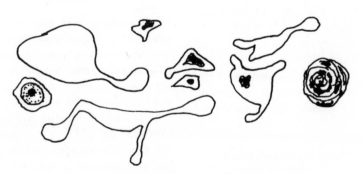

figure 13.5   Cytological pattern of a vulval carcinoma

The most common histological pattern of vulval carcinoma is that of keratinising squamous cell carcinoma with pearl formation. The surface of the carcinoma is often covered with anucleate squames or with large highly keratinised cells. When the lesion ulcerates the surface is coated with fibrin and cellular debris.

Usually the pattern of the cervical smear is that of a keratinising squamous cell carcinoma with anucleate squames, parakeratotic cells, malignant pearls and malignant cells of bizarre shapes. In addition there may be cells with a pale central nucleus, a macronucleolus and a thin rim of cytoplasm (figure 13.5). When the smear is taken from the superficial keratinised part of the tumour, it will contain mainly anucleate squames, often with parakeratotic cells. Frequently these anucleate squames are irregularly shaped, which is typical of a squamous cell carcinoma. In such a case the clinician might be requested to prepare another smear and to scrape more forcefully (preferably with a scalpel). Growths of the vulva may be endophytic or exophytic (for example, the verrucous carcinoma). It is the squamous cell carcinoma that metastasises quickly to the superficial and deep inguinal lymph nodes as well as to the hypogastric and iliac lymph nodes and can invade the rectum and the urethra. Vulval carcinoma develops predominantly in older women after the menopause (Novak and Woodruff, 1974).

13.3.2.3 Paget's Disease of the Vulva

This lesion is usually limited to the skin rather than the glandular ducts, in contrast to Paget's disease of the breast. The squamous epithelium contains the classical large pale cells with abundant finely granular cytoplasm.

If the macroscopically abnormal region is scraped firmly (preferably with a scalpel), it will be found that the smear contains large pale cells with clear cytoplasm and without squamous differentiation. Often the nuclei have a prominent nucleolus.

13.3.2.4 Adenocarcinoma of Bartholin's Gland

Adenocarcinoma can develop in Bartholin's gland although it is a rare lesion. If the tumour extends to the surface, it can be diagnosed cytologically. In most cases the cytological pattern is that of a well-differentiated adenocarcinoma.

13.3.2.5 Malignant Melanoma

Malignant melanoma is a malignant tumour originating in the melanin-producing cells of the skin. There is a predilection for the vulva since 5 per cent of all malignant melanomas develop in the vulval region, whereas the vulva accounts for only 1 per cent of the total body surface. There is an amelanotic form of malignant melanoma. Melanotic malignant melanoma may metastasise as amelanotic malignant melanoma.

The smear contains malignant cells with large eccentric nuclei, macronucleoli and in some cases cytoplasmic granules of melanin. The cells lie flat when in clusters but are rounded when solitary. They may also be spindle-shaped. Histiocytes loaded with melanin pigment may also be present.

13.4 Diseases of the Vagina

The proximal part of the vagina arises from the müllerian ducts, the distal part from the urogenital sinus. This pattern of development is significant for the haematogenous and lymphatogenous dissemination of malignant tumour cells. The vagina is lined with nonkeratinising stratified squamous epithelium.

13.4.1 Benign Abnormalities: Adenosis

In the vagina there may be islets of glandular epithelium of the endocervical type; it may also resemble endometrial or fallopian tubal epithelium (Hart *et al.*, 1976). This condition is called vaginal adenosis. It is encountered mainly in young girls, and often the mother received oestrogen medication such as diethylstilbestrol (DES) during pregnancy (Vooys *et al.*, 1973). The columnar epithelium of the glandular inclusions can be replaced by metaplastic squamous epithelium producing transformation zones similar to those in the cervix. The metaplastic areas may show dysplastic changes (Bibbo *et al.*, 1975). It is possible for vaginal adenocarcinoma to develop in a focus of vaginal adenosis (see section 13.4.2.3) (Herbst and Scully, 1970).

13.4.2 Malignant Tumours of the Vagina

13.4.2.1 Squamous Carcinoma *in situ* and Invasive Squamous Cell Carcinoma

The histological pattern of a *squamous carcinoma in situ* of the vagina resembles that of cervical squamous carcinoma *in situ*. The vaginal epithelium can show complete replacement by anaplastic cells or it may demonstrate two zones: a deep zone with poorly differentiated round cells and a superficial zone with squamoid abnormal cells. The cytological pattern may resemble that of cervical carcinoma *in situ*, or may display many small keratinised cells with relatively large, dense, hyperchromatic nuclei. These cells originate from the keratinised superficial layer (Merchant *et al.*, 1974).

The *invasive squamous cell carcinomas* are usually moderately differentiated (as compared with large cell nonkeratinising squamous cell carcinomas of the cervix) although invasive squamous cell carcinoma with keratinisation can also occur (Novak and Woodruff, 1974). The cytological pattern of invasive squamous cell carcinoma is similar to that of large cell non-keratinising squamous cell carcinoma of the cervix or, in a few cases, keratinising squamous cell carcinoma.

Primary carcinoma of the vagina constitutes only 1–2 per cent of all genital cancers. It pursues a highly malignant course and responds poorly to therapy. Squamous carcinoma *in situ* of the vagina is seen more frequently in patients who had squamous carcinoma *in situ* of the cervical epithelium. In a series of 539 patients (McIndoe and Green, 1969) with cervical squamous carcinoma *in situ*, follow-up examination after hysterectomy revealed five cases of carcinoma *in situ* of the vagina. Carcinoma *in situ* of the vagina in combina-

tion with cervical carcinoma is less 'aggressive' than primary vaginal carcinoma *in situ* (Geelhoed *et al.*, 1976). As previously mentioned (see section 10.2.3) carcinoma *in situ* is frequently a multifocal lesion. These neoplastic foci may develop simultaneously or dysynchronously. The simultaneous presence of *in situ* and infiltrating lesions at different sites in the vagina may be regarded as various stages of response to a carcinogenic agent (Kanbour *et al.*, 1974). Clinical and cytological follow-up of patients with carcinoma *in situ* of the vagina is essential.

Invasive squamous cell carcinoma occurs more frequently in the vulva than in the vagina. It is most likely to develop in women over sixty years of age. There is a predilection for the upper half of the posterior wall of the vagina. When the speculum is inserted to obtain a cervical smear, the posterior blade may mask a vaginal carcinoma so that it is not seen. It is therefore extremely important to conduct a complete visual examination of the vaginal vault, especially in older patients.

13.4.2.2 Invasion of the Vagina by Squamous Cell Carcinoma of the Cervix

Invasive squamous cell carcinoma of the cervix may extend into the vagina. The cytological pattern is, of course, that of the cervical carcinoma.

13.4.2.3 Adenocarcinoma

Primary adenocarcinoma of the vagina can develop in young girls if their mothers were treated with high doses of oestrogen during pregnancy (Vooys *et al.*, 1973). The cervix may also be involved. In smears the adenocarcinoma cells are generally similar to cells of an endocervical adenocarcinoma (see section 11.2.2.1). In some cases typical 'clear cells' will be found which are carcinoma cells with central nuclei, large nucleoli and abundant clear cytoplasm (Rosati and Jarzynksi, 1973). Clear cell adenocarcinoma has an age incidence curve with two peaks, ages 20–30 and 60–70. It is suggested that DES (being an oestrogen) interferes with the normal process of differentiation and degeneration of Müllerian epithelium in the foetal vagina (Nordquist *et al.*, 1976).

Adenocarcinoma of the vagina may also develop in foci of endometriosis. The cytological picture does not have any specific characteristics. Carcinomas of the vagina include those which have not arisen there but which spread to it by contiguity or metastasis such as carcinomas of the cervix, endometrium, ovary, rectum, bladder and breast. Metastasis from a neoplasm arising outside the pelvis may also take place.

13.4.2.4 Malignant Melanoma of the Vagina

Primary malignant melanoma of the vagina is a very infrequent lesion. Masubuchi *et al.* (1975) reported four cases with a positive cytological report. The cytological picture displayed the classical features as described in section 13.3.2.5.

13.5 Other Tumours and Related Lesions of the Genital Tract

13.5.1 Malignant Mesenchymal Tumours

The cytological samples may contain cells from malignant mesenchymal tumours localised in the cervix or the uterine corpus. The earliest manifestation of these tumours will be clinical so that early cytological diagnosis is rare. In contrast to epithelial tumour cells, cells from mesenchymal tumours are always *isolated*. The cytoplasm is not as dense as in keratinising cancer. Moreover, nuclear pyknosis is absent, and chromatin clumping less pronounced. Tumour diathesis is quite variable (Patten, 1978).

13.5.1.1 Leiomyosarcoma

This uncommon malignant tumour originates in nonstriated muscle. The cells are spindle-shaped or club-like; the cytoplasm may contain fibrillary structures. The cells do not show epithelial organisation. The nuclei are sometimes hyperchromatic, often with nuclear clearing. They almost always have prominent nucleoli; the Nc/N ratio is usually high (figure 13.6).

Leiomyosarcoma cells must be distinguished

from:
(1) decidual cells (see section 3.3.3). These cells are never spindle-shaped.
(2) repair cells (see section 7.5.2). In these cells no nuclear clearing occurs and the Nc/N ratio remains low.
(3) dysplastic cells and malignant squamous epithelial cells. The cytoplasm of these cells is more dense, with often hyperchromatic nuclei.
(4) choriocarcinoma cells or cells from an amelanotic malignant melanoma. This differentiation is not possible in most cases.

13.5.1.2 Rhabdomyosarcoma (Botryoid Sarcoma)

This is a malignant embryonic tumour originating in striated muscles. Botryoid sarcoma is seen in the vagina of very young girls. It probably originates in a remnant of a müllerian duct. It has a grape-like gross appearance and grows in the lumen of the vagina. The cytological picture is characterised by solitary cells with cigar-shaped and pleomorphic hyperchromatic nuclei. The cytoplasm may display characteristic cross-striations (Hajdu and Hajdu, 1976). It is highly malignant and spreads widely by contiguity and metastasis.

13.5.1.3 Mesodermal Mixed Tumour

This is a rare malignant tumour, composed of epithelial as well as connective tissue such as muscle and sometimes cartilage. The cytoplasm of the malignant cells may be fibrillar (muscular tissue differentiation) (Riotton and Christopherson, 1973).

13.5.1.4 Mesenchymal Sarcoma

This low malignant tumour originates in the stroma of the endometrium. The malignant cells are fairly small, may be slightly spindle-shaped and have large nucleoli (high Nc/N ratio) (figure 13.7).

13.5.1.5 Carcinosarcoma

These uterine tumours are composed of a malignant glandular component and a sarcomatous

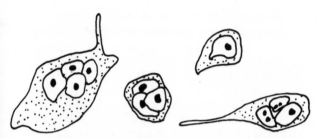

figure 13.6   Cytological pattern of a leiomyosarcoma

component. The malignant stromal cells may be confused cytologically with malignant squamous cells, leading to an erroneous diagnosis of adenosquamous carcinoma.

13.5.2 Malignant Lymphomas

Malignant lymphomas are defined as neoplasms of the reticulo-endothelial system, involving the lymph nodes, liver, spleen and bonemarrow. A quarter of these neoplasms are of extranodal origin, and occur in organs in which otherwise lymph follicles may develop. Involvement of the female genital tract is not rare (Katayama *et al.*, 1973). Also lesions limited to the uterus may occur (Krumerman and Chung, 1978).

In general the cytological pattern of these tumours is characterised by cells that always lie separated from each other and never in groups. The background of the smear is often relatively clean. For further classification we prefer air-dried Giemsa-stained smears.

13.5.2.1 Reticulum Cell Sarcoma (Histiocytic Lymphoma)

Occasionally cells of a reticulum cell sarcoma (histiocytic lymphoma) will be found in a cervical smear. The nuclei can show some polymorphism (lobulated, indented, bulging nuclei); the chromatin pattern is coarse and nucleoli are present. Krumerman and Chung (1978) reported that the presence of cells with conspicuous proboscis-like nuclear protrusions are highly characteristic.

We have seen one case of a localisation of histiocytosis X in the vagina (see Atlas section).

13.5.2.2 Lymphosarcoma and Leukaemia

In exfoliative cytology cells from leukaemia and from a lymphosarcoma cannot be distinguished from each other in the Papanicolaou stain. In both cases the smear contains solitary' cells which resemble lymphocytes but are somewhat larger. There is some nuclear polymorphism and occasionally a nucleolus is visible (Ceelen and Sakurai, 1962). There may be much blood in the smear, and in such a case leukaemia cells may be found even when there is no leukaemic infiltration of the uterus (Israel and Mutch, 1956).

Although it is often impossible to recognise the various types of lymphoreticular tumours with the Papanicolaou stain, one can discriminate between lymphoreticular tumours on the one hand and follicular cervicitis on the other. The cytological pattern of chronic lymphocytic cervicitis (see section 7.2.3.1) is highly varied (a mixture of lymphocytes, lymphoblasts, reticulum cells and plasma cells), in contrast to the monomorphic pattern of lymphoreticular tumours (Colmenares and Naib, 1965).

13.5.2.3 Multiple Myeloma

We found one report in the literature concerning a patient with diffuse multiple myeloma (plasma cell sarcoma or Kahler's disease), who had malignant plasma cells in the cervical smear (Figueroa *et al.*, 1978). The malignant cells were large and isolated, with hyperchromatic acentral nuclei and deeply basophilic cytoplasm. The nucleoli were prominent. It is not always easy to distinguish benign from malignant plasma cells. An important differential diagnostic criterion is the size of the nucleolus (Figueroa *et al.*, 1978). Multinucleation alone is not enough for a positive diagnosis (Qizilbash, 1974).

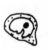

figure 13.7   Cytological pattern of a mesenchymal sarcoma

References

Beyer-Boon, M. E. (1974). Psammoma bodies in cervico-vaginal smears: an indicator of the presence of ovarian carcinoma. *Acta Cytol.,* **18**, 41–4

Bibbo, M., Ali, I., Al-Naquib, M., Baccarini, I., Climaco, L. A., Gill, W., Sonek, M. and Wied, G. L. (1975). Cytologic findings in female and male offspring of DES treated mothers. *Acta Cytol.,* **19**, 568–72

Boxer, R. J. and Skinner, D. C. (1977). Condylomata acuminata and squamous cell carcinoma. *Urol.,* **1**, 72–8

Ceelen, G. H. and Sakurai, M. (1962). Vaginal cytology in leukemia. *Acta Cytol.,* **6**, 370–3

Colmenares, R. F. and Naib, Z. M. (1965). Significance of lymphocytic pools in the routine vaginal smears. *Obstet. Gynec.,* **26**, 909–12

Dance, E. F. and Fullmer, C. D. (1970). Extrauterine carcinoma cells observed in cervicovaginal smears. *Acta Cytol.,* **14**, 187–92

Differding, J. T. (1967). Psammoma bodies in a vaginal smear. *Acta Cytol,* **14**, 199–201

Ferenczy, A., Talens, M., Zoghby, M. and Husain, S. S. (1977). Ultrastructural studies on the morphogenesis of psammoma bodies in ovarian serous neoplasia. *Cancer,* **39**, 2451–9

Figueroa, J. V., Hufakker, A. K. and Diehl, E. J. (1978). Malignant plasma cells in cervical smears. *Acta Cytol.,* **22**, 43–6

Geelhoed, G. W., Henson, D. E., Tayler, P. T. and Ketcham, A. S. (1976). Carcinoma in situ of the vagina following treatment for carcinoma of the cervix: distinctive clinical entity. *Am. J. Obstet. Gynec.,* **124**, 510–16

Geier, G., Kraus, H. and Schuhmann, R. (1974). *Aspiration Biopsy in Ovarian Tumours,* American European Conference on the ovary, Montreux

Graham, J. B. and Graham, R. M. (1967). Cul-de-sac puncture in the diagnosis of early ovarian cancer. *J. Obstet. Gynaec. Br. Commw.,* **74**, 371–8

Graham, R. M. and van Niekerk, W. A. (1962). Vaginal cytology in cancer of the ovary. *Acta Cytol.,* **6**, 496–500

Hajdu, S. I. and Hajdu, E. D. (1976). *Cytopathology of Uterine Sarcomas,* Saunders, Philadelphia and London

Hart, W. R., Townsend, D. E., Aldrich, J. O.,

Henderson, B., Roy, M. and Benton, B. (1976). Histopathologic spectrum of vaginal adenosis and related changes in stilbestrol exposed females. *Cancer,* **37**, 763–75

Herbst, A. L. and Scully, R. E. (1970). Adenocarcinoma of the vagina in adolescence. A report of seven cases including six clear-cell carcinomas (so-called mesonephromas). *Cancer,* **25**, 745–57

Highman, W. J. (1971). Calcified bodies and the intrauterine device. *Acta Cytol.,* **15**, 473–6

Israel, S. L. and Mutch, J. C. (1956). Leukemic infiltration of female genitalia. A gynecologic entity. *Obstet. Gynec.,* **7**, 425–32

Kanbour, A. I., Klionsky, B. and Murphy, A. I. (1974). Carcinoma of the vagina following cervical cancer. *Cancer,* **34**, 1838–41

Katayama, I., Hajian, G. and Evjy, J. T. (1973). Cytologic diagnosis of reticulum cell sarcoma of the uterine cervix. *Acta Cytol.,* **17**, 498–502

Kern, W. H. (1969). Benign papillary structures with psammoma bodies in culdocentesis fluid. *Acta Cytol.,* **13**, 178–81

Koss, L. G. (1968). *Diagnostic Cytology and its Histopathologic Bases,* Lippincott, Philadelphia

Krumerman, M. S. and Chung, A. (1978). Solitary reticulum cell sarcoma of the uterine cervix with initial cytodiagnosis. *Acta Cytol.,* **22**, 46–51

Masubuchi, S., Nagai, I., Hirata, M., Kubo, H. and Masubuchi, K. (1975). Cytologic studies of malignant melanoma of the vagina. *Acta Cytol.,* **19**, 527–32

McIndoe, W. A. and Green, G. H. (1969). Vaginal carcinoma in situ following hysterectomy. *Acta Cytol.,* **13**, 158–63

Meisels, A. and Ayotte, D. (1976). Cells from the seminal vesicles: Contaminants of the V-C-E smear. *Acta Cytol.,* **20**, 211–20

Merchant, S., Murad, T. M., Dowling, E. A. and Durant, J. (1974). Diagnosis of vaginal carcinoma from cytologic material. *Acta Cytol.,* **18**, 494–503

Nordquist, S. R. B., Fidler, W. J. Jr, Woodruff, J. M. and Lewis, J. L. (1976). Clear cell adenocarcinoma of the cervix and vagina. A clinicopathologic study of 21 cases with and without a history of maternal ingestion of estrogens. *Cancer,* **37**, 858–71

Novak, E. R. and Woodruff, J. D. (1974). *Gynecologic and Obstetric Pathology,* Saunders, Philadelphia and London

Patten, S. F. Jr (1978). *Diagnostic Cytopathology of the Uterine Cervix*, Karger, Basel

Picoff, R. C. and Meeker, C. I. (1970). Psammoma bodies in the cervicovaginal smear in association with benign papillary structures of the ovary. *Acta Cytol.*, **14**, 45–8

Qizilbash, A. H. (1974). Chronic plasma cell cervicitis. A rare pitfall in gynecological cytology. *Acta Cytol.*, **18**, 198–200

Riotton, G. and Christopherson, W. M. (1973). *Cytology of the female genital tract. International histological classification of tumours. no. 8,* World Health Organization, Geneva

Rosati, L. A. and Jarzynski, D. J. (1973). Clear cell (mesonephric) adenocarcinoma of the vagina. A case report. *Acta Cytol.*, **17**, 493–8

Song, Y. S. (1955). The cytological diagnosis of carcinoma of the fallopian tube. *Am. J. Obst. Gynec.*, **70**, 29–32

Umiker, W. and Skeen, M. (1953). Carcinoma of the ovary with malignant cells in the vaginal smear of an asymptomatic patient. *Am. J. Obstet. Gynec.*, **66**, 674–7

Vooys, P. G., Ng, A. B. P. and Wentz, W. B. (1973). The detection of vaginal adenosis and clear cell carcinoma. *Acta Cytol.*, **17**, 59–64

Wagman, H. and Brower, C. L. (1974). *Cytology of ovarian surface cells with reference to ovarian cancer,* American European Conference on the ovary, Montreux

Cytopathology of Iatrogenic Lesions

14.1 Introduction

Chemotherapy or administration of hormones may induce cellular changes which cannot always be distinguished from premalignant or malignant conditions. Therefore, for a correct cytological interpretation complete clinical data are indispensible. It is sometimes necessary to discontinue a therapeutic regimen in order to determine whether observed cellular abnormalities are reversible, and thus probably induced by the therapy. In this chapter several aspects of this problem will be considered in more detail.

14.2 Changes Induced by Hormones

14.2.1 Hormonal Contraceptives

Hormonal contraceptives can influence both the squamous epithelium and the glandular epithelium.

14.2.1.1 Influence on Squamous Epithelium

(1) The influence of hormonal contraceptives on the squamous epithelium can be evaluated by means of the K.I. at different moments of the menstrual cycle resulting in a vaginal cytogram (figure 14.1) Various formulations have different effects, with or without an ovulatory peak.

(2) In a number of cases inhibition of the hypothalamus is so marked that when the oral contraceptive is discontinued the cycle does not start up again. The vaginal smear then shows an atrophic pattern.

(3) In exceptional cases (75 out of 47 231 women who used the pill) the smear becomes atrophic when the oral contraceptives are still being used. It is possible to discern two patterns:

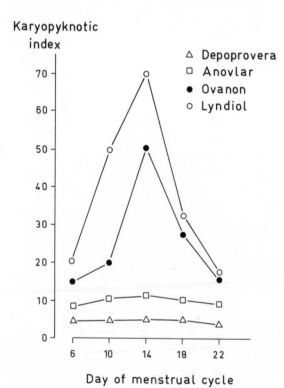

figure 14.1   K.I. curves of women using different hormonal contraceptives

table 14.1 The occurrence of 'pill atrophy' related to the use of various hormonal contraceptives (Leiden Cytology Laboratory, 1976)

Name of oral contraceptive	Distribution of atrophy among the various trade names (percentage)	Prevalence per trade name $\times 10^{-3}$
Depoprovera	32	16.94
Lyndiol	17	0.93
Stederil D	19	2.01
Neogynon	3	0.22
Eugynon	5	3.96
Ovanon	3	0.47
Orthonovum	3	1.19
Anovlar	3	4.76
Gynovlar	1	1.58
Exluton	1	0.40
Unknown	13	2.29
Total	100	1.58

'moist atrophy', where the smears are rich in cells, including glycogen-containing parabasal cells with red cytoplasm (compare with the post-partum pattern) (see section 6.2.1.6), and 'dry atrophy', characterised by a scarcity of cells and the presence of parabasal cells or only reserve cells. Not all oral contraceptives cause the same degree of atrophy (table 14.1). Depoprovera in particular has been shown to cause atrophy in a relatively large number of cases (table 14.1).

14.2.1.2 Influence on the Endocervical Columnar Epithelium

Under the influence of oral ·contraceptives the columnar epithelium may become tall columnar: the smear then contains cells with long strands of cytoplasm. Very large vacuoles of mucus (hypersecretion) may also be seen. Occasionally a pronounced atypia may also be induced, sometimes to such a degree that the diagnosis of malignancy must be considered. We have had two such cases, involving patients on Kombikwens and Depoprovera, respectively. In both patients it was noted that

almost all cells in the smear were more or less abnormal. The epithelial changes consisted of marked enlargement of the nucleus, prominent nucleoli and coarsening of the chromatin pattern. The nuclei, however, retained their smooth oval—round shape. After discontinuation of the contraceptives these cellular changes disappeared completely within several months.

14.2.1.3 Influence on the Presence óf Columnar Epithelial Cells and Metaplastic Epithelial Cells in the Smear

An investigation of the presence of columnar and metaplastic epithelial cells in smears taken from women, divided into those who had taken oral contraceptives and those who had not, revealed that significant differences exist between these two groups. The percentage of columnar and metaplastic epithelial cells was significantly lower for the women who took the 'pill' than for those who did not (table 14.2). Columnar epithelial cells and metaplastic epithelial cells were both absent in a significantly larger percentage of the users than

table 14.2   The presence of columnar and metaplastic epithelial cells in the smears of pill-users and non-users (material from the Leiden Cytology Laboratory)

Age	Non-users				Pill-users			
	C	M	A	Number	C	M	A	Number
		(percentage)		of smears		(percentage)		of smears
20—24	54	25	43	151	55	25	37	1250
25—29	75	46	19	156	60	29	33	2829
30—34	79	41	16	153	65	35	34	2787
35—39	86	45	11	430	61	35	30	1993
40—44	80	43	15	313	59	36	31	1370
45—49	81	51	14	412	63	42	27	935
Total	79	45	16	1615	61	33	32	11164

C, columnar cells; M, metaplastic cells; A, columnar and metaplastic cells absent

the nonusers (Beyer-Boon and Boon, 1977). In the smears from patients with a carcinoma *in situ*, however, these differences were absent (table 14.3); the presence of metaplastic cells among both pill-users and non-users is twice as high in the positive smears as in the negative smears. Since metaplastic cells can be recognised cytologically only when they are relatively immature, this find-

table 14.3   The presence of columnar epithelial and metaplastic epithelial cells in the positive smears (cytological and histological diagnosis: carcinoma *in situ*) of pill-users and non-users (material from the Leiden Cytology Laboratory)

	C	M	A	Number
		(percentage)		of smears
Nonusers	71	88	8	50
Pill-users	75	85	8	100
Both groups	73	86	8	150

C, columnar cells; M, metaplastic cells; A, columnar and metaplastic cells absent

ing underlines the importance of the immature metaplastic epithelium as neoplastic potential. In pregnant women columnar epithelial cells and/or metaplastic epithelial cells are rarely encountered in the smear.

14.2.2 Hormonal Treatment for Climacteric Symptoms

Hormone preparations used to treat climacteric symptoms contain predominantly oestrogen. After treatment the smears will show a high K.I. and often contain groups of endometrial cells which may be so atypical that it is difficult to distinguish them from the cells of a well-differentiated endometrial carcinoma (see section 12.2.2.4).

14.2.3 Hormonal Treatment to Induce Ovulation

For women with anovulatory cycles resulting in sterility, the ovaries can be stimulated by treatment with clomiphene citrate or gonadotropine. With the help of vaginal cytograms or urocytograms the hormonal effect can be evaluated (see section 6.3.2).

14.2.4 Hormonal Treatment to Prevent Abortion

If a pregnant woman is treated with high doses of artificial oestrogen and delivers a daughter, adenosis of the vagina may develop in the child (see section 13.4.1).

14.2.5 Influence of Other Drugs on the K.I.

Various non-hormonal preparations exert an influence on the maturation and exfoliation of squamous epithelium. Digitalis stimulates maturation, sometimes leading to a very high K.I. Tetracycline causes accelerated exfoliation (see section 10.3.4) so that in some cases only parabasal cells are found in the smear within several days after the drug has been administered (Koss, 1968).

14.3 Influence of an Intrauterine Contraceptive Device (IUD) on the Smear

An IUD may cause changes in the endometrial and endocervical epithelium. Endometrial cells may appear in the smear which cannot be explained physiologically; occasionally the endometrial cells may display swollen nuclei and coarse vacuolisation of the cytoplasm (Fornari, 1974). An erroneous diagnosis of endometrial adenocarcinoma may be given in such cases. The columnar epithelial cells of the endocervix sometimes show pronounced enlargement, prominent nucleoli and numerous mitotic figures. The smear can also contain fibroblasts, foreign-body giant cells and histiocytes with phagocytised spermatozoa (Sağiroğlu and Sağiroğlu, 1970). An inflammatory pattern with actinomycetes is common (Gupta *et al.*, 1976). Calcification of the IUD can result in psammoma bodies in the smear (Rethmeier-Croon and Beyer-Boon, 1975).

14.4 Effect of Surgical Intervention, Electrocoagulation and Cryotherapy

After surgical procedures such as conisation, hysterectomy or curettage, 'repair' cells may appear in the smear (see section 7.5.2), sometimes with slight nuclear atypia (that is, coarsening of the chromatin). Electrocoagulation, laser treatment and cryotherapy may cause changes in the cells which are highly similar to those seen in dysplasia (Koss, 1968; Butler, 1976). After cryotherapy cells may be found which resemble atypical reserve cells of the monomorphic type with small nuclei (Butler, 1976) but also repair cells with large nucleoli and abundant cytoplasm. In all cases atypical cells are found within the four weeks following cryosurgery. In most cases the smears are usually normal within eight weeks (Hasegawa *et al.*, 1975).

14.5 Changes Due to Ionising Irradiation

Under the influence of ionising radiation, benign as well as malignant cells can change markedly. The radiation reaction (RR) of benign squamous cells includes:

(1) cytoplasmic vacuolisation.

(2) cellular enlargement: both nuclei and cytoplasm increase in volume; the N/C ratio remains within normal limits.

(3) bizarre cellular shapes.

(4) The 'two-tone' effect in the cytoplasm: basophilic at the margins and eosinophilic around the nucleus.

(5) the nuclei acquire a peculiar wrinkled appearance.

(6) multinucleation.

(7) often clearly enlarged and even pleomorphic nucleoli are visible; the Nc/N ratio remains, however, low.

(8) karyorrhexis.

Malignant cells show:

(1) irregular distribution of the chromatin.

(2) high N/C ratio.

The cytological pattern during radiotherapy is, in general, characterised by numerous leucocytes, cellular debris and blood. Often, in addition to squamous epithelial cells showing RR, there will be many histiocytes and histiocytic giant cells as well as repair cells. As much as twenty years after radiotherapy an RR effect may still be apparent in the epithelial cells; usually, however, RR disappears within a short period. Radiosensitive malignant cells generally disappear during radiotherapy. After irradiation the smear becomes atrophic. The changes due to irradiation must be distinguished from:

(1) atrophy caused by hormones.
(2) inflammation.
(3) effect of cytostatic agents.
(4) folic acid deficiency.

Here too the cellular changes include vacuolisation of the cytoplasm, extreme cytomegaly, multinucleation and abnormal nuclear shapes (von Niekerk, 1966). Differentiation from irradiation effects is not always possible.

14.5.1 Radiation Dysplasia

The smears from patients who have received radiotherapy may develop cellular abnormalities which, morphologically speaking, resemble those of dysplasia. The 'dysplastic' cells may be found either as isolated cells or in sheets. The shapes of the cells vary from polygonal to oval or round. The cytoplasm is usually eosinophilic but it may also stain an indefinite colour. The nuclei are often slightly enlarged, and oval or round. Hyperchromatism and coarsening of the chromatin are common. Sometimes there is a nucleolus, but never a macronucleolus (Patten *et al.*, 1963). Radiation dysplasia can develop after a latent period varying from several months to twenty years. Radiation dysplasia must be differentiated from acute changes due to irradiation and from a new (or recurrent) carcinoma. According to the literature, radiation dysplasia will develop in 20 per cent of patients who have received radiotherapy. The chance that radiation dysplasia will change progressively into a carcinoma *in situ* is twice that of 'normal' dysplastic epithelium. A distinction should be made between a radiation dysplasia which develops within three years of treatment and one that develops later; the latter has a considerably better prognosis (Patten *et al.*, 1963).

14.5.2 Persistent and Recurrent Carcinoma

Patients who after radiotherapy display a high K.I. are more likely to have persistent or recurrent cervical cancer than patients with a low K.I. (Wachtel, 1964; Rubio, 1966). The posttreatment K.I. can forecast clinical cure: 87 per cent of the cured patients had K.I.s below 10, whereas only 32 per cent of the patients with recurrent cancer had such low indices. The K.I. during radiotherapy is of little prognostic value, however.

If a cervical carcinoma is treated with radiotherapy and malignant cells showing RR are found in the smear during and after this treatment, then it can be assumed that the carcinoma is not (or barely) sensitive to ionising radiation. An example of a persistent carcinoma is the undifferentiated carcinoma that exfoliates very small cells (about the size of lymphocytes or histiocytes) which are often naked nuclei. The smears from these patients must be screened very carefully during and after irradiation for such cells. Sometimes malignant cells with RR are seen after radiotherapy is terminated. Histological examination is then indicated. Carcinomas of the cervix which recur or develop after irradiation generally exfoliate cells which do not show irradiation effect (Koss, 1968).

14.6 Cytotoxic Effect

Treatment with cytostatic preparations (for example, for leukaemia) can lead to cellular changes which are highly similar to those seen in the epithelium as a result of radiotherapy. Bisulfan therapy, for example, gives rise to cells with markedly enlarged, highly abnormal nuclei and abundant cytoplasm (Gureli *et al.*, 1963). Multinucleation is common. The cytological and histological patterns may be similar to those of con-dylomatous dysplasia (see section 10.2.2.1).

In the past few years it has been reported with increasing regularity that prolonged administration of cytotoxic drugs enhances the development of carcinomas (Walker and Bole, 1971). Therefore, when the presence of abnormal cells due to cytotoxic drugs has been noted, intensive follow-up is essential.

14.7 Effect of Immunodepressants

Drugs which inhibit the immunological defence of the body (kidney transplant patients) increase the risk of cancer. These drugs have been used on a fairly large scale in the past few decades. In these patients abnormalities of the ectocervical epithel-ium have also been demonstrated (Gupta *et al.*, 1969).

References

Beyer-Boon, M. E. and Boon, L. M. (1977). The influence of hormonal anticonceptives on the presence of metaplastic and cylindrical endo-cervical cells in cervical smears, *7th European Congress of Cytology, Luik*

Butler, E. B. (1976). The cytology of the cervix after cryosurgery, *6th European Congress of Cytology, Weimar*

Fornari, M. L. (1974). Cellular changes in the glandular epithelium of patients using IUCD — a source of cytologic error. *Acta Cytol.*, **18**, 341–5

Gupta, P. K., Hollander, D. H. and Frost, J. K. (1976). Actinomycetes in cervicovaginal smears: an association with IUD usage. *Acta Cytol.*, **20**, 294–8

Gupta, P. K., Pinn, V. M. and Taft, P. D. (1969). Cervical dysplasia associated with azathioprine (Imuran) therapy. *Acta Cytol.*, **13**, 373–7

Gureli, N., Denham, S. W. and Root, S. W. (1963). Cytologic dysplasia related to bisulfan (myleran) therapy. *Obstet. Gynec.*, **21**, 466–70

Hasegawa, T., Tsutsui, F. and Kurihara, S. (1975). Cytomorphologic study on the atypical cells following cryosurgery for the treatment of chronic cervicitis. *Acta Cytol.*, **19**, 533–8

Koss, L. G. (1968). *Diagnostic Cytology and its Histopathologic Bases*, 2nd edn, Lippincott, Philadelphia

Niekerk, van W. A. (1966). Cervical cytological abnormalities caused by folic acid deficiency. *Acta Cytol.*, **10**, 67–73

Patten, S. F., Reagan, J. W., Obenauf, M. and Ballard, L. A. (1963). Postirradiation dysplasia of uterine cervix and vagina: an analytical study of the cells. *Cancer*, **16**, 173–82

Rethmeier-Croon, V. M. and Beyer-Boon, M. E. (1975). Psammoma bodies in cervicovaginal smears of women without ovarian carcinoma, *5th European Congress of Cytology, Milan*

Rubio, C. A. (1966). Prognostic value of the karyopyknotic index in carcinoma of the cervix. *Obstet. Gynec.*, **28**, 228–31

Sağiroglu, N. and Sağiroğlu, E. (1970). The cytol-ogy of intrauterine contraceptive devices. *Acta Cytol.*, **14**, 58–65

Wachtel, E. G. (1964). *Exfoliative Cytology in Gynaecological Practice*, Butterworths, Washing-ton

Walker, S. E. and Bole, G. G. (1971). Augmented incidence of neoplasia in female New Zealand black/New Zealand white mice treated with long-term cyclophosphamide. *J. Lab. clin. Med.*, **78**, 978–9

Technical Procedures

15.1 Introduction

The morphological appearances described in the preceding chapters are only possible when the cellular specimens are of the highest technical quality. Proper preparation, fixation and staining techniques are essential prerequisites to cyto-diagnosis. The laboratory techniques described in this chapter are not, of course, the only worthwhile techniques; however, we have found them to be entirely satisfactory.

15.2 Preparation of a Cellular Sample

For an accurate evaluation of a cellular sample, the following points are necessary.

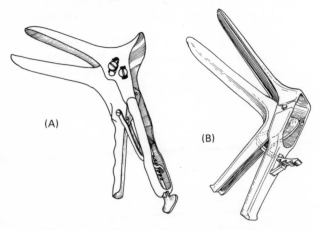

figure 15.1   The speculum. A. Classical speculum; B. plastic 'disposable' speculum (Continental Pharma, Zutphen, the Netherlands)

(1) The sample must be smeared evenly over the glass slide. For this purpose the spatula is drawn along the entire glass slide as smoothly as possible. To prevent drying, the sample must be smeared only once.

(2) The smear should not be too thick. Excess material appears macroscopically as 'blobs' on the slide. If the preparation is too thick, mounting with the coverslip as well as microscopic evaluation will be difficult.

(3) The smear should not contain too little material on the slide.

15.3 Taking a Cellular Sample

15.3.1 Ectocervix

Cervical smears are taken by a physician or an assistant who has been properly trained. The following are required:

(1) The speculum, which is used to expose the cervix (figure 15.1).

(2) A modified Ayre spatula with a long tip (figure 15.2), for scraping part of the ectovervix as well as squamocolumnar junction.

(3) Glass slides with frosted ends where the name and any other identifying information of the patient are written in lead pencil.

(4) Fixative.

It is recommended that a modified Ayre type cervical spatula with a blunt and a pointed end be used. An extensive erosion can best be sampled with

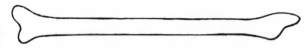

figure 15.2   Modified Ayre spatula with long tip

the blunt end of the spatula; the other end is used when the squamocolumnar junction lies deep in the endocervical canal. In the latter situation a sterile cotton swab can also be used (see section 15.3.2.1).

15.3.1.1 The Ectocervical Smear

After the cervix is exposed with the speculum (figure 15.3), both the ectocervix and the squamocolumnar junction are scraped with the spatula. The sample thus obtained is smeared over the glass slide, which is then either submerged immediately in a jar of 96 per cent ethanol or sprayed with a fixative spray (see section 15.4.1.2). Smears of atrophied squamous epithelium and samples taken after pelvic irradiation dry out very quickly; therefore for these smears rapid fixation is especially important. After the smear has been made, manual vaginal examination can be carried out. Should this be done before the smear is made, glove powder and lubricant contaminate the cell sample and may hamper evaluation. Excessive

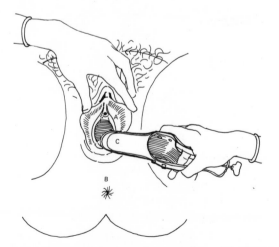

figure 15.3   Introduction of a speculum. (A) Spread labia majora; (B) anus; (C) speculum

mucus and pus must be removed from the cervix prior to taking the sample.

15.3.1.2 The Combination Smear

For detection of carcinomas of the ectocervix (squamous cell carcinoma *in situ* and invasive squamous cell carcinoma) the ectocervical smear produces good results as far as the number and type of cells is concerned (MacGregor *et al.*, 1966). An 'ideal' smear will, in general, contain little blood and mucus and few leucocytes and will contain squamous epithelial cells as well as columnar and/or metaplastic squamous epithelial cells. This ideal is not always achieved (see section 7.4.2.2).

It is possible to combine a vaginal, cervical and endocervical smear on one slide, the so-called 'V-C-E' smear. The vaginal smear will contain the smallest number of malignant squamous cells, the endocervical smear the largest (Bibbo *et al.*, 1976). When the modified Ayre spatula with a long tip is used, the ectocervical smear is in our opinion quite satisfactory; for women above 50 years of age we make a combined ectocervical and endocervical smear, the so-called 'C-E' smear (detection of endometrial carcinoma). For a spray-fixed C-E smear the ectocervical sample is first smeared and fixed on one half of the slide while the other half of the slide is covered with a piece of paper. Subsequently the endocervical scraping or aspirate (see section 15.3.2) is smeared on the other half of the glass and fixed.

15.3.2 Endocervix

15.3.2.1 The Endocervical Smear

The cervix is exposed with the speculum. A sterile cotton swab moistened in physiologic saline solution is inserted into the endocervical canal and rotated clockwise. The material obtained is smeared on the glass slide by rolling the cotton swab anticlockwise across the slide (figure 15.4).

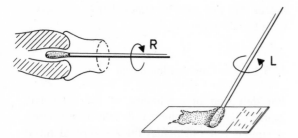

figure 15.4   Taking an endocervical sample

15.3.2.2 The Endocervical Aspirate

It is also possible to aspirate material from the endocervical canal. An instrument that appears to be suitable for this purpose is the 'endocervical aspirator', a disposable sterile Pasteur pipette which is attached to a rubber bulb. The cervix is exposed with the speculum and the pipette is inserted into the cervical canal. The aspirated material is expelled on to a slide and fixed immediately.

15.3.3 Endometrium

Various methods to obtain endometrial specimens can be used.

(1) *Endometrial aspiration.* After the cervix is exposed with the speculum, a sterile cannula is introduced into the endometrial cavity and material is aspirated (a *sterile* cannula is essential). After aspiration the cannula is withdrawn and flushed with physiologic saline solution ('pistolet' method; Wyss *et al.*, 1975) to force out the cells.

(2) *Endometrial washing.* Another method, used in the first half of this decade particularly in the USA, is the 'Gravlee Jet Wash' technique (Bibbo *et al.*, 1972; Lukeman, 1974; So-Bosita *et al.*, 1970). However, not every gynaecologist was dexterous with it and, due also to the high costs involved, it is no longer marketed.

(3) *Endometrial* (and endocervical) *brushing.* A promising method seems to be brushing with the Medosha or Citosmed brushing cannula (figure 15.5) (Jiménez-Ayala *et al.*, 1975).

15.3.3.1 Laboratory Preparation of Aspirated Endometrial Material

The sample obtained can be handled in the following manner.

(1) After centrifugation for 3 minutes (1500 rpm) part of the sediment is smeared for cytological examination. While still wet these smears are placed in Carnoy fixative for 30 minutes. After

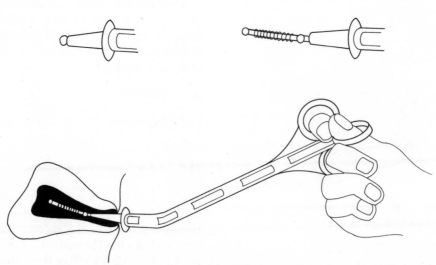

figure 15.5   Citosmed brushing cannula for endometrial cytology. It can also be used for endocervical cytology

rinsing in 70 per cent alcohol the preparations can be stained.

The remaining sediment is also fixed in Carnoy fixative for 30 minutes. It is then stored in 70 per cent ethyl alcohol until it is processed for histology.

(2) Instead of centrifugation the cellular sample can be concentrated using a Millipore or Nucleopore membrane filter with pores 5–8 μm in diameter. Upon request the manufacturers of these filters will provide a manual of instructions. After mounting, a lead weight is put on the coverslip until the mounting medium has dried, in order to flatten the membrane filter.

15.3.4 Vagina

15.3.4.1 Smear of the Posterior Fornix

To make a smear of the posterior fornix the cervix is exposed with the speculum and the posterior fornix is scraped with a spatula. For further details see ectocervical smear (section 15.3.1.1).

15.3.4.2 Aspiration of the Secretions in the Posterior Fornix

In this case the cervix need not be exposed. A pipette with a suction bulb is inserted into the vagina until the tip lies in the posterior fornix. The secretions are then aspirated.

15.3.4.3 Smear of the Upper Third of the Lateral Wall of the Vagina

The lateral wall of the vagina is scraped with a spatula. The sample thus obtained is suitable for evaluation. Beware of contaminating the specimen with squamous epithelial cells from the vulva or the skin, which could make the hormonal determination unreliable.

15.3.5 Purpose of the Various Methods for Acquiring Cellular Samples

Scraping of the ectocervix: detection of squamous carcinoma *in situ*, invasive squamous cell carcinoma, and endocervical adenocarcinomas.

Scraping or aspiration of the endocervix: detection of squamous cell carcinomas higher in the cervical canal and endocervical or endometrial carcinoma.

Endometrial aspiration: detection of endometrial carcinomas.

Scraping or aspiration of the posterior fornix: detection of endometrial carcinoma and (metastasis of) ovarian carcinomas.

Scraping of the upper third of the lateral wall of the vagina: hormonal evaluation.

15.3.6 Urine for Urocytograms

Urine for urocytograms should be processed immediately, or fixed with equal amounts of 50 per cent ethyl alcohol, or pretreated with Merthiolate (Beyer-Boon *et al.*, 1979a).

The cells in the urine must be concentrated (1) by centrifuging the whole sample at 2000 rpm for 10 minutes, followed by spreading one drop of the sediment over a slide; (2) by using the cytocentrifuge; (3) by using filter techniques.

After centrifugation or filtering, the cells must immediately be covered with a spray fixative (see section 15.4.1.2) and stained with the Papanicolaou method (see section 15.5.1) or the Shorr method (see section 15.5.3). The cell harvest with spray-fixed smears is approximately ten times larger than 96 per cent ethyl-alcohol-fixed smears (Beyer-Boon and Voorn-den Hollander, 1978).

15.4 Fixation

Fixation preserves the cells and prepares them for staining. A fixative must be able to kill bacteria and moulds as well as inactivate enzymes. The fixation method should suit the staining method. Gynaecological preparations – and in general all preparations containing mucus such as sputum, gastric contents, etc. – are best stained by the Papanicolaou method.

For this staining method, fixation with fast-acting dehydrating agents is preferable. In air-dried specimens, which are best suited for the

May-Grünwald—Giemsa method, the process of dehydration is a slow one. In the Papanicolaou method fast-acting fixatives (alcohol solutions) are commonly used (in cervical cytology 96 percent ethanol) or spray fixatives, commercially available or self-made (see section 15.4.1.2). Both methods are referred to as wet fixation methods. However, in the wet fixation methods some involuntary air drying may occur if the fixative is applied too slowly or covers the smear incompletely. The chromatin pattern of these cells is influenced by the air drying process, and will not be altered by subsequent wet fixation. In smears fixed with spray fixatives these air-dried cells may occur only in areas where the cells were not covered with fixative, whereas in partially dried 96 per cent ethyl alcohol fixed smears all of the cells appear air dried. In the literature the ill-conceived term 'poorly fixed' is used for cells with air-drying effects. Equally strange is the term 'air-drying artifact', which suggests that the chromatin patterns of the wet fixation methods are not real!

When the cells are air dried, the staining properties of the cytoplasm are different from wet-fixed cells: the cytoplasm of nonkerantinised cells is red in the Papanicolaou stain, often with two-tone patterns (blue at the periphery, red in the centre). The cytoplasmic borders are ill defined, and the cytoplasm of otherwise vacuolated cells is homogeneous.

The various fixation techniques result in different chromatin patterns. Wet fixation techniques result in a large difference between heterochromatin and euchromatin, and condensation of chromatin beneath the nuclear envelope. The alcohol fixed cells have, compared to cells fixed with a spray fixative, more chromatin condensation beneath the nuclear envelope and less distinct euchromatin. The nuclei of atypical reserve cells are often 'empty' with almost all chromatin near the nuclear envelope (see nuclear pattern 15, section 9.5.2). This phenomenon is almost never encountered in smears fixed with spray fixatives.

Air-dried cells do not have condensed chromatin beneath the nuclear envelope, and therefore the nuclei in the Papanicolaou staining appear ill-defined. Compared to wet-fixed cells the staining of the nuclei is weaker and the difference between euchromatin and heterochromatin is much less pronounced, resulting in a 'blurred' nuclear pattern.

The speed with which cell nuclei air dry depends on the environment of the cell (for example, slowly in mucus-containing material) and the type of cells. Nuclei of cells with squamoid differentiation are relatively resistant to some degree of air drying, whereas the nuclei of reserve cells are extremely susceptible to air drying. This explains the fact that, especially in smears fixed with a coating fixative, many reserve cells display some air-drying effects.

The various fixation techniques result in both smaller and larger nuclear and cytoplasmic sizes compared to unfixed, unstained cells, and also influence the three-dimensional appearance of the nuclei. In air dried smears the area of the nucleus can be 50 per cent larger; that of the cytoplasm 30 per cent larger (Beyer-Boon *et al.*, 1979b). This explains the expression 'blown-up' nuclei in air dried (or 'poorly fixed') areas of Papanicolaou stained smears. In wet fixed cells the nucleus can be 10—30 per cent and the cytoplasm 15—55 per cent smaller (Beyer-Boon *et al.*, 1979b). The shrinkage is dependent on the concentration of the ethyl alcohol used. As far as the three-dimensional appearance of the nuclei is concerned there are also striking differences: air dried nuclei are flat, and wet fixed nuclei more spherical. This phenomenon is amply illustrated by the photomicrographs in which, for instance, the large nuclei of atypical reserve cells cannot be brought into full focus with a 40 x objective.

15.4.1 Fixatives

15.4.1.1 Ethyl Alcohol

For the Papanicolaou stain 96 per cent ethyl alcohol is usually used as fixative. Fixation is excellent. After at least 10 minutes in the fixative the preparations can be stained. However, they may remain in the fixative several days before staining. A disadvantage of alcohol fixation is that the slides waiting to be stained must be carried to the laboratory in alcohol filled containers, which increases the work load.

In some laboratories a mixture of ethanol and ethyl ether (1:1) is used as a fixative. The method is not to be recommended since certain risks are involved in the use of ether: it is highly flammable, explosive, stupefactive and toxic. Furthermore, the fixation provided by this mixture is not superior to that of 96 per cent ethanol.

15.4.1.2 Spray Fixatives

Smears can be fixed with spray fixatives; they then are allowed to air dry (in a matter of seconds) and can be sent to the laboratory already in racks or they may be mailed to the laboratory in slide containers. This eliminates having to use containers of liquid fixative (see under section 15.4.1.1). Be sure to shake the spray can thoroughly before use. The glass slide must be sprayed with the fixative immediately after the smear has been prepared, before any drying takes place.

There are numerous spray fixatives on the market today. They are relatively expensive. In our laboratory we make the following fixative (Beyer-Boon, 1977).

polyethylene glycol, mol. weight 300	80 ml
isopropanol	690 ml
acetone	170 ml
distilled water	60 ml

This fixative can be applied to the smears with a perfume atomiser or an automotive aerosol sprayer. It produces better results than 96 per cent ethyl alcohol, because there is less variation in chromatin pattern (see section 15.4).

Spray fixative can be removed with 96 per cent ethyl alcohol.

15.4.1.3 Carnoy's Fixative (Ganter and Jolles, 1970)

Carnoy's fixative can be used for fixing aspirates. It is made up of:

ethyl alcohol 100 per cent	60 ml
chloroform	30 ml
glacial acetic acid	10 ml

After rinsing in 70 per cent alcohol the prepara-

tions can be stained according to the Papanicolaou method.

15.4.1.4 Carbowax*

Carbowax, which is a coating fixative, is recommended for samples containing only a few cells or specimens which shed many cells during the staining process (such as urine). A disadvantage is the presence of ether in the solution.

2.5g Carbowax 1540 polyethylene glycol is measured into a 100 ml glass beaker. Place the beaker in a container of warm water. The carbowax will melt at about 60°C (do not place over direct heat). After cooling to body temperature, 25 ml 96 per cent ethanol are added drop by drop; then stir constantly while adding 25 ml ethyl ether. This mixture is stored in a brown bottle in a fume cabinet.

After the smear has been made several drops of the Carbowax solution are spread over the glass slide. The slide is placed in the fume cabinet where the volatile constituents of this solution can evaporate; finally, the Carbowax covers the preparation as a thin film. When the preparation is thoroughly dry, it is carefully dipped in water 3 times (beware of loss of material). The preparation is left in water for 10—15 minutes until the Carbowax dissolves completely. The preparation is then stained according to the Papanicolaou method. If the fixative is not removed entirely from the preparation microscopic evaluation will be difficult since this particular fixative also has an affinity for the stain.

15.5 Staining Procedures

15.5.1 The Papanicolaou Staining Methods

15.5.1.1 Preparation of the Slides Before Staining

Each slide receives a laboratory number which is written in lead pencil on the frosted end of the slide (if necessary a diamond can be used to scratch the number on the slide).

If the preparations have been fixed with a spray

* Carbowax 1540 (polyethylene glycol) – Cat. 08049, Applied Science Laboratories, State College, Pennsylvania 16801, USA

fixative, the smears are submerged in 96 per cent ethyl alcohol for 30 minutes to remove the coating. If they have been fixed with Carbowax this is removed by carefully dipping the smears in water 3 times and then immersing in water for 10–15 minutes. The nuclear stain may now be used – if necessary, after passing the slides through 70 per cent ethyl alcohol and distilled water.

15.5.1.2 Stains for the Papanicolaou Staining

(1) *Haematoxylin.* Haematoxylin is a nuclear stain in an aqueous solution and is a pH indicator. It is a natural product and is extracted from the wood of a Central American tree *Haematoxylon campechianum L.* In reality, haematoxylin itself is not a stain; only its oxidation product haematein and the haematein salts are. However, the derivates of haematoxylin are also referred to in the literature as 'haematoxylin'; in this chapter we will follow this confusing habit. The process of oxidation occurs naturally as *'ripening'* of the haematoxylin with air and sunlight, or may be evoked during preparation of the staining solutions, for instance, by adding mercuric oxide as in the Harris method. When haematein progresses to overoxidation products it is no longer useful as a dye. Haematein itself cannot become bound to cell structures without the presence of positively charged usually metallic ions (so-called 'mordants').

Harris' haematoxylin can be applied as a *regressive stain*, that is, the stain is first deposited excessively and diffusely in the cytoplasm and nuclei of the cells, and then the excess stain is differentially extracted by means of a dilute acid solution to achieve optimal nuclear staining and minimal cytoplasmic staining (Luna, 1968).

For optimal cytoplasmic staining in E.A. and Orange-G, *all* haematoxylin should be removed from the cytoplasm. It is advisable to check this by removing a slide after the water rinsing following the HCl dish, and seeing under the microscope whether any stain is left in the cytoplasm. If this is the case, the HCl concentration should be higher, or the dipping in the acid bath should be more thorough.

Blueing agents', such as 1.5 per cent ammonium hydroxide or lithium carbonate which reoxidise the dye to its blue form, are applied after the excess haematoxylin has been removed by the tap water rinse. Blueing can also be achieved by using tap water if it is mildly alkaline, or by using Scott's water.

(a) *Harris' haematoxylin* (Culling, 1963)

100 per cent ethyl alcohol	50 ml
distilled water	1000 ml
haematoxylin crystals	5.0 g
mercuric oxide	2.5 g
ammonium or potassium alum	100 g

Dissolve the haematoxylin crystals in the ethyl alcohol. Dissolve the alum in the water. Mix the 2 solutions, and boil for a few minutes. Take it from the heater and carefully add small quantities of mercuric oxide. Heat the solution again. Take it immediately from the heater when the colour is purple, and cool it rapidly, for instance, by placing it in cold water. It is ready when it is completely cold. One may add 2–4 ml glacial acetic acid.
Filter prior to using.

Haematoxylin can also be applied as a *progressive stain*, that is, directly deposited in the nucleus; the cytoplasm is only slightly stained and further stain removal, other than by rinsing, is unnecessary. If the pH of the tap water is under 8, it is advisable to add 1.5 per cent ammonium hydroxide to the first water dish following the haemotoxylin dish, otherwise the nuclei are less blue (see blueing agents).

In this method, only part of the haematoxylin is oxidised. The acetic acid is added to the stain to make it more resistant to oxidation and to stabilise the haematein-salt complexes. The less acidified the stain, the more 'agressive' and only usable as a regressive stain. Mercury is a toxic, corrosive and polluting heavy metal. Harris' haematoxylin should be handled and disposed of with proper precautions.

(b) *Mayer's haematoxylin* (Culling, 1963)

haematoxylin	1 g
distilled water	1000 ml
sodium iodate	0.2 g
ammonium or potassium alum	50 g
citric acid	1 g
chloral hydrate	50 g

Dissolve the alum in water and dissolve the haematoxylin in the solution with a little heating. Then add the sodium iodate, citric acid and chloral hydrate (oxidant). Stir until all chemicals are completely dissolved. No boiling is required. The final colour is reddish violet. The stain can be kept for months. *Filter the stain prior to use.*

(c) *Gill's half-oxidised haematoxylin* (Gill *et al.*, 1974)

distilled water	730 ml
ethylene glycol	250 ml
haematoxylin, anhydrous, certified (CI No. 75290)	2.0 g
sodium iodate	0.2 g
aluminium sulphate, A/2 $(SO_4)_3$ $18H_2O$	17.6 g
glacial acetic acid	20 ml

The chemicals are combined in the given order, and stirred for one hour at room temperature. The staining solution can be stored for over one year.

In this method approximately half of the haematoxylin is oxidised by sodium iodate to the active staining components haematein and its salts. The initially unoxidised haematoxylin will oxidise slowly as time passes, thus replacing the haematein that is removed during staining (Gill *et al.*, 1974).

Gill's haematoxylin has a low concentration of haematein and an ideal proportion of mordant and, therefore, cannot overstain.

Filter the stain prior to use.

(d) *Commercial haematoxylins*

For smaller routine cytology laboratories commercial haematoxylins are to be preferred. The products of the different brands differ in staining capacities, and different batches from the same firm also vary. We have good results with DIFCO Haematoxylin Mayer 8550.88 and Harris 8556.88.

For Merck stains we use Harris 9253 and Mayer 9249.

(2) *E.A.*   E.A. (Eosin-Azur) stains predominantly the cytoplasm. The staining results are dependent on the proportion of the component Light-Green in the E.A., the pH of the cytoplasm and the fixation of the cytoplasm (see sections 15.4 and 15.7). Other components are Eosin Y CI 45380, Bismarck Brown Y CI 21000, Light-Green SF yellowish CI 42095, phosphotungstic acid and lithium carbonate.

Table 15.1 depicts the different shades of colour resulting from the different E.A.'s. It is advisable to buy these stains commercially. We prefer to use a 1:1 mixture of E.A. 50 and E.A. 65 (Merck E.A. 50 9272 and E.A. 65 9270; DIFCO E.A. 50 8613.88 and E.A. 65 8614.88).

The stains should be filtered prior to use.

(3) *Orange-G 6.*   Orange gold or orange-G is the stain which gives the cytoplasm of the cells a yellow-orange colour if keratin is present. It is dissolved in alcohol. The stain can be purchased commercially, or prepared as follows:

orange-G (CI 16230)	0.5 g
ethyl alcohol 95 per cent	100 ml
phosphotungstic acid	0.015 g

Dissolve the orange-G in the ethyl alcohol. Add the phosphotungstic acid, and stir until it is dissolved. We have good results with DIFCO 8615.80 and Merck 6887.

It is advisable to filter stains before use.

15.5.1.3 Water and Alcohol Dishes

In the water and alcohol dishes the excess stain is rinsed away. By passing the rack of slides in dishes of high percentages of alcohol the smears are dehydrated, or by passing it via lower percentages

table 15.1   Staining properties of wet-fixed cells

	E.A. 36	E.A. 50	E.A. 65
Basophilic cytoplasm	Intensive green	Blue green	Blue
Acidophilic cytoplasm	Rose	Rose	Red
Squamous cytoplasm	Orange/red	Orange/red	Orange/red

of alcohol into the distilled water the slides are hydrated. Usually, between the water-containing baths and the stains dissolved in ethyl alcohol, a series of graded percentage alcohol baths are used (see section 15.5.1.10). However, one-step hydration and dehydration can also be applied (see section 15.5.1.10, method III).

The distilled water should have pH of 7—7.5.

15.5.1.4 Rinsing

The rinsing process with tap water is essential, in particular in the progressive methods. Luke-warm water rinses most effectively (Gill *et al.*, 1974). If the pH of the tap water is under 8, 1.5 per cent ammonium hydroxide should be added (see section 15.5.1.2).

15.5.1.5 Last Phase of the Staining

(1) Dehydration in 100 per cent ethyl alcohol.
(2) Removal of residual alcohol with xylene. Xylene makes the cells transparent; however, a mixture of xylene with the slightest amount of water will produce a milky-white cloudiness. As a result numerous droplets will appear on the smear so that cytological evaluation becomes impossible. Xylene can be mixed with the mounting medium, in contrast to alcohol. Because of this it is exceedingly important to remove the alcohol entirely.

15.5.1.6 Interruption of the Staining Procedure

If the staining procedure has to be interrupted the smears can be left standing in the following solutions for reasonable periods (hours).

before haematoxylin	96%, 70% or 50% ethyl alcohol with water
after haematoxylin	water
after HCl	water
after lithium carbonate	water or 70% ethyl alcohol
after orange gold	ethyl alcohol 96%
after E.A.	ethyl alcohol 96%
after staining	xylene

15.5.1.7 Replacement and Filtering of Staining Solutions

When a staining circuit is used intensively (maxi-

mum 50 slides per 500 ml fluid), it is advisable to replace often all water baths, the HCl, the highly polluted 96 per cent ethyl alcohol and the last xylene dishes. All stains should be replaced after 1 week or a maximum of 350 slides. When the staining circuit is not used intensively the dishes of staining solution can, if necessary, be replenished with fresh solution.

It is recommended after every 3 days to prolong the staining time in the Mayer's and Gill's haematoxylin by 1 minute and in the Harris' haematoxylin by 0.5 minute. A prolongation of the staining times is not necessary for E.A. and orange-G.

Prior to use the stains should be filtered. We prefer to use normal filter paper 47 x 57 cm, which does not have to be analytical grade. The alcohol dishes should only be filtered if the danger of cross-contamination is large (urine, pleural fluid, sperm, etc.).

15.5.1.8 Staining Times

Harris' haematoxylin	1—15 minutes
Mayer's and Gill's haema- toxylin	2—5 minutes
Orange-G	1—1.5 minutes
E.A.	1—1.5 minutes

15.5.1.9 Several Comments Concerning the Technique of Staining

(1) Dip the racks gently in the dishes to prevent cell loss.

(2) Drain the staining racks well between the solutions to avoid excessive dilution of the following dish, but *do not allow the slides to dry*. The preparations must be dipped five times in all dishes to obtain intimate contact between the fluid and the specimen.

(3) The staining dishes must be covered whenever possible to prevent evaporation of the staining solutions.

(4) During staining cells from one slide may contaminate another. To keep this risk to a minimum the solutions must be replaced or filtered regularly. Because preparations of, for instance, urinary sediments shed cellular material easily, they

should not be placed together with cervical smears in one rack.

(5) At the end of a staining circuit, the rack of slides is in the xylene dish. Three or four slides should be taken out to be coverslipped. If more slides are taken out at one time, some of these will dry out before the mounting medium is applied. This results in brown granules in the cytoplasm.

(6) When a cytology laboratory handles a large number of preparations daily an automatic staining machine can increase efficiency. Other advantages are standardisation of the stain and elimination of human error. On the other hand, a machine may take longer and is expensive.

15.5.1.10 Various Papanicolaou Staining Methods

Papanicolaou staining method I
Progressive staining method
(Modification Koudstaal and Smid, 1974)

96 per cent ethyl alcohol
70 per cent ethyl alcohol
distilled water
Mayer's haematoxylin
tap water
70 per cent ethyl alcohol
96 per cent ethyl alcohol
96 per cent ethyl alcohol
Orange-G II
96 per cent ethyl alcohol
96 per cent ethyl alcohol
96 per cent ethyl alcohol
E.A. 50
96 per cent ethyl alcohol
96 per cent ethyl alcohol
100 per cent ethyl alcohol
100 per cent ethyl alcohol
100 per cent ethyl alcohol
xylene

Papanicolaou staining method II
Regressive staining method
(Modification Koss, 1968)

80 per cent ethyl alcohol
70 per cent ethyl alcohol

50 per cent ethyl alcohol
distilled water
Harris' haematoxylin,
    distilled water
0.5 per cent HCl
tap water
50 per cent ethyl alcohol
1.5 per cent amm. hydroxide in
    70 per cent ethyl alcohol
80 per cent ethyl alcohol
95 per cent ethyl alcohol
Orange-G
95 per cent ethyl alcohol
95 per cent ethyl alcohol
E.A. 65
95 per cent ethyl alcohol
95 per cent ethyl alcohol
100 per cent ethyl alcohol
100 per cent ethyl alcohol
100 per cent ethyl alcohol
xylene

Papanicolaou staining method III.
Progressive staining method
(Modification Gill *et al.*, 1974)

95 per cent ethyl alcohol
tap water
Gill's haematoxylin
tap water
tap water
Scott's water
tap water
tap water
95 per cent ethyl alcohol
95 per cent ethyl alcohol
Orange-G
95 per cent ethyl alcohol
95 per cent ethyl alcohol
95 per cent ethyl alcohol
E.A. 50
95 per cent ethyl alcohol
95 per cent ethyl alcohol
95 per cent ethyl alcohol
100 per cent ethyl alcohol
100 per cent ethyl alcohol
100 per cent ethyl alcohol
xylene

Papanicolaou staining method IV
Regressive staining method
(Modification Pundel, 1950)

96 per cent ethyl alcohol
70 per cent ethyl alcohol
50 per cent ethyl alcohol
distilled water
Harris' haematoxylin
distilled water
0.1 per cent HCl
distilled water
distilled water
distilled water
lithium carbonate
distilled water
50 per cent ethyl alcohol
70 per cent ethyl alcohol
96 per cent ethyl alcohol
Orange-G
96 per cent ethyl alcohol
96 per cent ethyl alcohol
E.A. 65
96 per cent ethyl alcohol
96 per cent ethyl alcohol
100 per cent ethyl alcohol
xylene

Papanicolaou staining method V
Regressive staining method
(Papanicolaou, 1942)

80 per cent ethyl alcohol
70 per cent ethyl alcohol
50 per cent ethyl alcohol
distilled water
Harris' haematoxylin
rinse with distilled water
HCl 0.25 per cent
rinse with tap water
50 per cent ethyl alcohol
70 per cent ethyl alcohol
80 per cent ethyl alcohol
95 per cent ethyl alcohol
Orange-G
95 per cent ethyl alcohol

95 per cent ethyl alcohol
E.A. 50
95 per cent ethyl alcohol
95 per cent ethyl alcohol
95 per cent ethyl alcohol
100 per cent ethyl alcohol
xylene

15.5.1.11 Decolourising Papanicolaou Stained Preparations

It is possible to decolourise Papanicolaou stained preparations, for instance, when another stain has to be applied to the same preparation.

The coverglass and mounting medium are removed by placing the preparation in xylene, until the coverslip drops off. It is essential to remove all of the mounting medium from the slide. This can be checked by hydrating the slide via 100 per cent ethyl alcohol and 96 per cent ethyl alcohol to distilled water. The mounting medium is not completely removed when in the water dish there is a milky film covering the slide. Then the slide must be redehydrated and replaced for a longer time in xylene. The process can be accelerated if the xylene bath is placed in a heating cabinet of 56°C. It may be very difficult to remove the mounting medium of old slides; especially the Continental Pharma mounting medium is difficult to remove.

When the mounting medium is removed, the slide is submerged successively in 100 per cent ethyl alcohol, 96 per cent ethyl alcohol (2x), 70 per cent ethyl alcohol and hydrochloric acid (1 per cent HCl in 70 per cent ethyl alcohol) until the preparation is decolourised. This process can take 3–5 minutes. Then rinse well in distilled water and check the results under the microscope while the slide is still wet.

It is important that the slide never dries out.

If the cells are not completely decolourised, the slide is placed via the dish with distilled water into the hydrochloric acid dish. Prior to restaining place the slide for 10 minutes in running tap water.

15.5.2 Quick Papanicolaou Staining Method
(Lopes Cardoze, 1975)

15.5.2.1 Preparation of the Slides before Staining

The preparations are fixed for a minimum of 10 seconds.

15.5.2.2 Staining Procedure

96 per cent ethyl alcohol	
50 per cent ethyl alcohol	
distilled water	
haematoxylin	1 minute
rinse in distilled water	
lithium carbonate solution	½ minute
50 per cent ethyl alcohol	
96 per cent ethyl alcohol	
Orange-G	15 seconds
2 x 96 per cent ethyl alcohol	
E.A.	1 minute
2 x 96 per cent ethyl alcohol	
1 x 100 per cent ethyl alcohol	
2 x xylene	
mount	

15.5.3 Shorr Staining Method (Shorr, 1941)

15.5.3.1 Preparation of the Slides before Staining

The slides must be *well fixed* with either 96 per cent ethyl alcohol or spray fixative.

15.5.3.2 Stain for the Shorr Method

S$_3$ solution:

50 per cent ethyl alcohol	100 ml
Biebrich Scarlet (aqueous)	0.5 g
Orange-G	0.25 g
Fast Green FCF	0.075 g
phosphoric acid	0.5 g
phosphomolybdic acid	0.5 g
acetic acid	1.0 g

15.5.3.3 Staining Procedures

Solution S$_3$	1 minute
70 per cent ethyl alcohol	

96 per cent ethyl alcohol
100 per cent ethyl alcohol
xylene
mount

15.5.3.4 Application of the Shorr Staining Method

This method is used for cytohormonal evaluation, principally to determine the eosinophilic index. The staining properties of air-dried cells (too slow wet fixation) differ from properly wet-fixed cells, and therefore make such evaluation unreliable.

15.5.4 Cresyl-Echt Violet Staining Method
(Amarose, 1974)

15.5.4.1 Preparation of the Slides before Staining

The slides must be very well wet fixed.

15.5.4.2 Staining Procedure

distilled water	5 minutes
Cresyl-Echt violet 1 per cent	7 minutes
96 per cent ethyl alcohol	3 minutes
96 per cent ethyl alcohol	3 minutes

Check results under microscope
100 per cent ethyl alcohol
2 x xylene
mount

15.5.4.3 Application of Cresyl-Echt Violet Staining Method

Assessment of Barr bodies. The chromatin and Barr body stain violet, the cytoplasm stains slightly.

15.5.5 Giemsa Staining Method

15.5.5.1 Preparation of the Slides before Staining

The smears must be well air dried, if necessary with a hairdryer. Lopes Cardozo (1975) prefers postfixation of the air dried smears for 10–15 minutes in methanol for his one-step Giemsa staining procedure.

15.5.5.2 Stains for the Giemsa Method

The May-Grünwald solution contains a combination of unoxidised methylene blue and eosin in methanol.

The Giemsa solution contains a combination of methylene blue, its oxidation products (the azures) and eosin γ. It is used by us in a 1:10 solution in buffer pH 6.8. The Giemsa solution should be filtered prior to staining.

15.5.5.3 Staining Procedure

One-step method (Lopes Cardoze, 1975)

rinse with tap water or phosphate buffer (pH 6.8)

Giemsa staining solution	20 minutes
rinse with tap water	2 minutes

air dry

Two-step method

May-Grünwald solution	1–3 minutes
rinse in phosphate buffer (pH 6.8)	1 minute
Giemsa solution	12 minutes thin smears;
	20 minutes medium smears;
	30 minutes thick smears

air dry

15.5.5.4 Application of the Giemsa Method in Gynaecological Cytology

We prefer the Giemsa method over the Papanicolaou method if:

(1) a malignancy of the RES is suspected. Here the comparison with blood films and/or lymph node aspirates, stained with the Giemsa method, can be of vital importance.

(2) the tumour cells must be distinguished from malignant urothelial cells, in cases of ingrowth of extension of bladder carcinomas. In the Giemsa stain, the cytoplasm of malignant urothelial cells have a characteristic 'lace collar' appearance.

15.6 Mounting Stained Preparations

After staining, the preparations are mounted with a mounting medium and covered with a coverglass.

The mounting medium must meet the following requirements.

(1) It must have a perfect viscosity and dry quickly.

(2) It must remain clear after drying.

(3) It must be neutral and chemically inactive.

(4) It must have approximately the same refractive index as glass.

The mounting medium may be a natural resin, although nowadays synthetic resins are frequently used, for example, Malinol, Histoclad, Entallan, Permount, Continental Pharma mounting medium. The synthetics are preferable because they harden quickly. Because the mounting medium is not miscible with alcohol, the preparations must first be immersed in xylene (see staining procedures, section 15.5).

Coverglasses protect the material against damage. It is important that they do not affect the microscopic examination adversely; therefore, they must be optically homogeneous and their two surfaces must be plane and in parallel. The size of the coverglass depends upon the size of the preparation. In our laboratory the coverglasses are 24–40 mm across. Ideally, coverslips should be 0.17 mm thick, usually sold as No. 1.5.

15.6.1 Mounting

The preparation is removed from the xylene bath and placed on a flat surface. Then a drop of mounting medium is applied to the still moist preparation and the coverglass is placed on top. The slides should never be allowed to dry (see section 15.5.1.6). To remove excess mounting medium apply light pressure in the middle of the coverglass and then press firmly along the edges. If the sample has been smeared too thickly air bubbles develop under the coverglass. These can be removed from a preparation which has just been coverslipped as follows.

(1) Exert extra pressure at the point where the air bubble is located.

(2) If the preparation is too thick, remove the coverglass and carefully scrape the excess material with a metal spatula.

(3) A weight can be placed on the coverglass during the drying period.

If after hardening of the mounting medium air bubbles are still present the coverglass must be soaked loose by placing the preparation in xylene. The preparation can then be coverslipped again, this time using more of the mounting medium.

A variety of mounting machines are appearing on the market using glass or plastic coverslips. As with staining machines, their practicality depends on the volume of work handled.

15.7 Pitfalls

(1) *The chosen staining method* should always suit *the fixation method.* The best example of a disastrous combination in gynaecological cytology is the Papanicolaou staining method with (involuntary) air-dried fixation (slide is not fixed fast enough). The nuclear pattern is blurred, the nuclei are more spread (see section 15.4) and they take up less haematoxylin. The cytoplasm is ill defined, and stains red in nonkeratinised cells. As a result the nuclei seem reddish and there is less contrast between nuclei and cytoplasm, giving the cells a 'dull' appearance.

(2) *The staining results should always be checked under the microscope* and the staining times changed accordingly.

(3) Nuclei are easily overstained in Harris' haematoxylin, especially when the differentiation is incomplete.

(4) Nuclei in too thick cell groupings are not fixed properly with 96 per cent ethyl alcohol, and do not take up the stains well.

(5) If the Harris' haematoxylin is not filtered, it will result in blueish contaminants on the smear.

(6) There will be red nuclei when the water dishes are too acid, or when not completely neutralised.

(7) If the smear is dried before the mounting medium is applied, the result will be brown granules in the cytoplasm (see section 15.5.1.9).

(8) Air bubbles can develop, especially when the smear is thick or when the mounting medium contains air bubbles.

(9) If the xylene is mixed with water, the result will be droplets on the smear (see section 15.5.1.5).

(10) Beware of contamination with air-borne fungi, pollen, etc.

(11) If the smear was sprayed from too close a distance, it will result in vacuolisation of the nuclei.

(12) Understaining of the nuclei will result from too old or exhausted haematoxylin, from too short a staining time, when the haematoxylin is not well prepared, and when the differentiation is too long (see section 15.4 and section 9.5.2, nuclear pattern 16).

Addendum

Commercial Spray Fixatives

(1) Cyto-dri Fix: Paragon C + C Co. Inc., 2540 Belmont Avenue, New York, USA
(2) Cyto-fixer: Lba-Tex Plastic Co., 30 East Burlington Street, Westmont, III, USA
(3) Pro-fix: Scientific Products, 1210 Leon Place, Evanston, III, USA
(4) Cytology—Fixative (water soluble): Richard Allan, Med. Industries Inc., 1335 Dodge Avenue, Evanston, III, USA
(5) Spray-Cyte: Clay Adams, East 25th Street, New York, USA

Millipore and Nucleopore Filters

Shandon Nucleopore, lab. center B. V., Loolaan 5c, Apeldoorn, Netherlands.
Millipore Benelux S.A./N.V. Heliotropenlaan 10, Brussels, Belgium.

References

Amarose, A. P. (1974). *Compendium on Cytopreparatory Techniques* (ed. C. M. Keebler, J. W. Reagan and C. L. Wied), Tutorials of Cytology, Chicago

Beyer-Boon, M. E. (1977). *Urinary Cytology,* Springer, Heidelberg, pp. 15—40

Beyer-Boon, M. E. and Voorn-den Hollander,

M. J. A. (1978). Cell yield obtained with various cytopreparatory techniques for urinary cytology. *Acta Cytol.,* 22, 589–94

Beyer-Boon, M. E., Arentz, P. W. and Kirk, R. S. (1979a). A Comparison of Merthiolate and 50 per cent alcohol as preservatives in urinary cytology, *J. clin. Path.,* in press

Beyer-Boon, M. E., van der Voorn, M. J. A., Arentz, P. W., Cornelisse, C. J., Schaberg, A. and Fox, C. H. (1979b). Effect of various routine cytopreparatory techniques on normal urothelial cells and their nuclei. *Acta Path. Microbial. Scand.,* in press

Bibbo, M., Bartels, P. H., Chen, M., Harris, M. J., Truttman, B. and Wied, G. L. (1976). The numerical composition of cellular samples from the female reproductive tract. *Acta Cytol.,* 20, 249–54, 565–72

Bibbo, M., Shanklin, D. R. and Wied, G. L. (1972). Endometrium cytology on jet wash material. *J. reprod. Med.,* 8, 90–6

Culling, C. F. A. (1963). *Handbook of Histopathological Techniques,* Butterworths, London

Ganter, P. and Jolles, G. (1970). *Histochimie, Normale et Pathologique 2,* Gauthier-Villars, Paris.

Gill, G. W., Frost, J. K. and Miller, K. A. (1974). A new formula for a half-oxidized hematoxylin solution that neither overstains nor requires differentiation. *Acta Cytol.,* 18, 300–11

Jiménez-Ayala, M., Vilaplana, E., Becerro de Bengoa, C. and Zomeno, M. (1975). Endometrial and endocervical brushing techniques with a Medosha Cannula. *Acta Cytol.,* 19, 557–60

Koss L. G. (1968). *Diagnostic Cytology and its Histopathologic Bases,* 2nd edn Lippincott Philadelphia

Koudstaal, J. and Smid, L. (1974). Variant van de cytodiagnostische kleuring volgens Papanicolaou. *Tijdschrift voor medische Analisten,* 11, 397–8

Lopes Cardozo, P. (1975). *Atlas of Clinical Cytology,* Targa B. V. 's Hertogenbosch, Holland

Lukeman, J. M. (1974). An evaluation of the negative pressure "Jet Washing" of the endometrium in menopausal and postmenopausal patients. *Acta Cytol.,* 18, 462–71

Luna, L. G. (1968). *Manual of Histologic Staining Methods of Armed Forces Institute of Pathology,* 3rd edn, McGraw-Hill, New York

MacGregor, J. E., Fraser, M. E. and Mann, E. M. F. (1966). The cytopipette in the diagnosis of early cervical carcinoma. *Lancet,* i, 252–6

Papanicolaou, G. N. (1942). A new procedure for staining vaginal smears. *Science,* 95, 438–9

Pundel, J. P. (1950). *Les Frottis Vaginaux et Cervicaux,* Masson, Paris

Shorr, E. (1941). New technic for staining vaginal smears. III. Simple differential stain. *Science,* 94, 545–6

So-Bosita, J. L., Lebherz, T. B. and Blair, O. M. (1970). Endometrial jet washer. *Obstet. Gynec.,* 36, 287–93

Wyss, R., Vassilakos, P. and Riotton, G. (1975). *Beschreibung einer neuen Aspirations Methode mit 'Pistolet',* 4th edn, Arbeitstagung für klinische Zytologie, Wengen

The Cytological Diagnosis

A correct cytological diagnosis is dependent on an adequate specimen, properly fixed and stained (see chapter 15) and accurately screened. For a good understanding between clinician and cytologist the method of reporting is essential. The importance of uniformity and consistency cannot be overstressed. The cytological report should state the facts the doctor needs and should not include all the data the cytologist has collected (for example, relative proportion of cells with inflammatory changes). If a repeat smear is needed the time interval must be stated and whether any treatment should be given (for example, for trichomonas infection) before the smear is repeated.

In our laboratory we use a standard form for cytological reporting (figure 16.1). The form is devised for computerised data processing. The report to the doctor will include only the marked entries. For example a cytological report may read: 'Severe leucocytosis with trichomonads and dirty background. Conclusion: negative for epithelial atypia and malignancy.

When more than one disease is present, such as atypical reserve cells and dysplastic cells, both entries can be marked. The report to the doctor would then read: 'Atypical reserve cell hyperplasia *and* dysplasia'. When a differential diagnosis is appropriate, as between undifferentiated carcinoma and adenocarcinoma, the cytologist can put question marks after the entries. The report will read: 'Undifferentiated carcinoma *or* adenocarcinoma'. The novice cytologists will use many question marks and will thus issue many differential diagnoses. When they have gained more experience they will give more definite diagnoses, thus risking many mistakes. After this they will return to giving differential diagnoses, but now exclusively in those cases in which by their experience it is known that a definite cytological diagnosis is unwarranted.

We recommend

Repeat smear in 9–12 months for
C6 slight atypical reserve cell hyperplasia
C7 slight dysplasia
C15/16 slight atypia of endocervical or endometrial cells
Colposcopy and repeat smear in 6 months for
C8 moderate atypical reserve cell hyperplasia
C9 moderate dysplasia
Repeat smear in 3 months, colposcopy and biopsy for
C10 severe atypical reserve cell hyperplasia
C11 severe dysplasia
C17/18 moderate atypia of endocervical or endometrial cells.
Immediate histological investigation and colposcopy for
C11 severe dysplasia, keratinising type
C12 carcinoma *in situ*
C13/14 suspected invasive squamous carcinoma
C19/20 severe atypia of endocervical or endometrial cells

C21/22 suspected adenocarcinoma or adenocarcinoma
C24/25/26 cases with suspected or definite
undifferentiated malignancy

Both endocervical *and* endometrial histology
should be requested for
C15/16 slight or moderate atypia of endocervical cells
C17/18 slight or moderate atypia of endometrial cells

The method of reporting must be consistent and
understood by all users. Care must be taken that
there are no ambiguities which lead either to the
failure to understand that a lesion is malignant and
requires treatment or (equally bad) that a patient
with a benign lesion is treated for a non-existent
malignancy.

The doctor should be aware of the limitations
and pitfalls of cytology. For instance, the cytological diagnosis depends on the *scraping* of the
cervical epithelium. Cytological under-diagnoses
may occur when the lesion is ulcerated. Sometimes
the surface epithelium is not representative of the
true nature of the lesion. An illustrative example:
a 48-year-old woman without complaints had a
routine smear taken. Cytological diagnosis: carcinoma *in situ*. A biopsy, taken with the aid of
colposcopy, confirmed the diagnosis. In the cone
biopsy, however, a widespread invasive growth was
found. When the cytological diagnosis depends on
the spontaneous exfoliation of cells (endometrial
cells) gynaecological cytology is not efficient. This
is illustrated in the poor detection of endometrial

adenocarcinoma by cervical smears (see chapter
12). Perhaps the use of methods in which the
endometrial surface is scraped *directly* will be
more effective (see chapter 15). In some cases it is
not possible to predict whether the malignant cells
are from a carcinoma *in situ* or an invasive cancer.
In such cases it is wise to use the tentative diagnosis 'suspicious, for invasive carcinoma' and recommend a biopsy without delay.

The cytological diagnosis will be used by the
doctor in conjunction with the information from
the clinical history, physical examination, colposcopy, and other laboratory proceedures. A negative cytology report does not exclude malignancy.
Similarly, negative cytology is not a protection
against the development of cancer. The cytological
report should be viewed in perspective, that is,
realising that one is looking at one moment of an
unpredictable biological process. Cytology is well
suited for longitudinal studies, especially in conjunction with colposcopy, since it is simple, cheap
and non-invasive. These follow-up studies, however,
may cause anxiety. For many patients it is difficult
to understand that they have a lesion that is in
between cancer and non-cancer and that nobody
can as yet predict the course it will take. The
doctor has to play an important role in relieving
their anxiety and convincing them of the importance of returning for a repeat smear.

When cytology is handled in the right way and
interpreted with care it can be used as an indis-
pensable method for cancer control and as an
approach to the management of patients with
lesions of the uterine cervix.

A. Cytological Findings:

1. slight leucocytosis ☐
2. moderate leucocytosis ☐
3. severe leucocytosis ☐
4. trichomonads ☐
5. fungi, yeasts ☐
6. bacteria ☐
7. virus ☐
8. no columnar endocervical cells ☐
9. endometrial cells ☐
10. reserve cells ☐
11. atrophy ☐
12. metaplasia ☐
13. repair cells ☐
14. anucleate squames ☐
15. radiation effect ☐
16. too high karyopycnotic index ☐
17. inflammatory cell changes ☐
18. micropolyps ☐
19. nuclear enlargement ☐
20. necrosis ☐
21. lymphocytes, plasma cells
    reticulum cells ☐

B. Background:

1. clean background ☐
2. Proteinaceous diathesis ☐
3. with debris and fibrin ☐
4. with old blood ☐
5. fresh blood ☐
6. bacterial overgrowth ☐

C. Diagnosis:

1. neg. for atypia and malignancy ☐
2. no diagnosis: too sparse cellular material ☐
3. no diagnosis: no squamous cells ☐
4. no diagnosis: too severe leucocytosis ☐
5. no diagnosis: air-dried smear ☐

Changes of Squamous Epithelium:

6. slight atypical reserve cell hyperplasia ☐

7. slight dysplasia ☐
8. moderate atypical reserve cell hyperplasia ☐
9. moderate dysplasia ☐
10. severe atypical reserve cell hyperplasia ☐
11. severe dysplasia ☐
12. carcinoma *in situ* ☐
13. suspicious for squamous cell carcinoma ☐
14. squamous cell carcinoma ☐

Changes of Adenomatous Epithelium

15. slightly atypical endocerv. cells ☐
16. slightly atypical endometr. cells ☐
17. moderately atypical endocerv. cells ☐
18. moderately atypical endometr. cells ☐
19. severely atypical endocerv. cells ☐
20. severely atypical endometr. cells ☐
21. suspect for adenocarcinoma ☐
22. positive for adenocarcinoma ☐
23. positive for adenosquamous carcinoma ☐
24. atypical undifferentiated cells ☐
25. suspect for undiff. carcinoma ☐
26. positive for undiff. carcinoma ☐
27. other malignancy ☐

D. Recommended Investigations

1. endocervical aspiration ☐
2. endometrial aspiration ☐
3. histology ☐

E. Repeat

1. direct ☐
2. after treatment of inflammation ☐
3. after treatment with oestrogens ☐
4. after cessation of hormonal treatment ☐
5. after 12 months ☐
6. after 6 months ☐
7. after 3 months ☐

F. Other Findings

figure 16.1   A form for data input

Index

Part Two

Introduction

This atlas provides examples of the cytology encountered in routine practice and illustrates several of the less common patterns. We have not tried here to achieve completeness.
For the terminology, see *'Cytology of the Femal genital tract'* WHO, 1973. We hope the illustrations chosen will be a valuable aid in the classroom and a useful tool in daily cytodiagnostics.

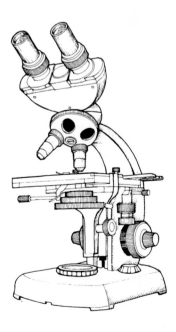

Contents

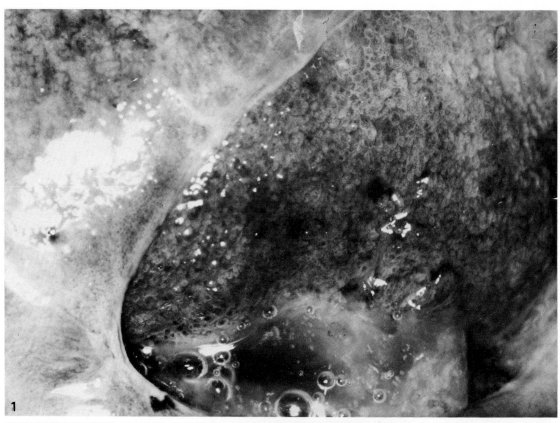

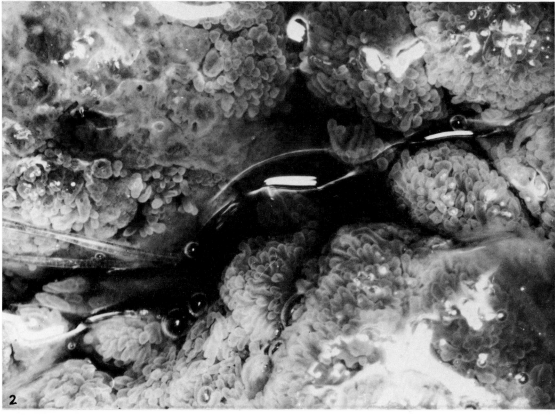

Colposcopy of the Normal Uterine Cervix

Ectocervix and external os (see section 2.2.3.1.).

1. The photograph shows a large portion of the anterior lip with the squamocolumnar junction (see section 2.2.3.2.). The area with columnar epithelium consists of fine villi (flocks). Careful inspection reveals that each villus has a fine regular net-like vascular pattern. To the left is the normal stratified squamous epithelium with fine subepithelial capillaries (lower left-hand corner) and a net-like vascular pattern (upper left-hand corner). (x 5)
Cytology and histology normal.

2. In this photograph the external os with the entrance to the endocervical canal is in the centre. Distinct folds (rughae) disappear within the endocervical canal. The flocks consist of columnar epithelium with a capillary in the middle which is masked by the acetic acid. In the upper left-hand corner metaplastic epithelium has appeared. (x 5)
After application of 3 per cent acetic acid.

Courtesy of Dr J.M. van Meir, Department of Gynecology and Obstetrics, Academisch Ziekenhuis, Rotterdam-Dijkzigt, The Netherlands.

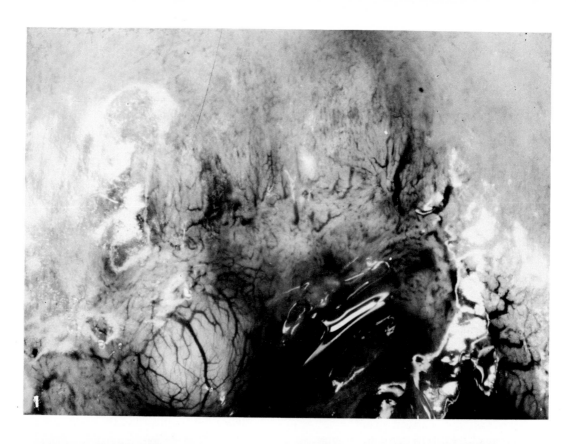

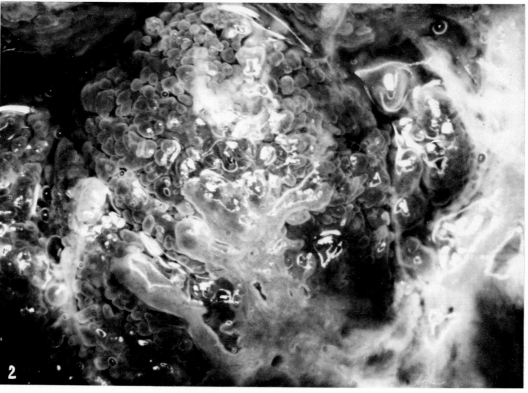

Colposcopy of Benign Changes in the Uterine Cervix

1. The photograph shows a portion of the anterior lip. The dark area (right) is the external os. The swelling on the left covered by a regular branched vascular pattern is a *Nabothian* or a *retention cyst* (see section 7.6.4.). The other pronounced, sometimes dilated, capillaries either branch out or form a net-like vascular pattern. This distinct vascular pattern is limited to the transformation zone. In the upper part of the photograph is a very fine net-like vascular pattern caused by the capillaries in the stroma under the stratified squamous epithelium. (x 5)
Histology: chronic cervicitis.

2. The external os is partly visible in the upper left-hand corner. Here rughae can be recognised. Fine as well as somewhat thicker flocks are visible. Finger-like branches of metaplastic epithelium can be seen extending from the lower right. The metaplastic epithelium replaces the columnar epithelium (see section 2.2.3.2). (x 5)
Cytology: normal.

Courtesy of Dr J.M. van Meir, Department of Gynecology and Obstetrics, Academisch Ziekenhuis, Rotterdam-Dijkzigt, The Netherlands.

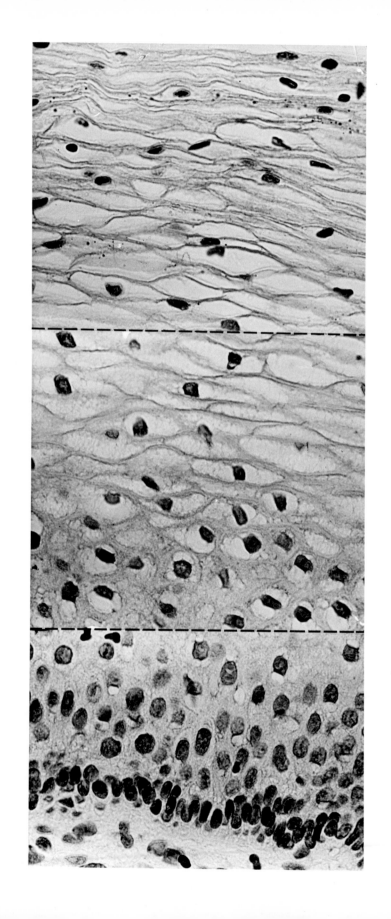

3

Benign Squamous Epithelium

Histology
Normal stratified squamous epithelium of the uterine cervix, fully matured (see section 2.3.1.1).

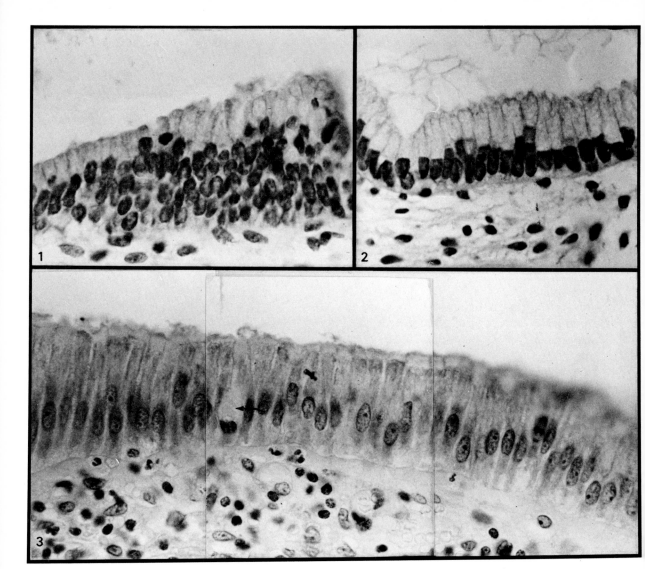

4

Benign Endocervical Epithelium

Histology
1. Reserve cell hyperplasia underneath endocervical columnar epithelium (see sections 2.3.2.1 and 7.4.1). (x 500)

2. Mucus-producing columnar endocervical epithelium. (x 500)

3. Columnar endocervical epithelium with ciliated cells. The arrow indicates a goblet cell.(x 500)

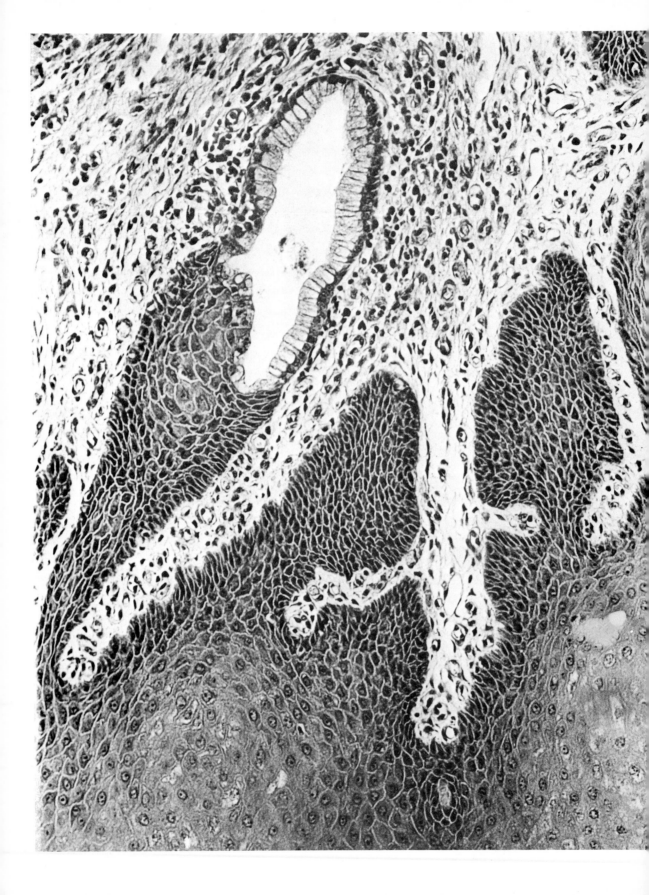

5

Metaplastic Epithelium

Histology
Maturing metaplastic epithelium extending
into endocervical gland (see section 7.4.2).
(x 500)

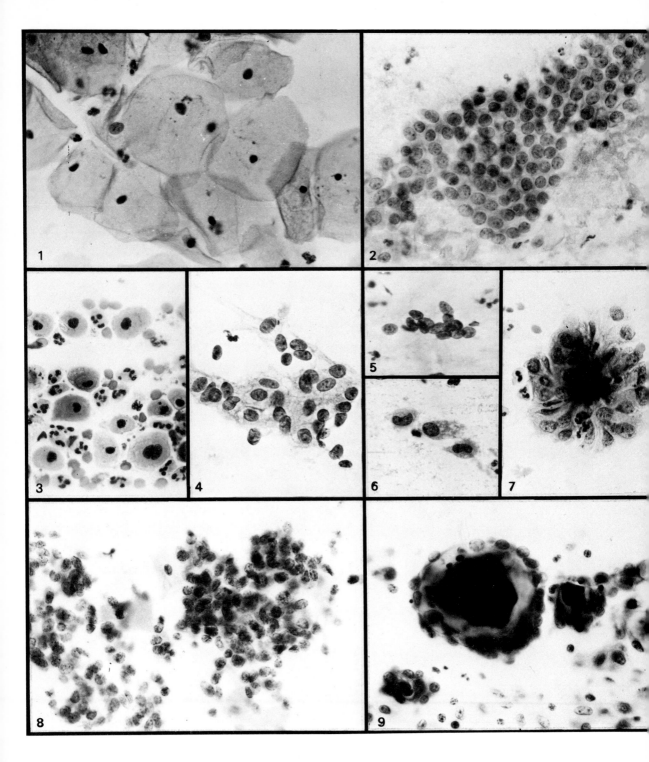

6

Benign Cells

1. Intermediate and superficial epithelial cells from the stratified squamous epithelium of the ectocervix (section 2.3.1.2). (x 500)

2. Endocervical columnar epithelial cells in a group; the nuclei form a typical regular honeycomb pattern (section 2.3.2.2). The group appears flat. (x 500)

3. Smear pattern of atrophic squamous epithelium (section 6.2.1.9). It consists mainly of parabasal cells; some cells have a pyknotic nucleus and markedly dense cytoplasm which stains orange, others have a pale enlarged nucleus and finely vacuolated cytoplasm. (x 500)

4. Primitive cells (reserve cells) such as often encountered in an atrophic smear pattern (vaginal as well as cervical) (sections 2.3.1.2 and 6.2.1.9) [A]. These cells have sparse poorly defined cytoplasm; the cell borders cannot be identified [B]. Compare with the cytoplasm of the cells in figures 5 and 6 of Plate 33. (x 500)

5. Reserve cells in an atrophic smear pattern. The cells are arranged in a row with ramifications. These cells have the characteristic reserve exfoliation pattern of cells (section 2.3.1.2). (x 500)

6. Histiocytes with a kidney-shaped nucleus and finely vacuolated cytoplasm with poorly defined borders. The nuclei contain obvious chromocentres. (x 500)

7. Histiocytes arranged around haematoidin crystals (cockleburrs) [C]. This could be incorrectly interpreted as a group of epithelial cells. (x 500)

8. Menstrual phase: numerous endometrial cells in the smear, some solitary and some arranged in groups. The highly irregular nuclei show a disorderly arrangement in contrast to the nuclei of endocervical epithelial cells. (x 500)

9. Menstrual phase. The endometrial cells lie in groups characterised by a dark zone in the centre surrounded by a lighter zone. (x 500)

[A] Graham, R.M. (1964). *The Cytologic Diagnosis of Cancer*. Saunders, Philadelphia and London, p.6

[B] Patten, S.F. (1969). *Diagnostic Cytology of the Uterine Cervix*. Williams and Wilkins, Baltimore, p.68

[C] The term 'cockleburr' is used by Hollander for haematoidin crystals in cervical smears. The typical cockleburr is a rosette-shaped crystalline aggregate of radially arranged needles which stain either pinkish or orange-red. These structures are usually surrounded by or lie among histiocytes. (Hollander, D.H. *et al.* (1974). Hematoidin Cockleburrs in cervico-vaginal smears. *Acta Cytol.*, **18**, 268–270)

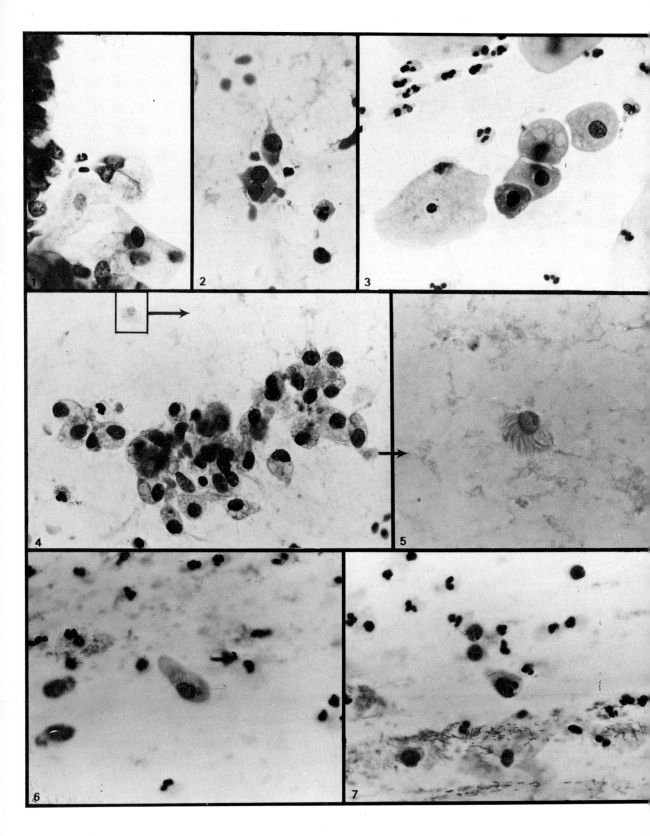

7

Benign Cells

1. Mucus-producing endocervical columnar cells (see section 2.3.2.2). (x 500)

2. Ciliated endocervical cells, one is binucleate. (x 500)

3. Metaplastic cells with mucus-containing vacuoles in the cytoplasm (see section 7.4.2.2). (x 500)

4. Endocervical cells with finely vacuolated cytoplasm and several ciliated tufts ciliacytophtoria or (C.C.P.) (see section 7.2.2.2). (x 500)

5. One tuft (see box in figure 4) magnified. (x 1000)

6, 7. Histiocytes, one with phagocytised material (see section 3.1.4). (x 500)

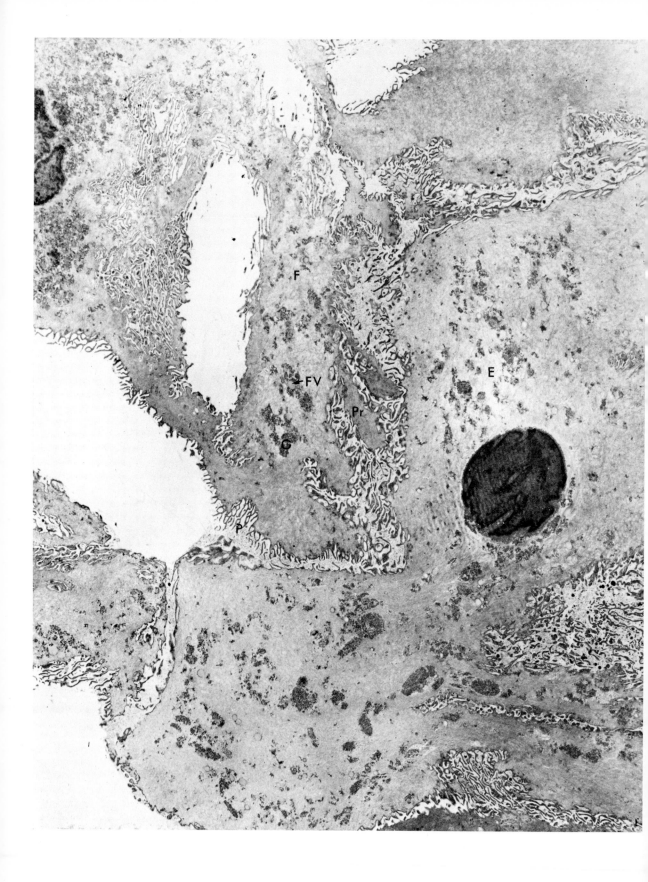

8

Transmission Electron Microscopy of Benign Cells

Electron micrograph of *superficial squamous cell* (see section 2.3.1.3). (x 4000) Polygonal cells that show numerous remnants of plasmodia (P) and plump cytoplasmic projections (Pr). The cytoplasm is poor in organelles but consists mostly of densely packed, fine fibrillar material (F) in which fatty vacuoles (FV), partly associated with electrondense granular (probably keratohyalinous) material (G) are seen. Around the nucleus the cytoplasm seems oedematous (E). The nucleus (N) is pyknotic, and shows indentations. Note the lack of a nuclear envelope.

Courtesy of Dr D.J. Ruiter and B.J. Mauw, Department of Pathology, University Medical Center, Leiden, The Netherlands.

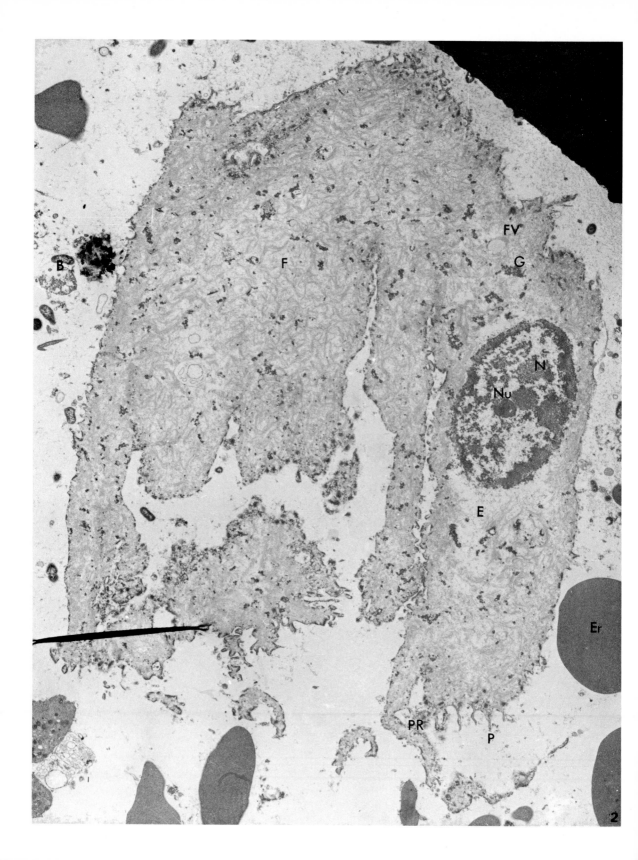

Transmission Electron Microscopy of Benign Cells

Electron micrograph of *intermediate squamous cell* (see section 2.3.1.3). (x 6000) The resemblance with the superficial cells (see Plate 8) is evident. Some rodlike plump bacteria (B) and erythrocytes (Er) are seen. In comparison with superficial cells more intact plasmodia (P) are seen. The nucleus (N) is larger and clearly less pyknotic than the nucleus of a superficial cell. A small nucleolus (Nu) can be seen. As in the superficial cell a nuclear envelope is lacking. No glycogen could be demonstrated.

Courtesy of Dr D.J. Ruiter and B.J. Mauw, Department of Pathology, University Medical Center, Leiden, The Netherlands.

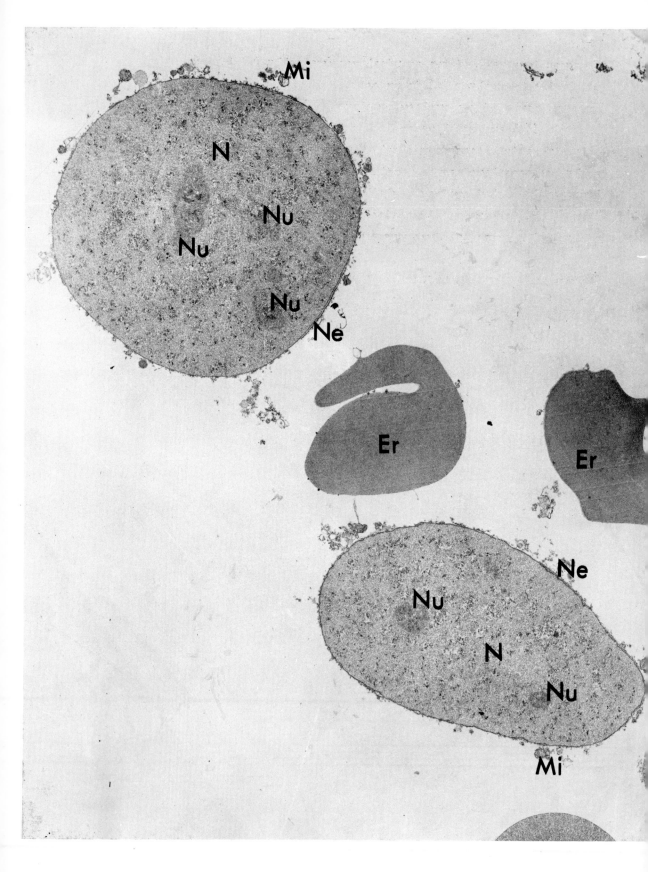

10

Transmission Electron Microscopy of Benign Cells

Electron micrograph of two reserve cells (see section 2.3.1.3). (x 10000) Only the nucleus (N) appears to be present. Further, parts of the nuclear envelope (Ne) and remnants of mitochondria (Mi) are recognisable. The nuclei consist completely of euchromatin. Nucleoli (Nu) are present. Compare the dimension of the nuclei of the two reserve cells with the two erythrocytes (Er).

Courtesy of Dr D.J. Ruiter and B.J. Mauw, Department of Pathology, University Medical Center, Leiden, The Netherlands.

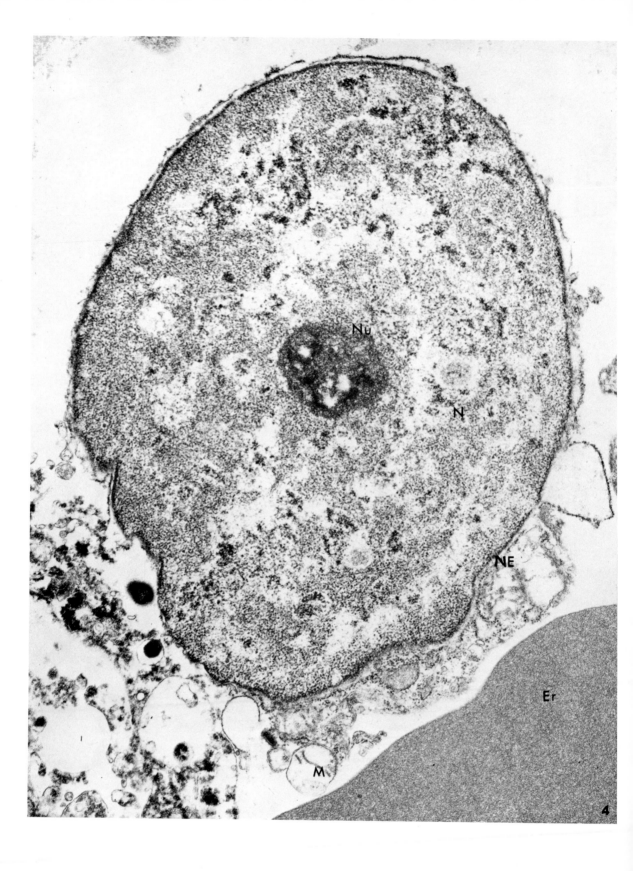

4

Transmission Electron Microscopy of Benign Cells

Electron micrograph of *reserve cell* (see section 2.3.1.3). (x 33000) Note remnants of cytoplasm with swollen mitochondria (M) and the intact nuclear envelope (NE). The nucleus (N) largely consists of euchromatin. The nucleolus (Nu) is inconspicuous.

Courtesy of Dr D.J. Ruiter and B.J. Mauw, Department of Pathology, University Medical Center, Leiden, The Netherlands.

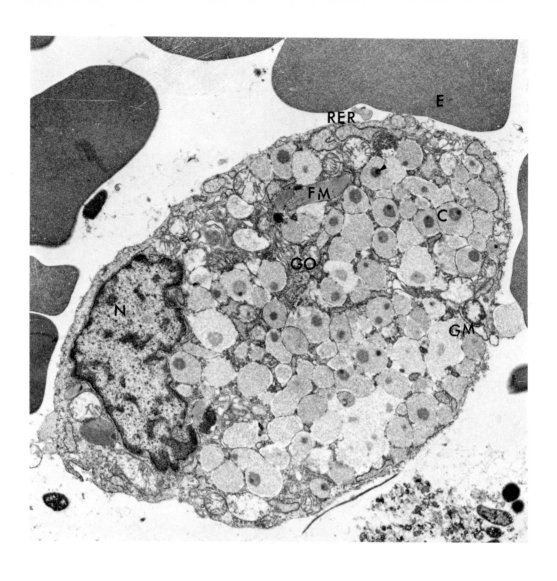

Transmission Electron Microscopy of Benign Cells

Electron micrograph of *endocervical colum-nar cell* (see section 2.3.2.3). (x 9250) Note oval cell shape, basally localised nuclues (N), numerous rounded vacuoles filled with granular mucinous material (GM) that fre-quently show an electron-dense core (C), sometimes with a still denser subcore (arrow). Another type of secretory material, that is, fibrillar mucine (FM) is seen. The rough endoplasmic reticulum (RER) is somewhat dilated.

Courtesy of Dr D.J. Ruiter and B.J. Mauw, Department of Pathology, University Medi-cal Center, Leiden, The Netherlands.

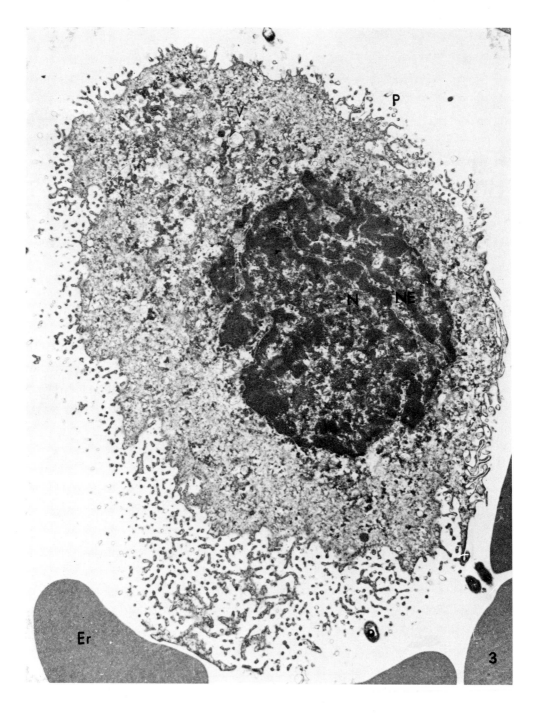

13

Transmission Electron Microscopy of Metaplastic Cells

Electron micrograph of a *metaplastic cell*. (× 12500) Note resemblance to superficial and intermediate squamous cells (section 7.4.2.4). A nuclear envelope is partly absent.

Courtesy of Dr D.J. Ruiter and B.J. Mauw, Department of Pathology, University Medical Center, Leiden, The Netherlands.

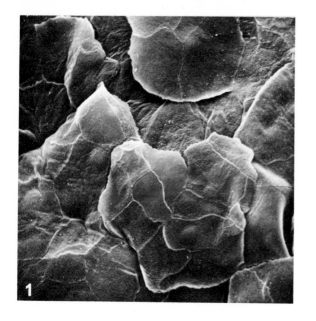

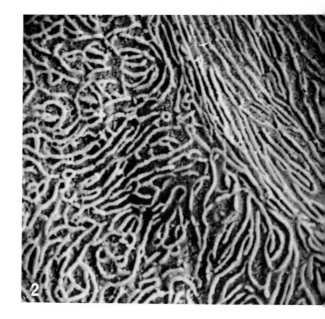

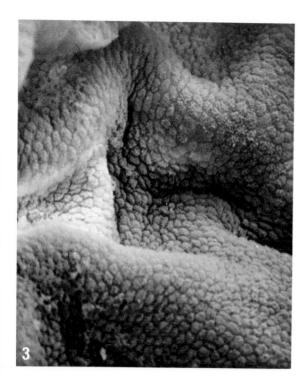

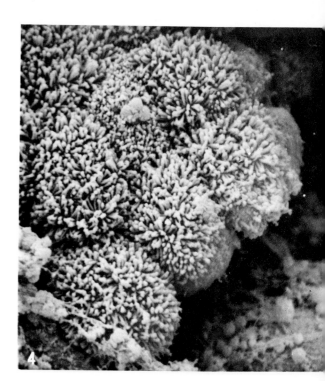

Scanning Electron Microscopy of the Exfoliating Surface of the Cervix

Benign squamous epithelium

1. The exfoliating surface of normal squamous epithelium is composed of cells arranged in flat polygonal mosaics. Some epithelial cells are on their way to being exfoliated. Note prominent nuclei in some cells. (x 400)

2. High-power view of the epithelial surface demonstrating a system of parallel, sometimes branched, convoluted microridges (see section 2.3.1.3). (x 9000)

Glandular epithelium

3. Surface of the natural glandular epithelium that covers the endocervical canal. The tightly-packed cells show a honeycomb arrangement. (x 400)

4. Detail of the surface of the glandular epithelium seen from the top at high magnification. (x 9000) Note the multiplicity of thin microvilli of similar size.

Courtesy of Dr C.A. Rubio, Department of Pathology, Karolinska Institute, Stockholm, Sweden.

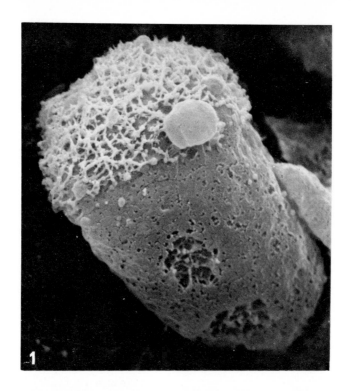

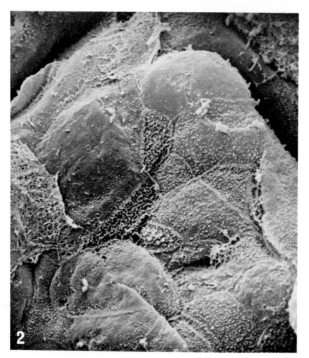

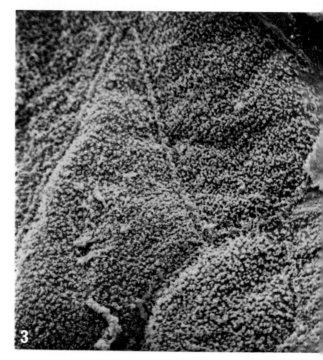

Scanning Electron Microscopy of the Exfoliating Surface of the Cervix

Glandular epithelium
1. Isolated columnar cell showing lateral walls and microvilli on top. One mucous 'ball' is apparent between the smooth and the villous zone. (x 10000)

Metaplastic epithelium (see section 7.4.2).
2. The surface of metaplastic epithelium has mosaic-like structures just like squamous epithelium. However, in the metaplastic epithelium the cells vary in size so the mosaics are irregular. Also sharp cellular borders are seen. (x 400)

3. High-power view of squamous metaplastic epithelium showing sparsely distributed rudimentary microvilli. (x 7000)

Courtesy of Dr C.A. Rubio, Department of Pathology, Karolinska Institute, Stockholm, Sweden.

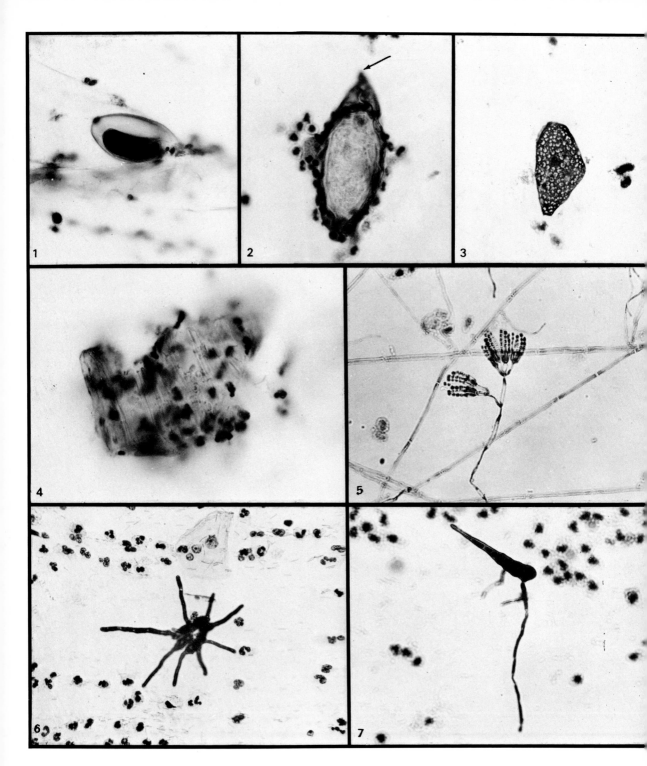

16

Contaminants

1. Ovum of *Enterobius vermicularis* (pinworm). Contaminant from the intestine [A]. (x 500)

2. Ovum of *Schistosoma haematobium*. The terminal spine of the ovum is indicated by an arrow. Contaminant from the urinary tract [A]. (x 500)

3. Pseudo-cyst contaminating the smear; patient had toxoplasmosis of the urinary tract. Note the small structures (the parasites) surrounded by a halo [B]. (x 500)

4. Part of a pubic louse (*Phthirus pubis*). Note the diagonal stripes across the body of the louse. These stripes stain bright yellow; the rest of the body is orange-pink with the Papanicolaou stain. Note the leucocytes clustered around the louse. The smear also contained legs belonging to this insect. Contamination from the external genitalia. (x 500)

5. Smear with many mycelia and conidophores, probably of a *Penicillium*. Note the bamboo structure of the hyphae. Contamination from the air. (x 500)

6, 7. *Alternaria*. Vivid brown macroconidia with hyphae [C] (section 3.2). Contimination from the air. (x 500)

[A] Koss, L.G. (1968). *Diagnostic Cytology and its Histopathologic Bases*. 2nd edn. Lippincott, Philadelphia, p. 161

[B] Cristobal, A. and Roset, G. (1976). Toxoplasma cysts in vaginal and cervical smears. *Acta Cytol.*, **20**, 285–286

[C] Soost, H.J. (1976). *Lehrbuch der klinischen Zytodiagnostik*, 2te aufl. Georg Thieme Verlag, Stuttgart, p. 54

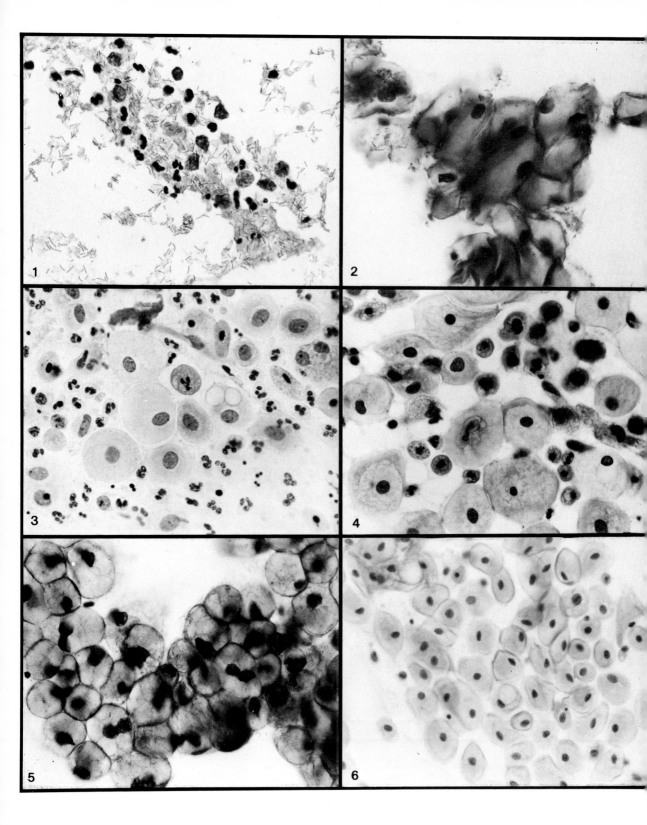

17

Hormonal Cytology

1. Pattern of cytolysis. Most of the cytoplasm of the intermediate cells has disappeared. Many *Lactobacilli vaginalis* (Döderlein's bacilli) are present. The naked nuclei lie separately in contrast to, for example, the nuclei of the reserve cells. (x 500)

2. Navicular cells in a smear from a pregnant woman. The intermediate cells appear squarish as a result of the concentration of glycogen in the cytoplasm. (x 500)

3. Smear containing predominantly parabasal cells from a 30-year-old woman who uses an oral contraceptive (see section (14.2.1.1). This type of smear is highly cellular. (x 500)

4. Atrophic smear pattern (section 6.2.1.9) from a 70-year-old female, 15 years after menopause. Compare with figure 3. (x 500)

5. Hypersecretion of endocervical cells in a smear of a woman who uses an oral contraceptive. Such hypersecretory cells are found mainly after hormonal stimulation (via drugs or during pregnancy [A]). (x 500)

6. Androgenic pattern. This smear was taken from a woman 5 years after menopause. The parabasal cells are rectangular; some cells contain glycogen. This woman showed other signs of virilisation, such as hair growth on the upper lip. (x 500)

[A] Novak, E.R. and Woodruff, J.D. (1974). *Gynecologic and Obstetric Pathology*. 7th edn, Saunders, Philadelphia, pp. 76–77

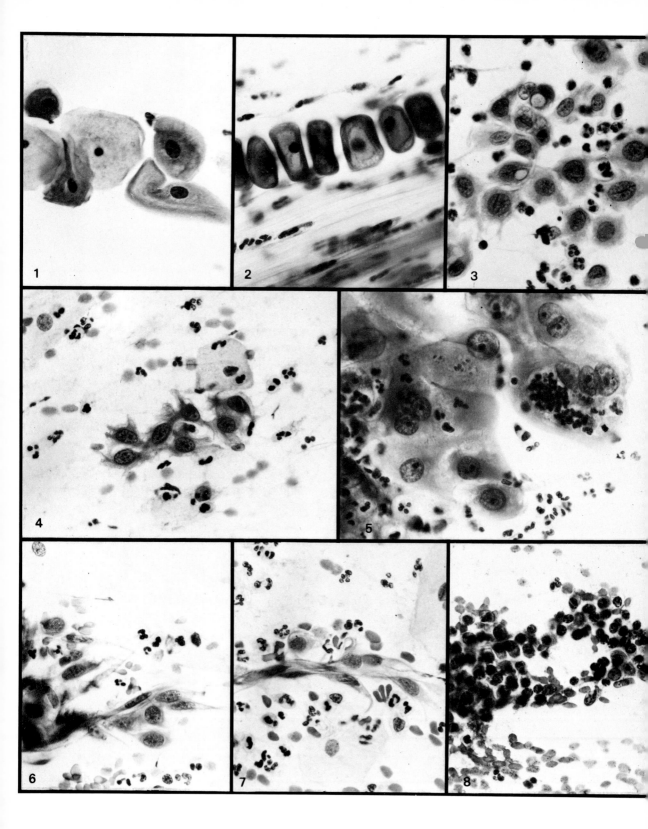

18

Metaplasia, Tissue Repair and Chronic Infection

1. Superficial squamous epithelial cells and several metaplastic squamous cells; the latter can be recognised by the dark outer zone and light inner zone in the cytoplasm. (x 500)

2. Metaplastic cells lying in a row. This exfoliation pattern is characteristic for metaplastic cells. (x 500)

3. Immature metaplastic cells, some with vacuolated cytoplasm. A mucous stain will domonstrate mucin in the vacuoles (section 7.4.2.2). (x 500)

4. Regenerative (primitve) cells in a smear one week after a hysterectomy. The nuclei have prominent nucleoli (section 7.5.2.2). (x 500)

5. Cells derived from a reparative process are conspicuous because of their prominent nucleoli. The cell borders are indistinct, the nuclear polarity is preserved [A]. The cells have abundant cytoplasm and the nuclei are large; multinucleation is frequent. Since the chromatin pattern has become slightly coarse, a repeat smear is recommended (for instance, within 6 months). (x 500)

6, 7. Fibroblasts from an ulceration. Note the oblong nuclei and the streaked appearance of the cytoplasm. (x 500)

8. Plasma cells and lymphocytes in a chronic infection. (x 500)

[A] Patten, S.F. (1969). *Diagnostic Cytology of the Uterine Cervix*. Williams and Wilkins, Baltimore, p. 40

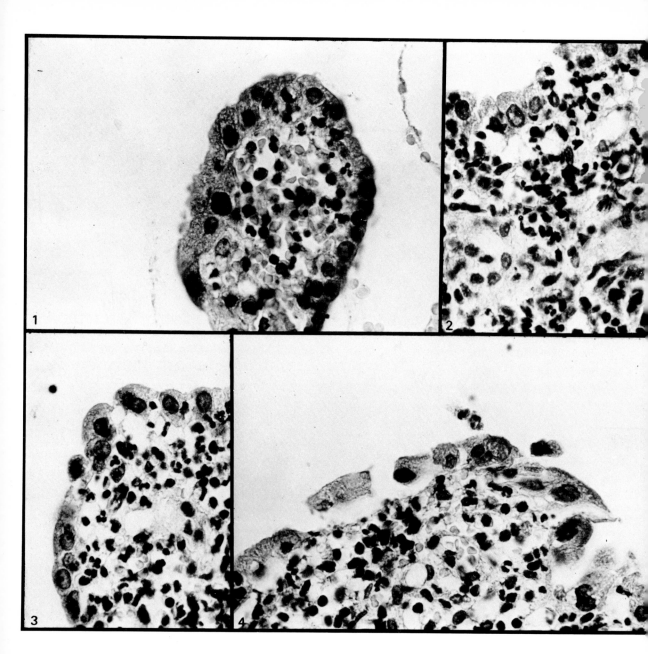

19

Endocervicitis

Histology

1, 2, 3, 4.   Atypia of endocervical columnar cells associated with repair in endocervicitis (see section 7.5.2). Note the
anisokaryosis, ample cytoplasm and
prominent nucleoli. (x 500)

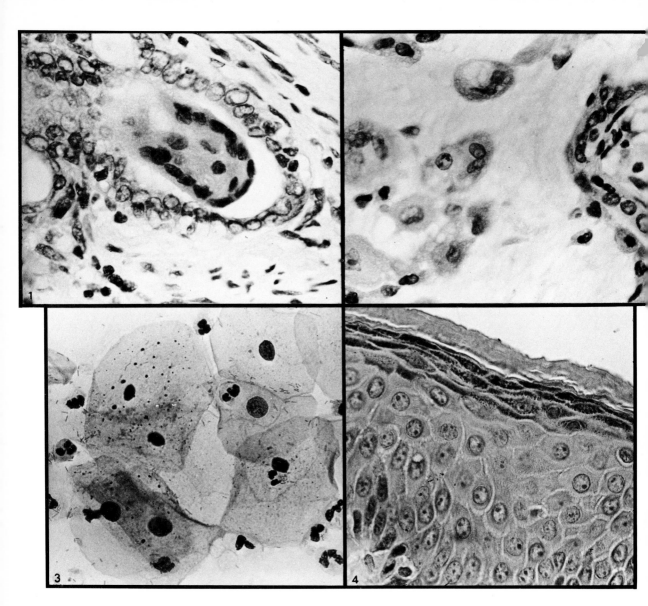

20

Benign Changes in the Cervix Uteri

1. Endocervical gland with a giant cell in the centre. (x 500)

2. A Nabothian cyst lined with flattened endocervical cells (right), and foam cells floating in the lumen (centre and left). These cells originate from the epithelial lining (see right) and change into foam cells in the mucous fluid of the cyst. (x 500)

3. Superficial cells with granulae derived from the granular cell layer (see sections 2.3.1.1 and 7.4.4.1) of hyperkeratotic squamous epithelium. A small number of these cells can be found in routine cervical smears (see section 2.3.1.2). (x 500)

4. Hyperkeratosis involving atrophic squamous epithelium (see section 7.4.4.3). Note granular cell layer. (x 500)

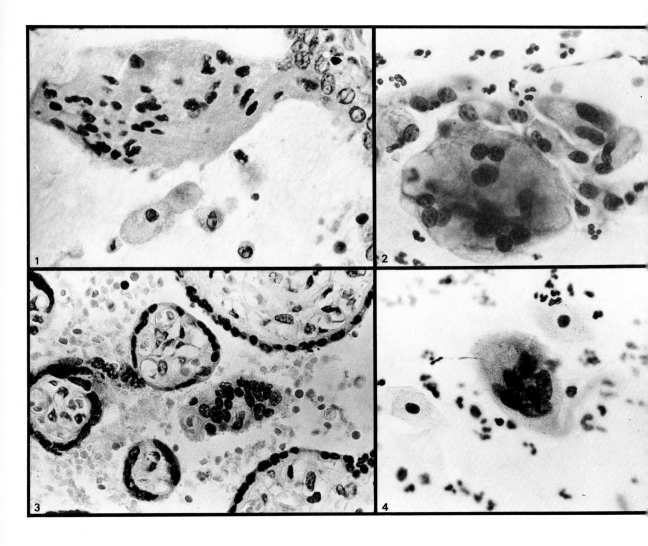

1

2

3

4

21

Giant Cells

1. The formation of a multinucleate cell in a Nabothian cyst (see section 7.6.4). Right: the epithelial lining from which the giant cell originates. Mononucleate cells with foamy cytoplasm can also be seen in the lumen. (x 500)

2. Cells from a Nabothian cyst. Note the foamy cytoplasm of the mononucleate cells (see section 7.6.4). (x 500)

3. Tissue section from an early placenta. Note syntrophoblast cell in the centre. (x 500)

4. Syntrophoblast cell in a cervical smear. Note the characteristic 'ground pepper' appearance of the chromatin (see section 3.3.1). (x 500)

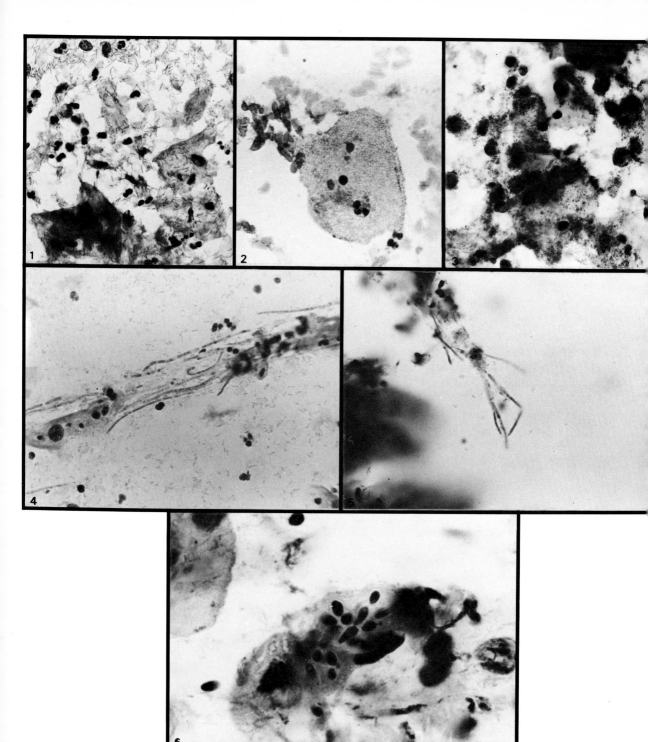

22

Inflammation

1. Döderlein flora (see section 7.3.1.1.). (x 500)

2. 'Clue cell' in *Haemophilus vaginalis* infection (see section 7.3.1.2). The squamous epithelial cell is covered with a cloud of bacteria, while relatively few bacteria are seen in the background. (x 500)

3. Coitus effect (see section 7.3.1.2). Prior to coitus there was a Döderlein flora, while the smear depicted here (taken 16 hours after coitus) displays an overgrowth of coccoid bacteria and a flase high karyopyknotic index. (x 500)

4, 5. Hyphae of *Candida vaginalis*. Note branching in figure 5 (see section 7.3.4). (x 500)

6. Magnification of spores of *Candida vaginalis*. (x 1250)

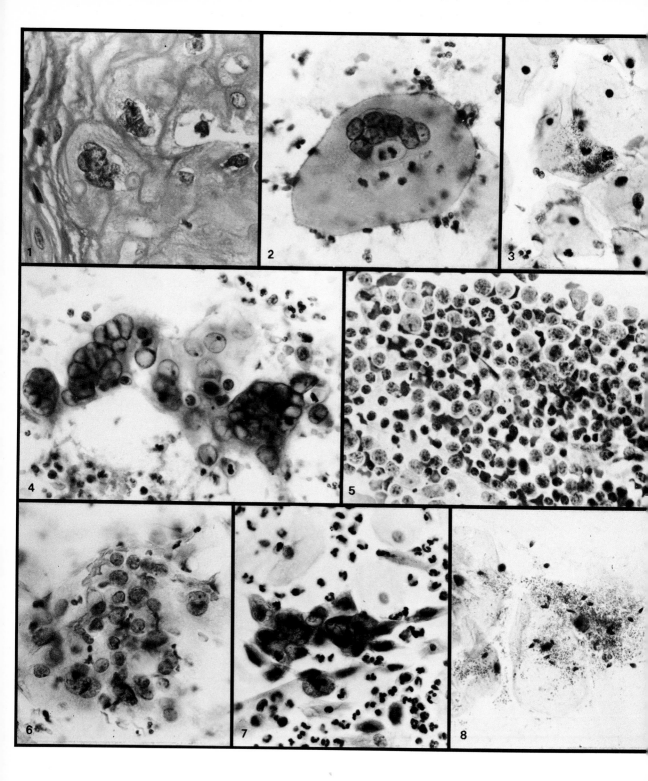

23

Inflammation

1. Cervical biopsy showing several multinucleated cells with abundant cytoplasm. Other portions of the biopsy which were not as deep showed koilocytotic atypia ('koilos' means hollow). These changes can be attributed to viral infection [A] (section 7.3.5.2). (x 500)

2. A similar multinucleated cell with abundant cytoplasm in the smear (same patient as in figure 1). The cytoplasm appears opaque and granular. (x 500)

3. Intracellular diplococci. In such a case, a specific culture for gonococci is recommended. (x 500)

4. Cellular changes in herpes simplex infection. Note the multinucleation, nuclear moulding and the ground-glass aspect of the nuclei. The ground-glass aspect is caused by invasion of the nucleus by the virus [B]. (x 500)

5. Chronic lymphocytic cervicitis (section 7.2.3.1). Numerous lymphoid cells, plasma cells and reticulum cells. Mitotic figures occur. (x 500)

6. Multinucleation and anisonucleosis of the columnar cells of the endocervix in a case of endocervicitis (section 7.2.2.2). (x 500)

7. Metaplastic cells with inclusions surrounded by halos in the cytoplasm. The inclusions are probably a manifestation of a *Chlamydia* infection (section 7.3.5.3). (x 500)

8. A smear with a normal cellular pattern and a 'clean' background contained a small spot filled with spermatozoa and many diplococci. It is possible that this woman's sexual partner has urethritis (gonococcal infection?). (x 500)

[A] Novak, E.R. and Woodruff, J.D. (1974). *Gynecologic and Obstetric Pathology*. 7th edn, Saunders, Philadelphia, pp. 94, 105

[B] Koss, L.G. (1974). *Diagnostic Cytology and its Histopathologic Bases*. 2nd edn. Lippincott, Philadelphia, p. 163

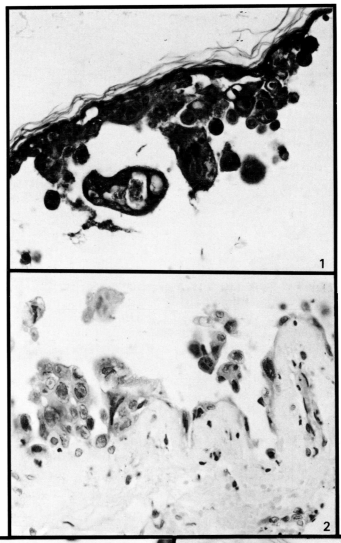
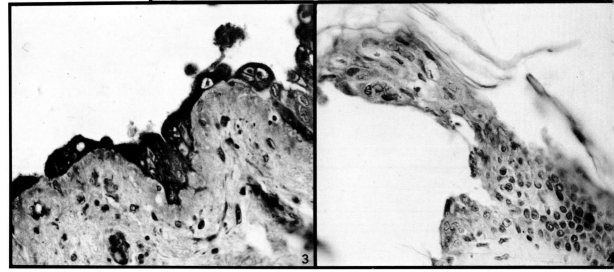

24

Herpesvirus Infection

Immunostaining on tisue sections

1, 3. Squamous epithelium immunostained for herpesvirus with perioxidase-labelled antibodies (black in this photography). 1. upper part of vesicle; 3. basal part of vesicle. (x 125)

2. Virus-affected cells in upper part of vesicle. Note ground-glass appearance of nuclei, inclusion bodies and multi-nucleated giant cells (see section 7.3.5.1). (x 125)

4. Outer border of vesicle. Note difference of nuclear pattern of affected and non-affected epithelial cells. (x 125)

Courtesy of Dr. J. Lindeman, Deprtment of Pathology, S.S.D.Z., Delft, The Netherlands.

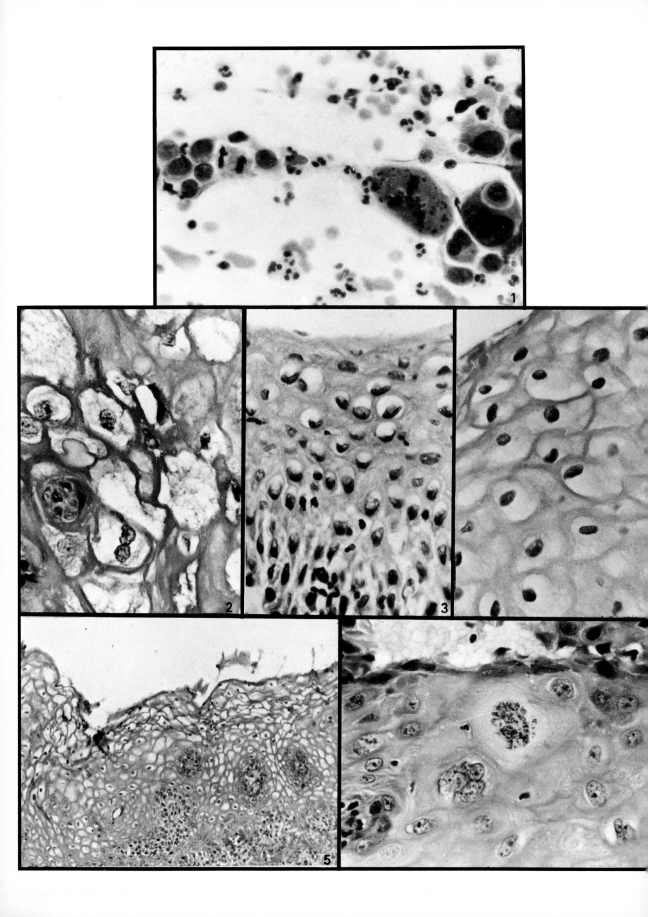

25

Condylomata Acuminata

Differential diagnosis of a koilocytotic halo

1. Tripolar mitotic figure (right) and bipolar mitotic figure (left) in smear from a patient with a condylomatous lesion concomitant with carcinoma *in situ*. Note the lagging chromosomes in the tripolar spindle. (x 500)

2. Koilocytosis in biopsy of condylomata acuminata. Note the multinucleation and the scalloped outline of the clear zone (see section 7.3.5.2). (x 500)

3. Perinuclear halo's due to tissue shrinkage. (x 500)

4. Perinuclear glycogen storage in the squamous epithelium in pregnancy. (x 500)

5. Lacy appearance of koilocytotic epithelium of flat condyloma. (x 125)

6. Polyploid mitotic figure in the smear of a patient with a condylomatous lesion. Note the abnormally large number of chromosomes. (x 500)

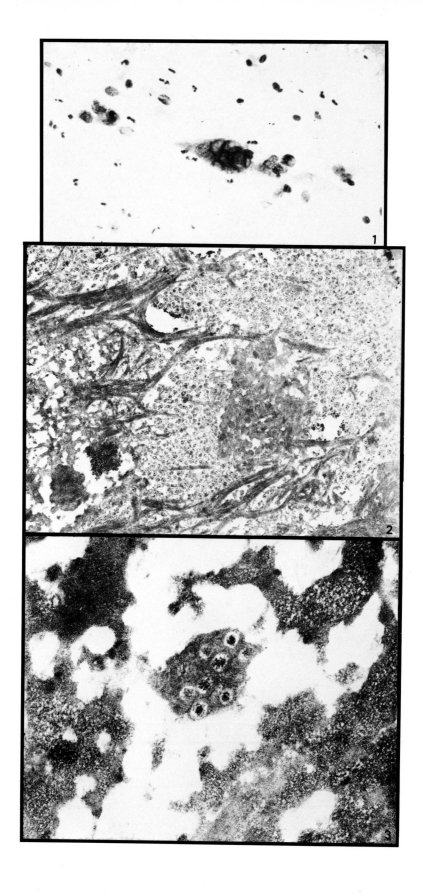

26

Transmission Electron Microscopy of Herpesvirus Particles

1. Multinucleated giant cell in a routine cervical smear consistent with the diagnosis of herpesvirus infection (see section 7.3.5.1). (x 500)

2. Herpesvirus particles in a cell reprocessed for electron microscopy from a routine cervical smear. (x 11 200)

3. Note the electrondense core in the centre of the virus particles and compare the morphology of these with the papilloma virus particles (plate 27). (x 69 500)

Courtesy of Dr C.R. Laverty, Department of Pathology, King George V Hospital, Sydney, Australia.

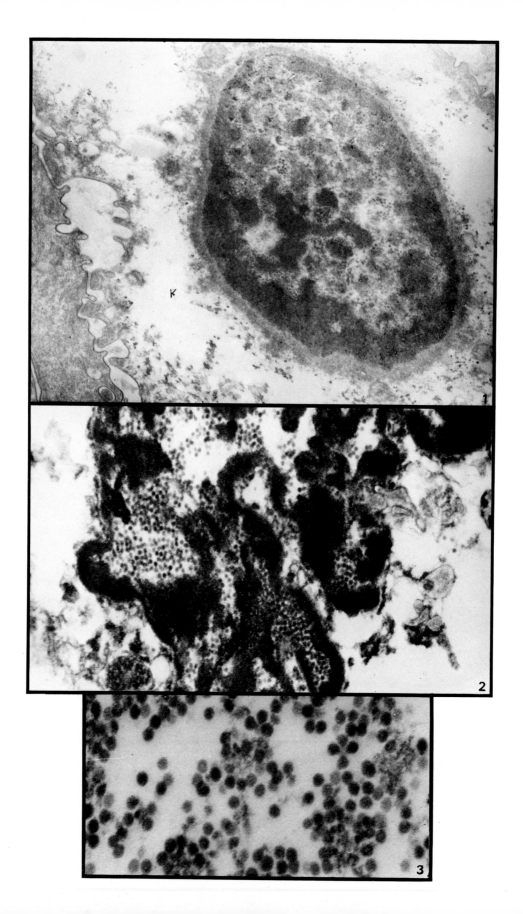

27

Transmission Electron Microscopy of Papillomavirus Particles

1, 2, 3.   Colposcopically selected biopsies fixed with glutaraldehyde from condylomatous flat cervical lesions. The viral infection was originally detected by the occurrence of koilocytotic cells in the routine cervical smear (see section 7.3.5.2).

1. Electron micrograph of the nucleus of a koilocytotic squamous epithelial cell. (x 18300). The koilocytotic halo is seen as a large clear zone (K) in the electron microscope, almost completely lacking cytoplasmic components. Note the occurrence of intranuclear virus particles (40–50 nm in diameter) either elongated or lobulated in shape, consistent with the diagnosis of papillomavirus.

2. Same cell x 50 000.

3. Same cell x 100 000.

Papillomavirus particles can also be demonstrated in alcohol-fixed routine cervical smears.

Courtesy of Dr C.R. Laverty, Department of Pathology, King George V Hospital, Sydney, Australia.

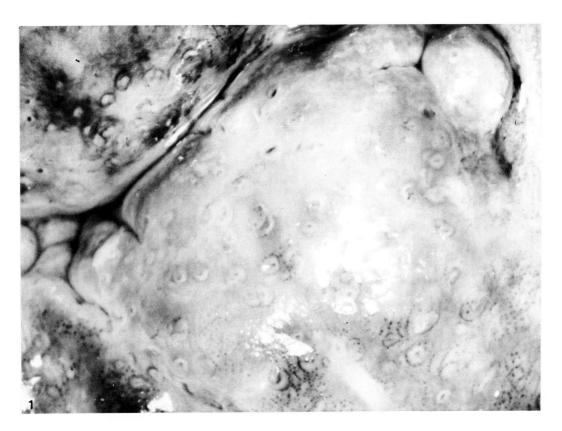

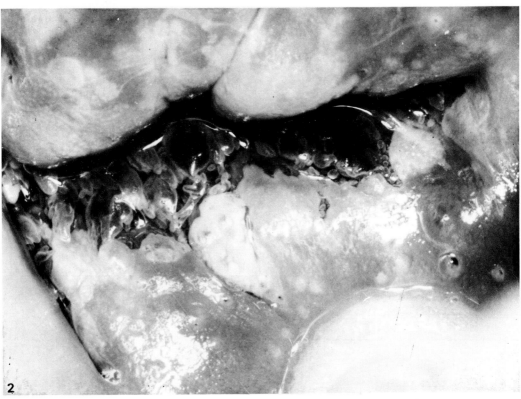

28

Colposcopy of Dysplastic Lesions

1. The external os crosses the upper left-hand corner, thus to the left is part of the anterior lip and to the right the posterior lip. A *punctuation pattern* is clearly visible at the bottom. It is striking that the entire region is completely white; this is compatible with an increased nuclear density of the epithelium. Close to the centre and also on the anterior lip are gland openings with a broad white rim and a strip in the middle which is the actual gland opening. The white epithelium with the gland opening indicates the presence of mature metaplastic epithelium. (x 5)

Cytological diagnosis: severe dysplasia. Biopsies taken from both the anterior and posterior lip close to the external os showed the histological pattern of a severe dysplasia. The portio was swabbed with 3 per cent acetic acid.

2. The photograph shows the external os with distinct thick flocks, which vary markedly in shape and size on the anterior lip. White epithelium is scattered over the posterior as well as the anterior lip. Biopsies were taken from both lips precisely at the transition from white (metaplastic) epithelium to columnar epithelium. (x 5)

Cytology: mild dysplasia. Histology: chronic cervicitis with mild dysplasia.

Courtesy of Dr J.M. van Meir, Department of Gynecology and Obstetrics, Academisch Ziekenhuis, Rotterdam-Dijkzg, The Netherlands.

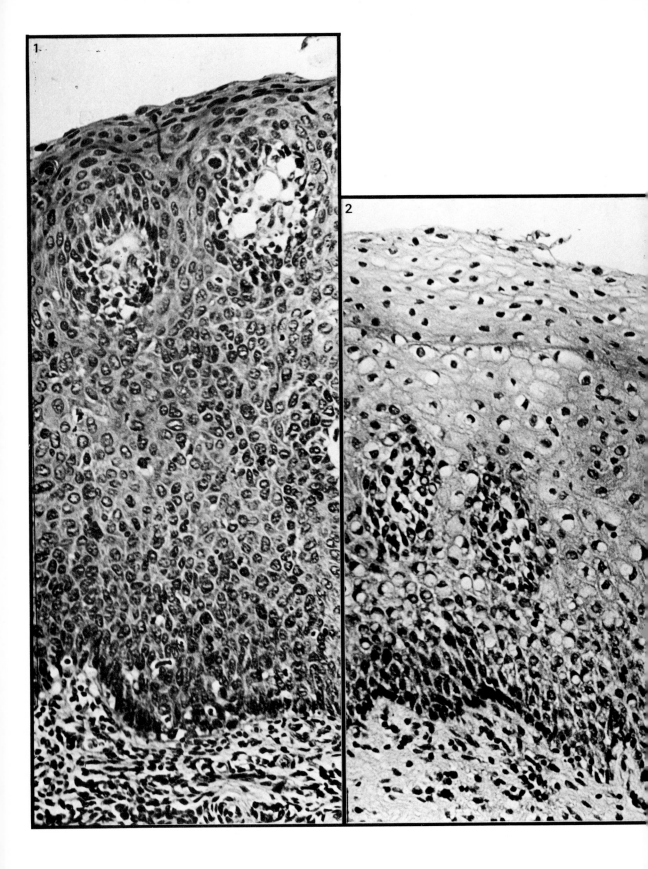

29

Vascularisation Patterns in Dysplastic and Metaplastic Epithelium

1. Stroma with small capillaries is found in the upper part of this dysplastic epithelium. The intraepithelial capillaries are seen with the colposcope as a punctate pattern (see section 10.5.2.2).

2. The stroma with small capillaries is only found in the lower half of this benign metaplastic epithelium. Tissue section from the transformation zone.

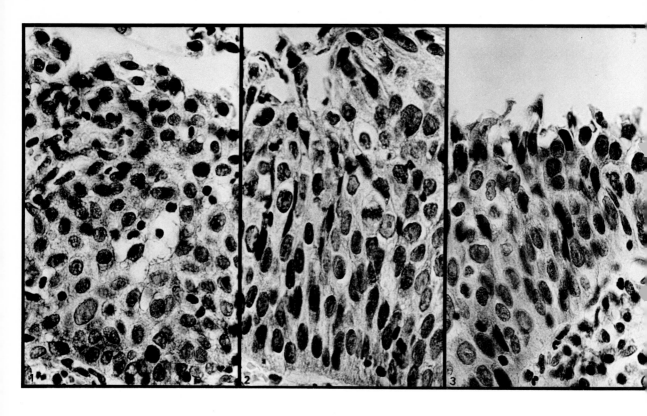

30

Atypical Reserve Cell Hyperplasia

Histology

1, 2, 3. Atypical reserve cell hyperplasia. All cell layers consist of primitive cells with hazy, ill-defined cytoplasm without signs of squamoid differentiation. (x 500)

1. Note the blandness of the chromatin pattern, the striking anisokaryosis and the prominent nucleoli.

2, 3. These cases will be undoubtedly classified as carcinoma *in situ* by some pathologists, by others as 'borderline' cases (see section 10.2.1.3). One can observe nuclei with bland chromatin patterns (compare with figure 1) adjacent to nuclei showing a granular chromatin pattern. Note mitotic figures.

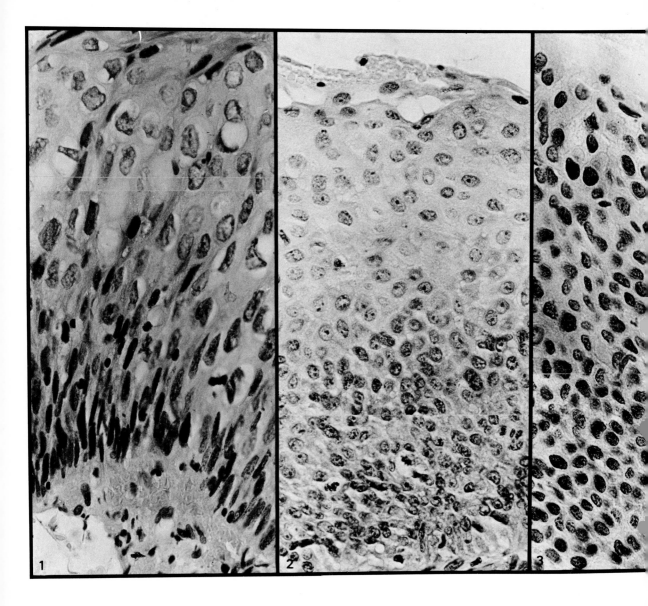

31

Dysplasia

Histology

1. Dysplasia, severe. Note the squamoid differentiation of the (dense) cytoplasm and the relatively favourable nucleo-cytoplasmic ratios in the upper layers (see section 10.2.2.1). (x 500)

2. Dysplasia, moderate. The cytoplasm is less dense in comparison with figure 1, but remains clearly defined. The nuclear density is high in the deep zone and low in the upper part of the epithelium. (x 500)

3. Dysplasia, severe. The cytoplasm resembles that seen in figure 2; however, hyperchromasia is more pronounced and the nuclear density in the superficial zone of the epithelium is high. (x 500)

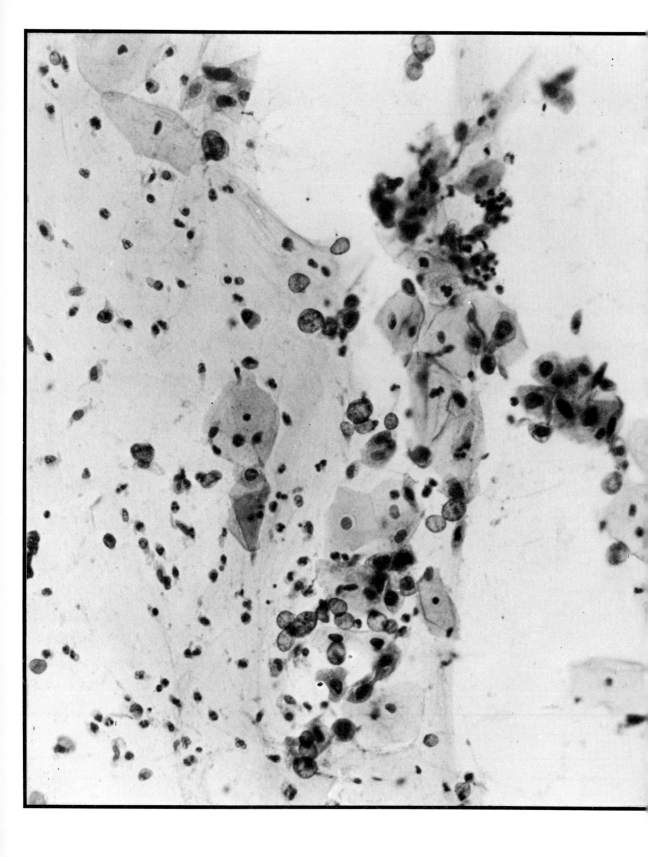

32

Exfoliation Pattern of Atypical Reserve Cells

Identification of atypical reserve cells in a cervical smear at screening magnification. Note the hypochromasia and the characteristic exfoliation pattern (see section 10.2.1.2). (x 125)

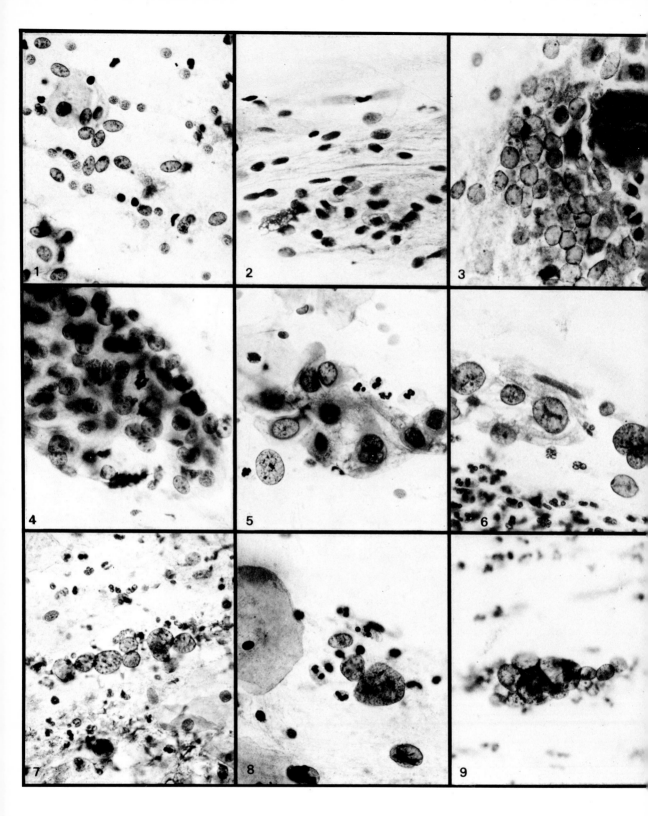

Atypical Reserve Cells

Cytology

1. Reserve cells in an atrophic vaginal smear from a 70-year-old female. Note the side-by-side arrangement of the naked nuclei and the lack of anisokaryosis. (x 500)

2. Naked degenerated nuclei; the chromatin structure is not visible. It is impossible to classify these cells [A]. (x 500)

3. Several endocervical columnar ciliated cells, including some reserve cells. The latter show mild anisokaryosis; they are slightly larger than those seen in figure 1. The arrangement in rows and clumps with nuclear moulding is characteristic for reserve cells (see plate 6) [A]. (x 500)

4. A group of slightly atypical reserve cells of the monomorphic type. We classify these cells as slightly atypical on the basis of the mitotic figures and the slight condensation of the chromatin network. The cytoplasm is sparse with ill-defined borders [A]. (x 500)

5. Atypical reserve cells with hazy cytoplasm or none at all. Anisokaryosis is rather pronounced here [A]. (x 500)

6. Atypical reserve cells with sparse cytoplasm which surrounds the nucleus like a veil. To the right are several naked atypical reserve cells [A]. (x 500)

7. Characteristic arrangement of naked atypical reserve cells in a row. The cells display anisokaryosis and slight clumping of chromatin [A]. (x 500)

8. Naked atypical reserve cells arranged side by side. Anisokaryosis and macronucleoli are conspicuous here [A]. (x 500)

9. Atypical reserve cells in a solid clump with a three-dimensional aspect (as a result some of the nuclei are not in sharp focus). There is marked anisokaryosis [A]. (x 500)

[A] Beyer-Boon, M.E. and Verdonk, G.W. (1975). Atypical reserve cell hyperplasia and the development of squamous cell carcinoma of the cervix. *5th European Congress of Cytology, Milan*

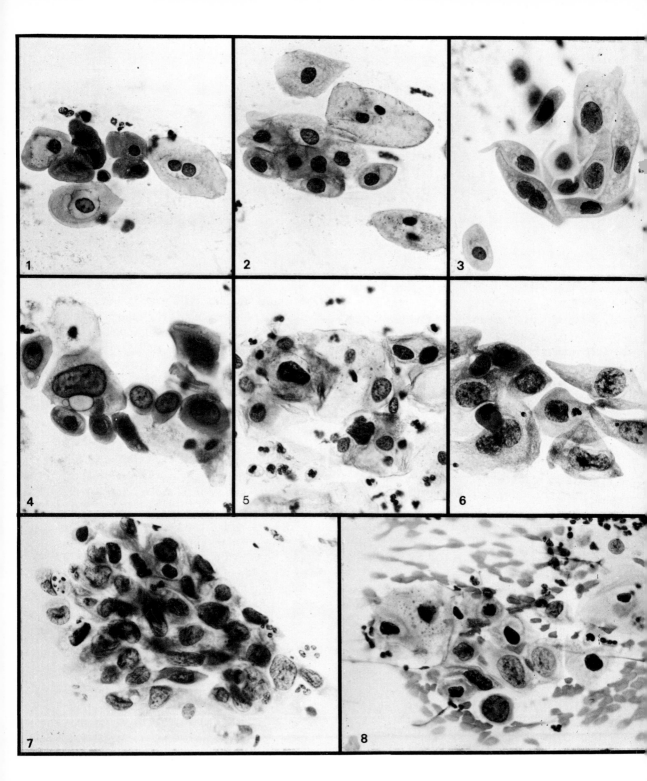

34

Dysplasia

Cytology

1. Mild dysplasia. There is slight coarsening of the chromatin, hyperchromasia and multinucleation. (x 500)

2. Mild dysplasia. There is some granulation of the chromatin. (x 500)

3. Mild dysplasia. The nuclei are enlarged. The chromatin pattern is, however, quiescent and there is little hyperchromatism. (x 500)

4. Moderate dysplasia. Several nuclei are markedly enlarged and there is some condensation of the chromatin at the nuclear border. (x 500)

5. Moderate dysplasia. There is obvious hyperchromatism and coarsening of the chromatin pattern. The clumps of chromatin are about equal in size. (x 500)

6. Moderate dysplasia. In addition to slight coarsening of the chromatin, small nucleoli can also be seen in the nuclei. (x 500)

7. Severe dysplasia. The cells have little cytoplasm; the cell boundaries are still clearly visible. Obviously polychromatic nuclei. (x 500)

8. Severe dysplasia. Varying amounts of cytoplasm and variable staining of the nuclei. (x 500)

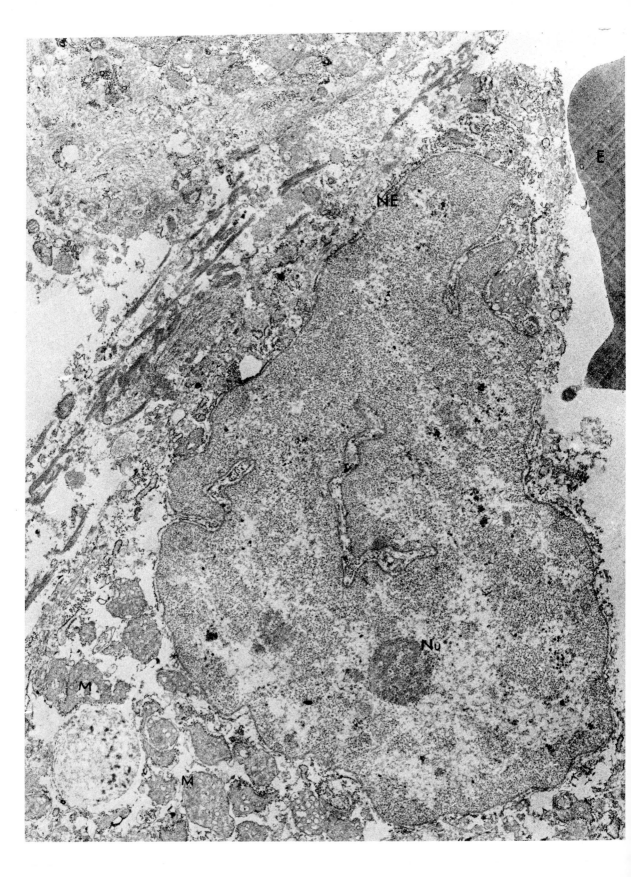

35

Transmission Electron Microscopy of Atypical Reserve Cells

Electron micrograph of a highly atypical reserve cell (x 1500); uranyl acetate and lead citrate. Note the irregular nuclear contour and the nucleolus (Nu) (see section 10.2.1.5. The nuclear envelope (NE) is intact. The cytoplasm is damaged due to the smear procedure. Mitochondriae (M) can be discerned. F = fibrin; E = erythrocyte

Courtesy of Dr D.J. Ruiter and B.J. Mauw, Department of Pathology, University Medical Center, Leiden, The Netherlands.

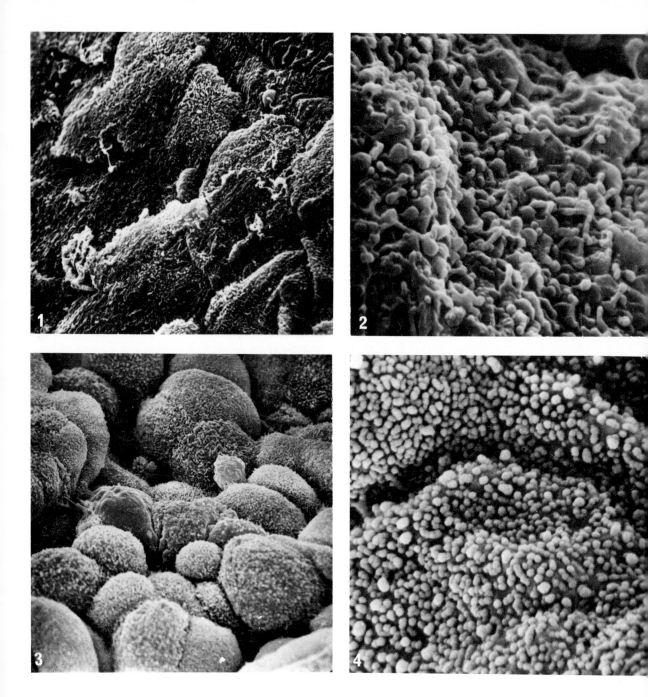

Scanning Electron Microscopy of the Exfoliating Surface of Dysplasia and Carcinoma *in situ*

Dysplasia
1. The dysplastic epithelium shows irregular, in contrast to the normal squamous or slightly emerging cobblestone-like structures and diffuse cellular borders. (x 900)

2. At high magnification the cellular surface shows clubbed appendages and fragmented microridges with thick free borders which resemble drumsticks. (x 10000)

Carcinoma *in situ*
3. The epithelial surface of carcinoma *in situ* demonstrates irregular spherical cobblestone-like structures. These are separated by deep furrows. (x 900)

4. At high power the cells are furnished with short, closely packed microvilli, sometimes in rows. (x 10000) It remains obscure whether these rows of microvilli are the expression of fragmented microridges.

Courtesy of Dr C.A. Rubio, Department of Pathology, Karolinska Institute, Stockholm, Sweden.

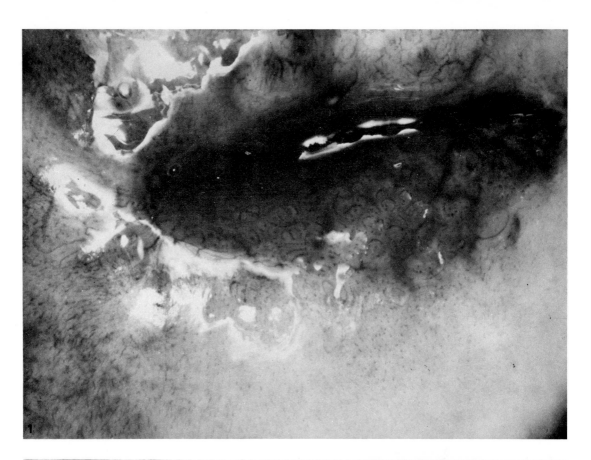

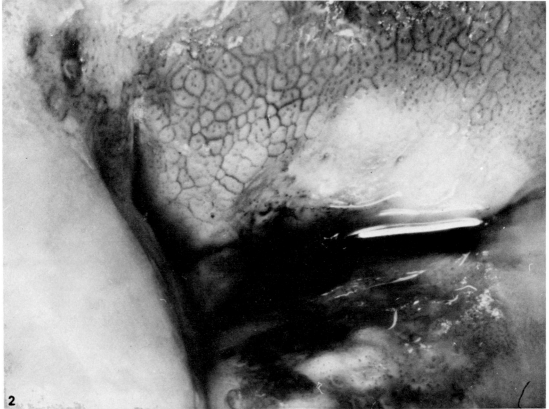

37

Colposcopy of Malignant Lesions

1. The photograph shows the external os, part of the posterior lip and a small part of the anterior lip. The interesting aspect of this photograph is the so-called *mosaic structure* and the punctation pattern in the transformation zone (posterior lip) which extends into the endocervical canal. Although less clearly defined, part of the transformation zone can be seen on the anterior lip. As far as the vascular pattern beneath the squamous epithelium is concerned, on the right it consists of very fine stipples which are in fact very fine capillaries perpendicular to the surface. Toward the left the course of these capillaries becomes more oblique. (x 5) Cytological diagnosis: carcinoma *in situ*. A biopsy taken from the posterior lip, the region containing the mosaic structure, showed a carcinoma *in situ*. A biopsy taken from the anterior lip close to the external os was found to contain metaplasia.

2. In the middle of the photograph is the split-shaped external os. Note the *mosaic structure and punctation pattern* on the upper lip. The mosaic structure is polygonal, sometimes diamond-shaped with a rather fine structure and a smooth surface. On the lower lip the punctation pattern in the white epithelium is not as distinct. (x 5) Cytological diagnosis: severe dysplasia. Three biopsies were taken. A biopsy from the posterior lip in the white area containing the fine punctation pattern yielded a diagnosis of carcinoma *in situ*. The other two biopsies were obtained from the mosaic structure of the anterior lip, specifically on the far left (11 o'clock) and the far right (12 o'clock). Both showed micro-invasive carcinoma with 2 mm invasion.

Courtesy of Dr J.M. van Meir, Department of Gynecology and Obstetrics, Academisch Ziekenhuis, Rotterdam-Dijkzigt, The Netherlands.

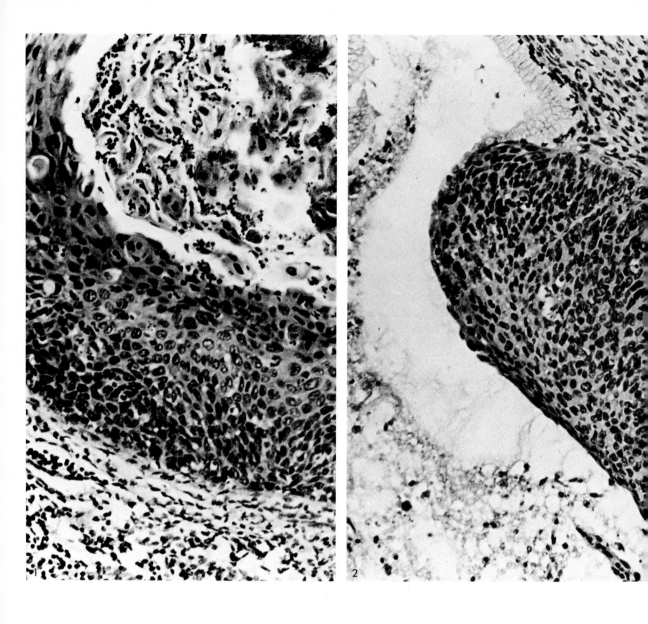

38

Epidermoid Carcinoma *in situ* of the Uterine Cervix

Involvement of the endocervical glands

1. The endocervical columnar epithelium is completely replaced by cells with abnormal hyperchromatic nuclei. The N/C ratio of these cells is high. In the superficial zone there is some squamous differentiation of the cytoplasm. Because of this some pathologists may classify this lesion as marked keratinising (pleomorphic) dysplasia [A] (see section 10.2.2.4). In the lumen abnormal cells exfoliate with hyperchromatic nuclei and squamoid cytoplasm, originating from the upper layers of the lining epithelium.

2. The endocervical epithelium is completely replaced by undifferentiated cells with abnormal, hyperchromatic nuclei without any signs of squamoid differentiation. These cells do not exfoliate spontaneously as easily as squamoid cells (only lower right part of the photograph).

[A] Patten, S.F. (1978). *Diagnostic Cytopathology of the Uterine Cervix*. Karger, New York

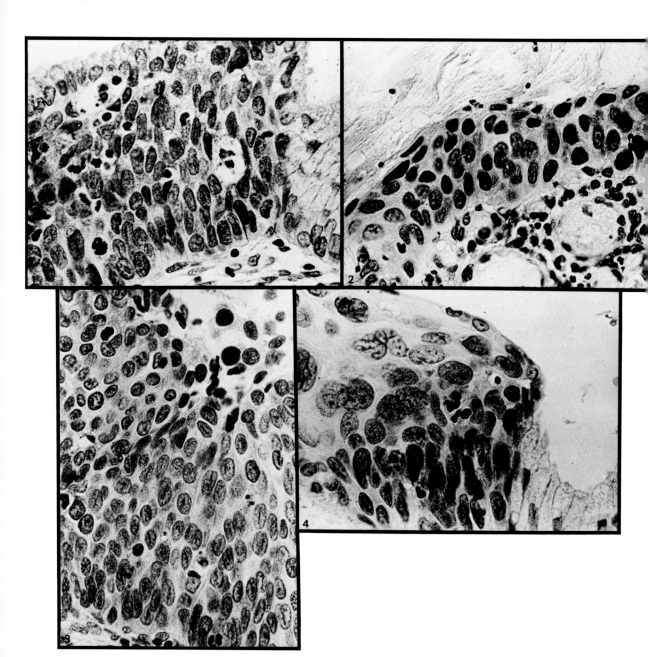

39

Epidermoid Carcinoma *in situ* of the Uterine Cervix

Histology

1. The benign columnar epithelium is pushed upwards by several rows of undifferentiated cells with hazy, ill-defined cytoplasm (see section 10.2.1.1) and hyperchromatic nuclei with coarsely granular chromatin. (x 500)

2. In this section the original benign columnar endocervical epithelium is completely replaced by cells with carcinomatous nuclei and sparse cytoplasm with some signs of squamoid differentiation (that is, dense). Carcinoma *in situ* (see section 10.2.3.). (x 500)

3. This photograph displays spontaneously exfoliating cells from the surface of carcinoma *in situ*. (x 500)

4. Dysplasia. Note the relatively abundant squamoid cytoplasm in the superficial zone of the lesion (see section 10.2.2.1). The cells in the deep zone of this epithelium resemble those in figures 1 and 3. (x 500)

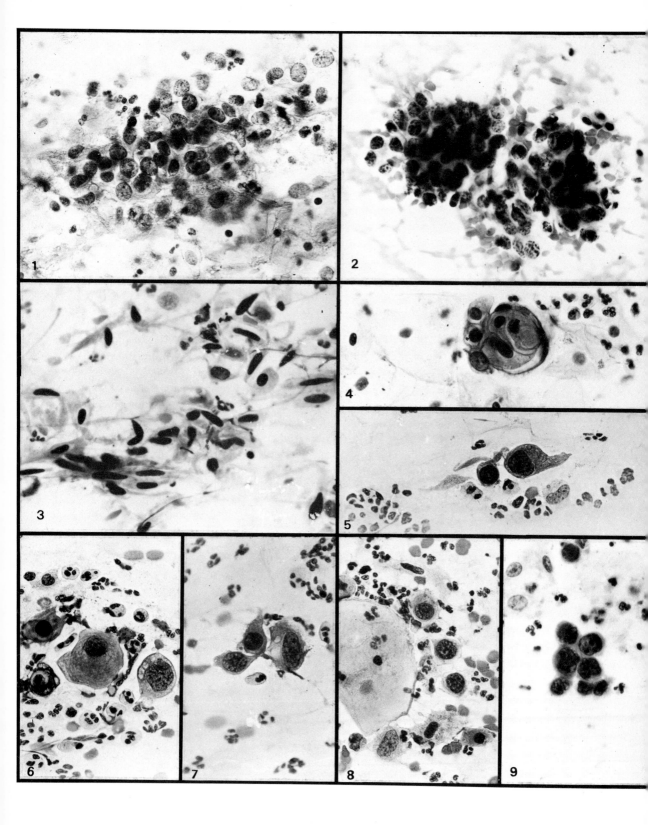

40

Epidermoid Carcinoma *in situ* of the Cervix Uteri

Cytology

1. Epidermoid carcinoma *in situ*. The cells lie in closely packed groups. The cell borders cannot be distinguished; the chromatin structure is coarse-grained. (x 500)

2. Carcinoma *in situ*. Nuclear overlapping in the centre of the cell group. The nuclei are markedly hyperchromatic. (x 500)

3. Keratinising carcinoma *in situ*. These cells come from the outermost layer. The nuclei are hyperchromatic, fusiform and uniform. (x 500)

4. Squamous pearl from a keratinising carcinoma *in situ*. (x 500)

5, 6, 7, 8. Cells from an epidermoid carcinoma *in situ*. The chromatin pattern is coarse and irregular. The shape of the cells resembles that of metaplastic cells. The cancer cells tend to lie separately. (x 500)

9. Cells of a microinvasive squamous cell carcinoma. The nuclei contain a clearly defined nucleolus. There is some nuclear clearing (section 10.2.4.1). (x 500)

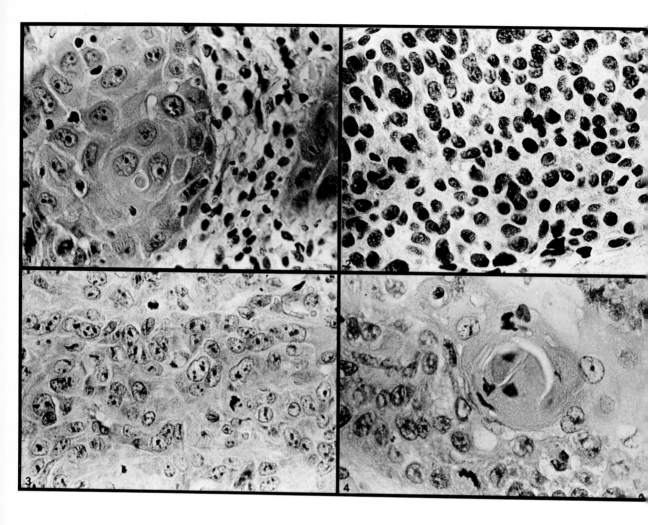

41

Squamous Cell Carcinoma

Histology

1. Focus of invasion in a case of micro-invasive carcinoma. Note the squamoid differentiation of the cytoplasm, the relatively abundant cytoplasm and the macronucleoli. At the site of invasion is a dense lymphocytic infiltrate (see section 10.2.4.1). (x 500)

2. Small cell nonkeratinising carcinoma (see section 10.2.4.2). The cells have coarsely granular chromatin, nucleoli and hazy ill-defined cytoplasm (compare with atypical reserve cell hyperplasia). (x 500)

3. Large cell nonkeratinising carcinoma (see section 10.2.4.2). Note prominent nucleoli. The cytoplasm is more dense than in figure 2. (x 500)

4. Keratinising squamous cell carcinoma (see section 10.2.4.2). In the centre are cells with squamoid cytoplasm in an epithelial pearl. (x 500)

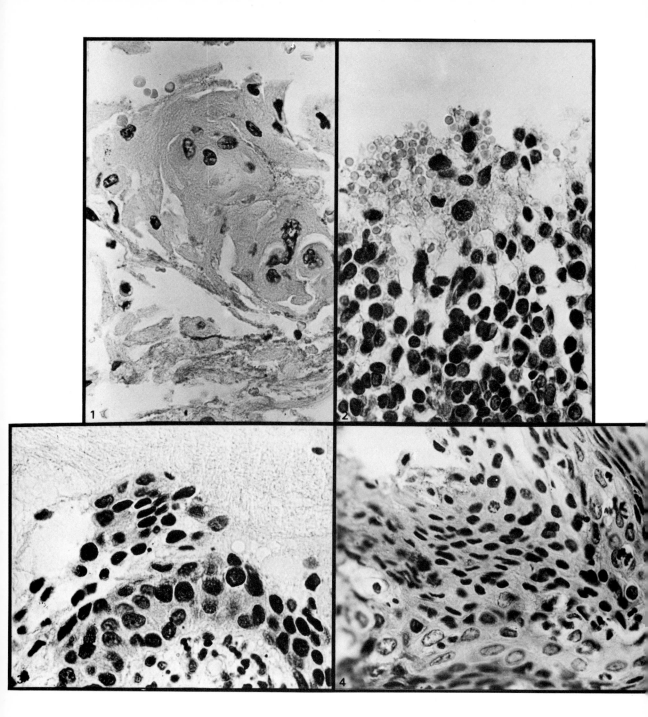

42

Exfoliating Epithelial Surfaces

1. Cells originating from a keratinising squamous cell carcinoma. Note abnormal cellular shapes and pronounced nuclear abnormalities (see section 10.2.4.2). (x 500)

2. Cells originating from small cell non-keratinising carcinoma (see section 10.2.4.2). Note granular chromatin, nucleoli and ill-defined or absent cytoplasm. (x 500)

3. Cells originating from large cell carcinoma *in situ* (see section 10.2.3.2). The cytoplasm is visible. (x 500)

4. The superficial zone of a dysplastic epithelium (see section 10.2.2.2). Cells from the surface layer will have hyperchromatic nuclei and ample squamoid cytoplasm. Cells from the intermediate or deep zone (if the epithelium is vigorously scraped) will show large, somewhat pale nuclei with irregularly distributed chromatin and ill-defined cytoplasm. (x 500)

All photographs were made of tissue sections.

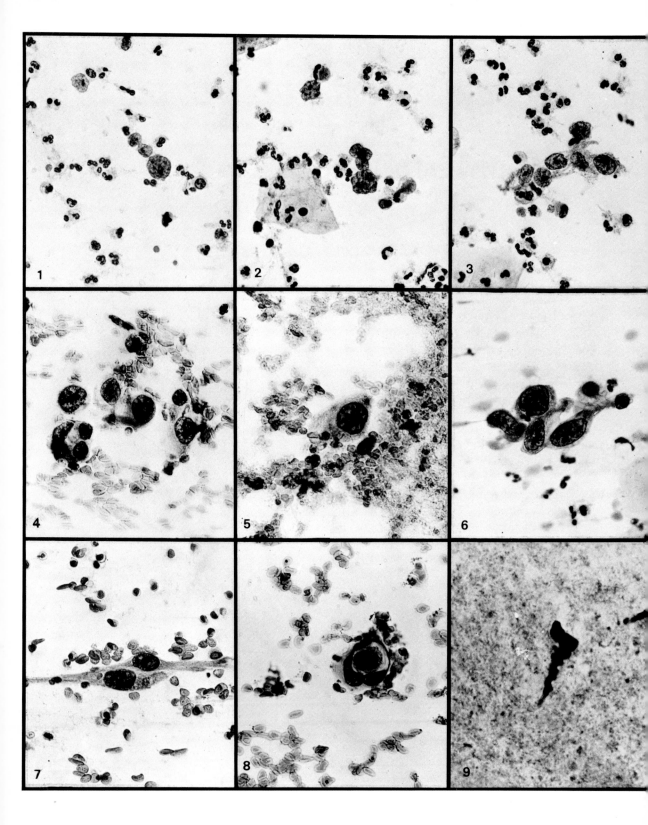

43

Epidermoid Squamous Cell Carcinoma of the Cervix Uteri

1, 2, 3. Malignant cells from a small-cell nonkeratinising carcinoma of the cervix uteri. The cells are arranged like atypical reserve cells. Some nuclei have a bizarre shape; the chromatin structure is slightly coarsened and the nucleolus/nucleus ratio is high. Sparse cytoplasm is still visible in figure 3. (x 500)

4, 5, 6. Cells of a large cell nonkeratinising carcinoma. The nuclei contain macronucleoli; there is nuclear clearing. The nucleocytoplasmic ratio is unfavourable. (x 500)

7. Fibre cells in a smear of a keratinising carcinoma of the cervix uteri. The nuclei show nuclear clearing and macronucleoli. (x 500)

8. Malignant epithelial pearl from a keratinising carcinoma of the cervix uteri. (x 500)

9. Corkscrew-shaped squame (stains bright orange with the Papanicolaou stain) from a keratinising carcinoma of the cervix uteri. The background contains necrotic material. (x 500)

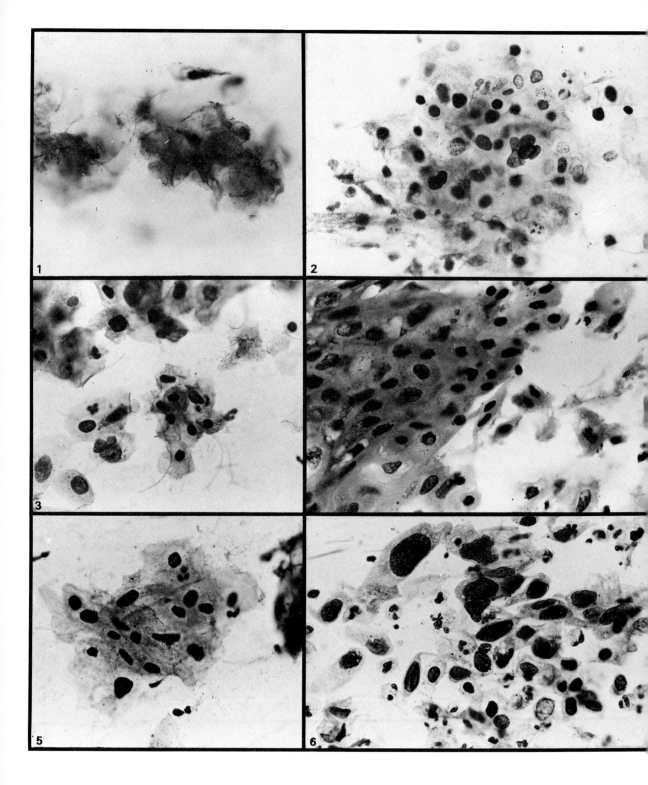

44

Comparison of Keratinising Dysplasia with Keratinising Squamous Cell Carcinoma

1, 2, 3.   Cells exfoliated from a keratinising dysplasia (see section 10.2.2.3). Only squames in figure 1. In figures 2 and 3 squamoid cells with cytoplasmic granulae and hyperchromatic nuclei. Compare nuclear size and N/C ratio with those in figures 5 and 6. (x 500)

4. Exfoliating surface of a keratinising dysplasia (biopsy). These cells have ample cytoplasm. (x 500)

5, 6.   Cells from a keratinising squamous cell carcinoma (see sections 10.2.4.2 and 10.2.4.3). Note chromatin pattern and nuclear shape in figure 6. (x 500)

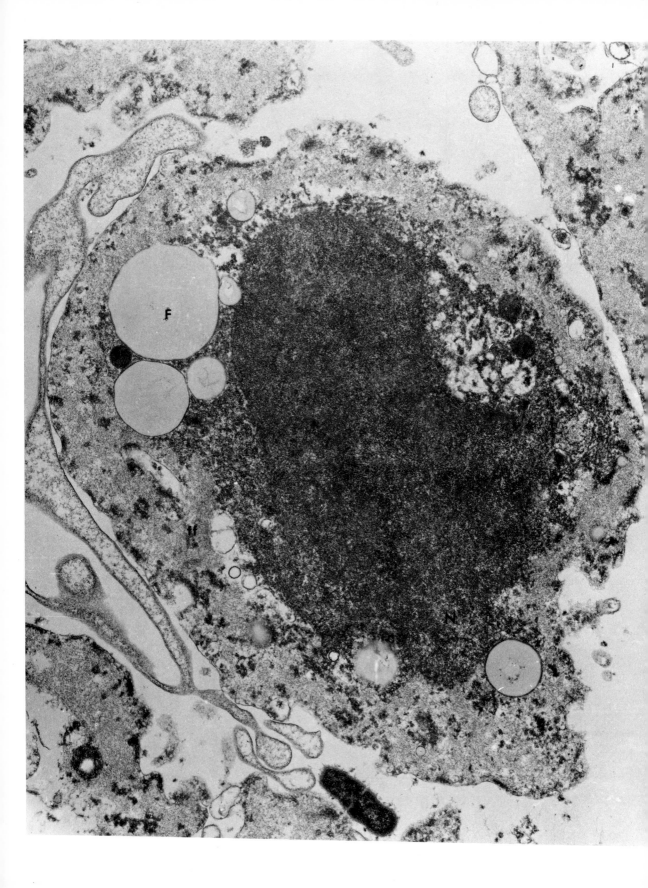

45

Transmission Electron Microscopy of a Malignant Squamous Cell

Electron micrograph of a carcinoma *in situ* cell (x 26000); acetate and lead citrate. Note the similarities of the cytoplasmic characteristics (fine filaments, ff) with the normal superficial and intermediate squamous epithelial cells (see plates 8 and 9). However, the fat droplets (F) are much larger than in the latter. The nucleus (N) is very large, irregular and highly electrondense. The nuclear envelope is partly absent. The cytoplasmic border is intact; mitochondria are absent.

Courtesy of Dr D.J. Ruiter and B.J. Mauw, Department of Pathology, University Medical Center, Leiden, The Netherlands.

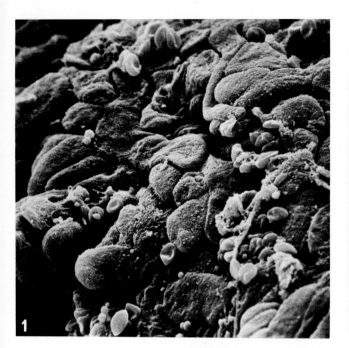 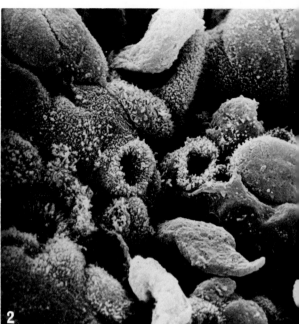

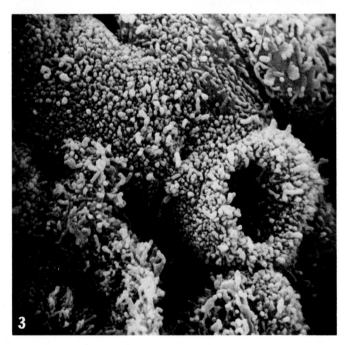

Scanning Electron Microscopy of the Exfoliating Surface of Squamous Cell Carcinoma

1. The appearance of the exfoliating surface in squamous cell carcinoma may be similar to that of carcinoma *in situ*. However, in the case of invasive carcinoma bizarre cancer cells may be seen overlapping other cancer cells. (x 600)

2. Invasive carcinoma may show crater-like formations, the surface being covered by irregular microvilli and tall finger-like protusions. (x 1000)

3. High-power view of the cells in figure 2 demonstrating the presence of anisovillosis (irregular microvilli of variable size) in the slopes of the crater. The crater probably represents the origin of ingestive vacuoles. (x 7000)

Courtesy of Dr C.A. Rubio, Department of Pathology, Karolinska Institute, Stockholm, Sweden.

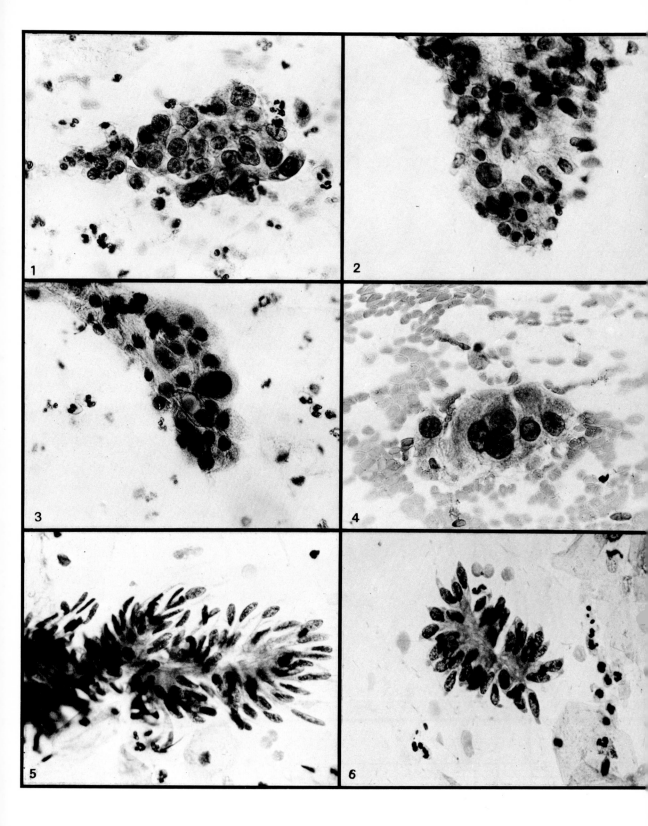

47

Atypia of the Endocervical Epithelium

Cytology

1. Group of endocervical cells showing slight atypia. The nuclei contain macronucleoli. (x 500)

2. Group of endocervical cells which are somewhat atypical. There are signs of pronounced anisokaryosis. (x 500)

3. Cells from the same smear as seen in figure 2. Anisokaryosis and hyperchromasia. (x 500)

4. Endocervical epithelial cells with pronounced atypia. Macronucleoli; some coarsening of the chromatin; some nuclear clearing. (x 500)

5. Atypical endocervical epithelial cells arranged in palisades; cigar-shaped nuclei and slight coarsening of the chromatin. The chromatin pattern is not as abnormal as that seen in figure 2 of plate 49 (adenocarcinoma of the endocervix). (x 500)

6. A group of cells from the same smear. These cells lie in an acinar arrangement. (x 500)

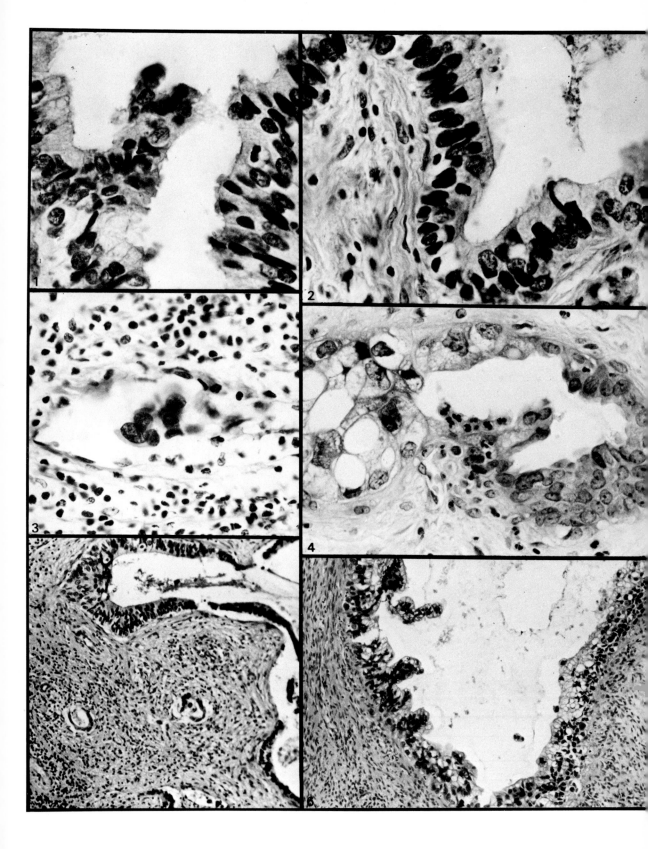

48

Adenocarcinoma of the Endocervix

Histology

1, 2. Adenocarcinoma *in situ* of the endo-cervix (see section 11.2.2.1). The nuclei are elongated and hyperchromatic with evenly distributed granular chromatin. Frequent mitoses. (x 500)

3. Adenocarcinoma cells in a lymphatic vessel in a case of microinvasive adeno-carcinoma. Note resemblance to cells in figures 1 and 2. (x 500)

4. Left: mucus-producing adenocarcinoma cells. Right: gland lined with reserve cells. (x 500)

5. The endocervical gland is lined with car-cinoma cells; in the lower half are foci of infiltrative growth surrounded by a dense lymphocytic infiltrate. (x 125)

6. Endocervical gland lined with mucus-producing carcinoma cells. (x 125)

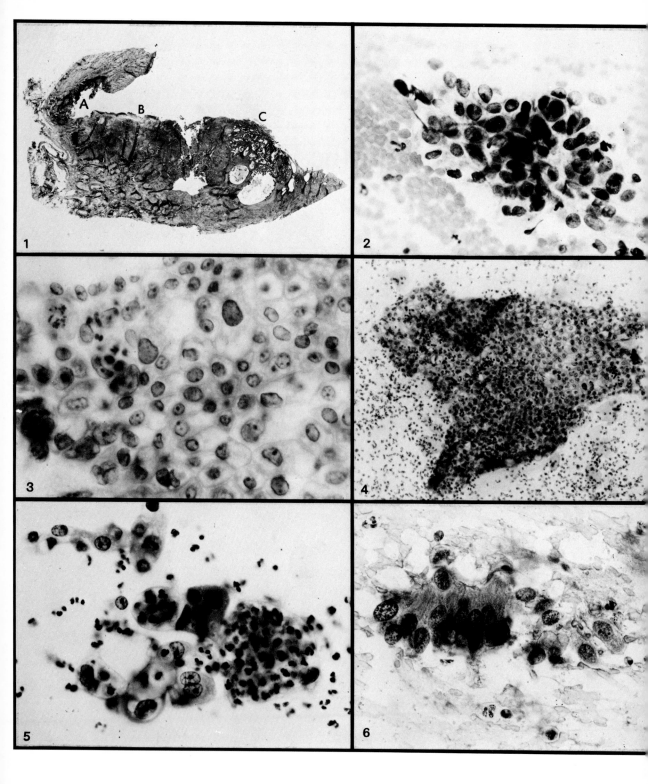

49

Adenocarcinoma of the Endocervix

1. Cone biopsy from a patient with an epidermoid carcinoma *in situ* (A) adjacent to a nonkeratinising epidermoid carcinoma (B) as well as a well-differentiated adenocarcinoma (C) of the endocervical epithelium. The adenocarcinoma is the most proximal of the three. (x 4)

2. Well-differentiated endocervical adenocarcinoma. Note the 'glandular' aspect of the cell group and the hyperchromatism of the oval nuclei. (x 500)

3. Well-differentiated mucus-producing endocervical adenocarcinoma. These cancer cells form a disorganised honeycomb because the mucous vacuoles differ greatly in size. (x 500)

4. The same pattern as seen in figure 3. (x 125)

5. Moderately differentiated endocervical adenocarcinoma. Cytologically it cannot be differentiated from an adenocarcinoma of the endometrium. (x 500)

6. Adenocarcinoma *in situ* of the endocervix. Note the palisade arrangement of the cells and the rice-like aspect of the chromatin. (x 500)

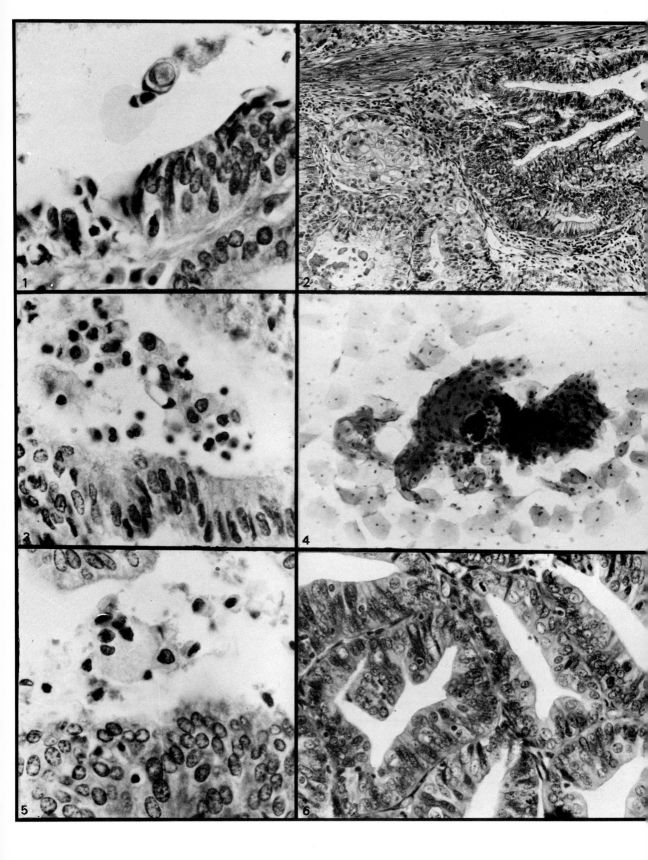

50

Endometrial Adenocarcinoma - Tissue Sections with Exfoliating Surfaces

1, 3, 5.   In the upper half of the photographs the spontaneously exfoliated tumour cells can be seen: in the lower half is the epithelium from which they originate. Note the difference in appearance. While exfoliating the cellular shape becomes spherical and the cytoplasm more vacuolated (see section 12.2.2.2). (x 500)

2. Adenoacanthoma (see section 12.2.2.3). Left: the (morphologically benign) squamous component. Right: the (morphologically malignant) glandular component. (x 125)

4. Smear from the same case as figure 2. The dark central part of this tissue fragment originates from the malignant glandular component, the adjacent squamous cells from the (morphologically benign) squamous component. The diagnosis adenoacanthoma can only be made on the basis of the cervical smear if entire tissue fragments with both components are shed. (x 125)

6. Adenocarcinoma of the endometrium. (x 500)

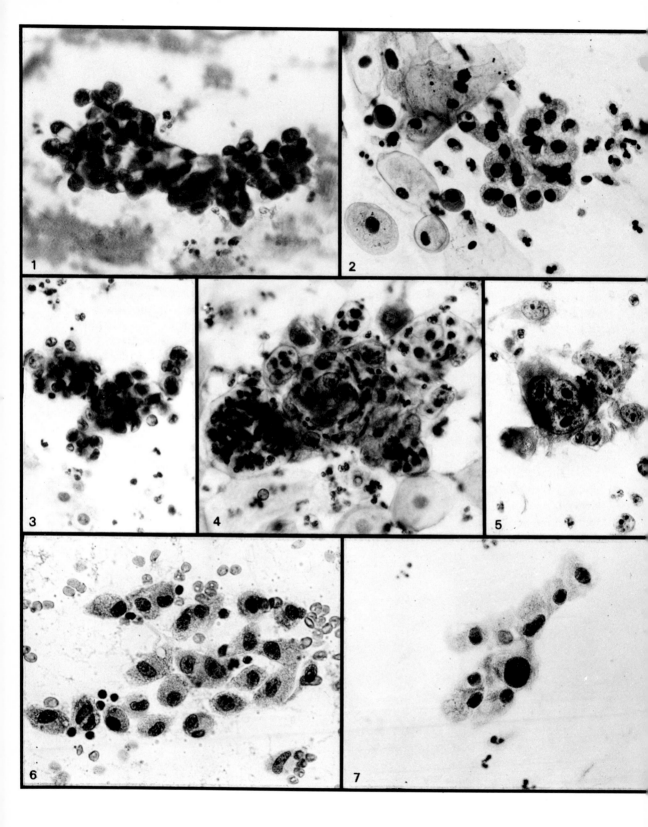

51

Adenocarcinoma of the Endometrium

1. Atypical endometrial cells with enlarged nuclei and nucleoli; the nuclei usually have one nucleolus. The cytoplasm is vacuolated. This smear was taken from a woman 3 years after menopause; she used lynoral. The cell changes disappeared after the drug was withdrawn. (x 500)

2. Slightly atypical cells, possibly from the endometrium, in the smear from a patient with an intrauterine device. (x 500)

3. Papillary arrangement of malignant cells from a well-differentiated adenocarcinoma of the endometrium. The nuclei are somewhat larger than normal and generally contain one nucleolus. Nuclear clearing also occurs. (x 500)

4. Cells of a moderately differentiated adenocarcinoma of the endometrium. The nuclei are larger than the nuclei of intermediate cells and contain prominent nucleoli. Note cytoplasmic vacuolisation with granulocytes. (x 500)

5. Cells of a poorly differentiated adenocarcinoma of the endometrium. The nucleoli are very big and abnormal in shape. (x 500)

6, 7. Cells from a clear cell carcinoma of the endometrium [A]. The cytoplasm is finely vacuolated; the nuclei are polychromatic and contain abnormal nucleoli. (x 500)

[A] Reagan, J.W. and Ng, A.B.P. (1965). *The Cells of the Uterine Adenocarcinoma*. Karger, Basel, p. 40

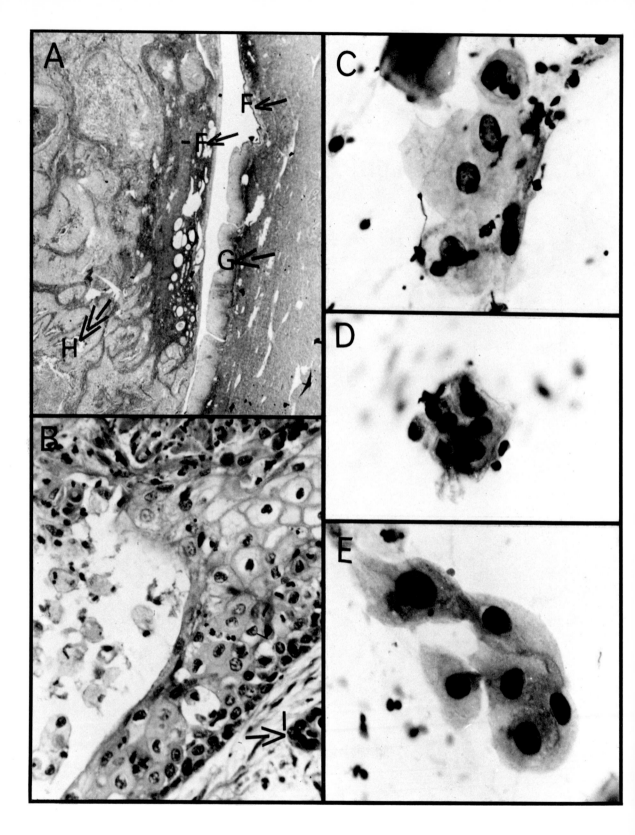

52

Primary Squamous Cell Carcinoma of the Endometrium

1. Tissue section of primary squamous cell carcinoma of the endometrium (H) (section 12.2.2.3), in conjunction with benign squamous metaplasia (G). (*not* in connection with the stratified squamous epithelium of the cervix). F is the atrophic endometrium. (x 6)

2. Higher magnification of an area with endometrial glands lined by squamous tumour cells, partly well differentiated, and a focus of infiltrative growth. (x 325)

3, 4, 5. Direct smears from the exfoliating tumour surface. In figure 5 the cells are well differentiated and lack diagnostic signs of malignancy. (x 500)

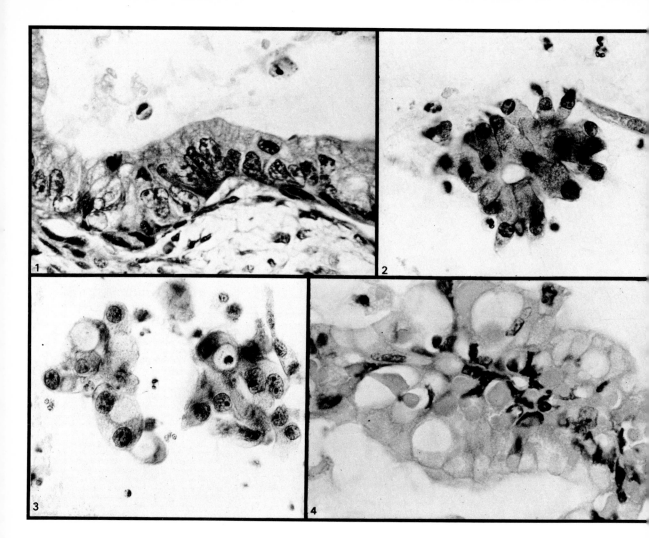

53

Adenocarcinoma of the Ovary

1. Serous ovarian adenocarcinoma (see section 13.1.1), histological section. Note single layer with nuclear crowding. The nuclei are large and contain macronucleoli. (x 500)

2. Malignant cells from a cervical metastatic lesion of mucinous ovarian adenocarcinoma. The cells are arranged in an acinous pattern (seldom seen in benign glandular cells). Note the unfavourable Nc/N ratio. (x 500)

3. Malignant cells from a serous adenocarcinoma of the ovary. These cells have vacuolated cytoplasm and contain huge nucleoli. Note the relatively bland chromatin pattern. (x 500)

4. Mucinous ovarian cyst adenocarcinoma (histological section). The nuclei are pushed aside by the mucin-filled vacuoles. (x 500)

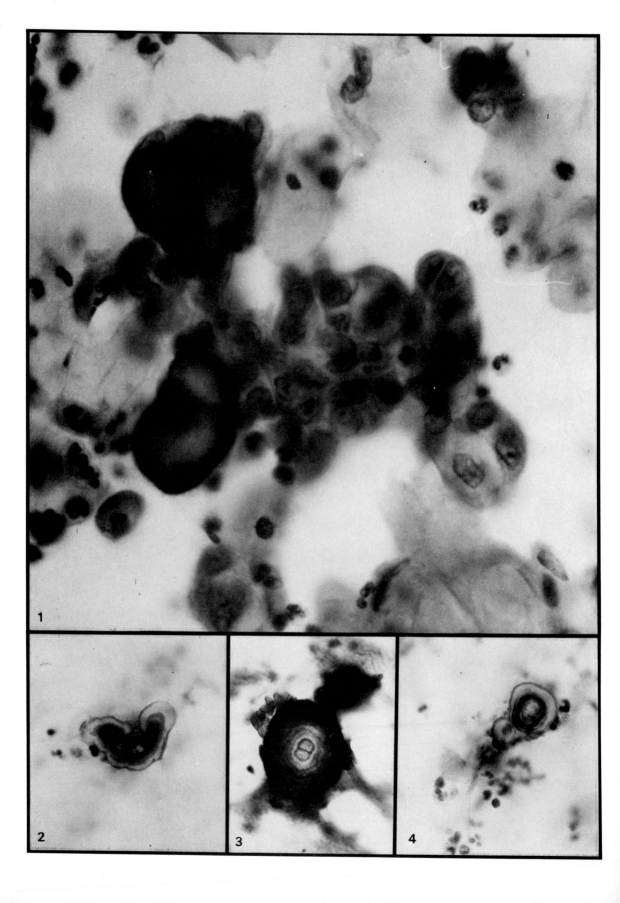

54

Adenocarcinoma of the Ovary and Psammoma Bodies

1. Papillary adenocarcinoma of the ovary. The cells lie in a papillary arrangement. The group of cells contains several psammoma bodies. (x 500)

2, 3, 4.   Psammoma bodies in a smear from a woman who used an intrauterine device.

In contrast to figure 1, no adenocarcinoma cells are seen [A]. (x 500)

[A] Highman, W.J. (1971). Calcified bodies and the intrauterine device. *Acta Cytol.*, 15, 473–475

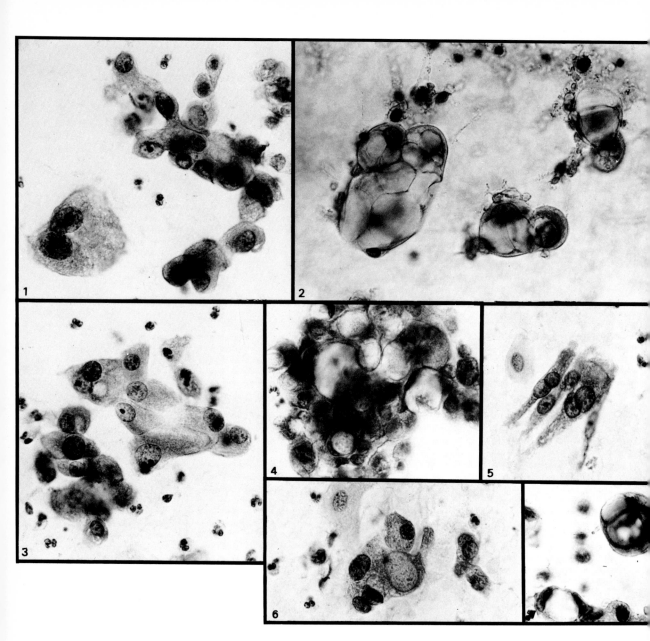

55

Metastasis of Ovarian Carcinoma in the Vagina

Mucinous cyst adenocarcinoma of the ovary (see section 13.1.1). Smears taken from metastasis in the vagina. All the epithelial cells photographed are malignant and are 'ortsfremd' in the vagina. (x 500)

1. The chromatin is fine and evenly distributed; however, there is severe anisokaryosis and (in the smaller nuclei) an unfavourable Nc/N ratio.

2, 4. In these photographs the nuclei are hardly visible because they lie in a different plane of focus. The vacuoles differ greatly in size (disorganised honeycomb; compare with adenocarcinoma of the endocervix, plate 49).

3, 5, 6. In these photographs it is very difficult to detect the malignant nature of cells. However, (1) the cells are alien to the vagina (ortsfremd), (2) they contain large nucleoli with unfavourable Nc/N ratios in the smaller nuclei and (3) they are slightly hyperchromatic with a prominent nuclear border (figure 5).

7. A mitosis in a vacuolated malignant cell. This is rarely observed in benign cells.

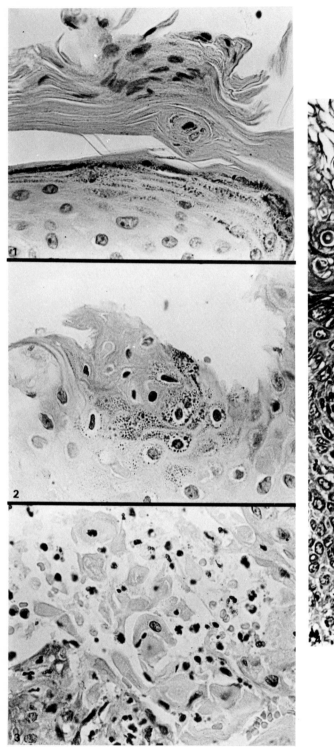
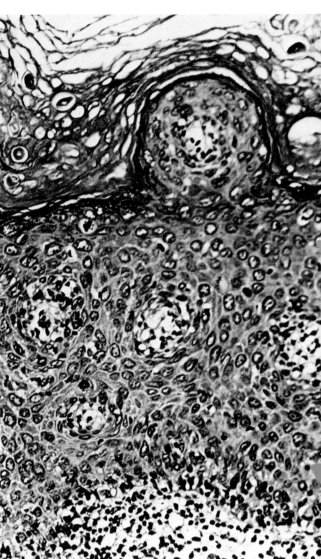

56

Exfoliating Surfaces in Hyperkeratotic Lesions of the Vulva

1. Benign hyperkeratosis of the vulva (see section 13.3.1.3). The anucleated squames are regularly shaped. (x 500)

2. Surface of a carcinoma *in situ* of the vulva (see section 13.3.2.1). The nuclei are hyperchromatic and large in comparison with normal superficial cells. Some abnormal cell shapes. (x 500)

3. Surface of keratinising squamous cell carcinoma of the vulva (see section 13.3.2.2). Note abnormal cell shapes. (x 500)

4. Full lesion of a keratinising carcinoma *in situ* of the vulva.

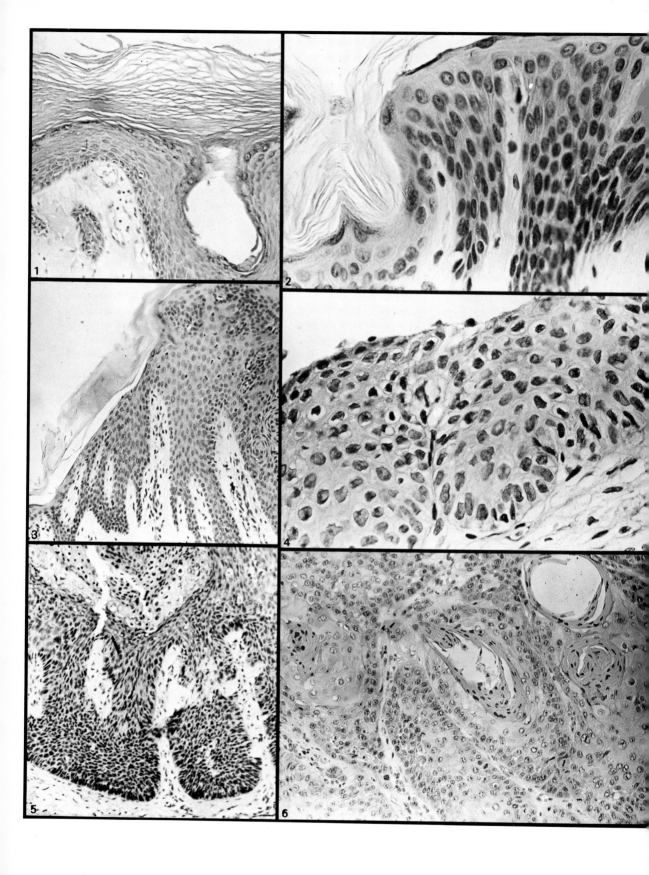

57

Histology of Vulvar and Vaginal Lesions

1. Vulvar epithelium with hyperkeratosis and dermal collagenisation, in a case of lichen sclerosis (see section 13.3.1.3). (x 125)

2. Vulvar epithelium with hyperkeratosis, irregular rete pegs and basal cell hyperplasia and atypia. This epithelium was found adjacent to invasive squamous cell cancer. (x 500)

3. Vulvar lesion with hyperkeratosis and irregular rete pegs on the left and invasive squamous cell cancer on the right. (x 125)

4. Carcinoma *in situ* of the vaginal epithelium diagnosed two years after conisation for cervical carcinoma *in situ* (see section 13.4.2.1). (x 500)

5. Early invasive squamous cell carcinoma of the vagina. Note the exfoliating immature surface cells. (x 500)

6. Keratinising squamous cell carcinoma of the vagina (see section 13.4.2.1). Note pearl formation. (x 325)

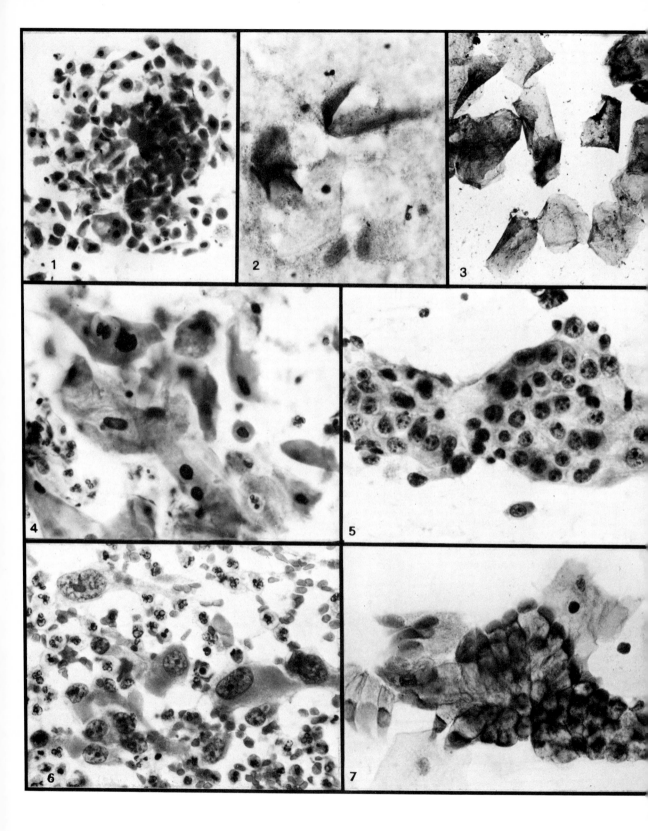

58

Carcinoma of the Vulva and Vagina

1. Epidermoid carcinoma *in situ* of the vagina. The malignant cells have markedly hyperchromatic nuclei and are fairly small [A]. (x 125)

2. Abnormally shaped squames in a smear of a keratinising squamous cell carcinoma of the vulva. The background of the smear contains considerable debris [B]. (x 500)

3. Normal squames from a hyperkeratotic lesion of the vulva. The squames are equal in size and shape; the background of the smear is 'clean' [C]. (x 500)

4. Squamous cell carcinoma of the vulva. These abnormally shaped cells have abundant cytoplasm; the nuclei are large and markedly hyperchromatic. (x 500)

5. Adenocarcinoma of Bartholin's glands. The carcinoma extended to the surface. The cells have finely vacuolated cytoplasm and prominent nucleoli [C]. (x 500)

6. Smear from a bulging tumour mass in the vagina. The nuclei of these highly abnormal cells are eccentric. The primary tumour was an adenocarcinoma of the endometrium [C]. (x 500)

7. Cylindrical cells in a vaginal smear ('ortsfremd'): adenosis of the vagina in a 7-year-old girl. Her mother took diethylstilboestrol during pregnancy [D]. (x 500)

[A] Koss, L.G. (1968). *Diagnostic Cytology and its Histopathologic Bases.* 2nd edn. Lippincott, Philadelphia, p. 271

[B] Koss, L.G. (1968). *Diagnostic Cytology and its Histopathologic Bases.* 2nd edn. Lippincott, Philadelphia, p. 272
Novak, E.R. and Woodruff, J.D. (1974). *Gynecologic and Obstetric Pathology.* 7th edn, Saunders, Philadelphia, pp. 38–40

[C] Novak, E.R. and Woodruff, J.D. (1974). *Gynecologic and Obstetric Pathology.* 7th edn, Saunders, Philadelphia, p. 40

[D] Novak, E.R. and Woodruff, J.D. (1974). *Gynecologic and Obstetric Pathology.* 7th edn, Saunders, Philadelphia, p. 59

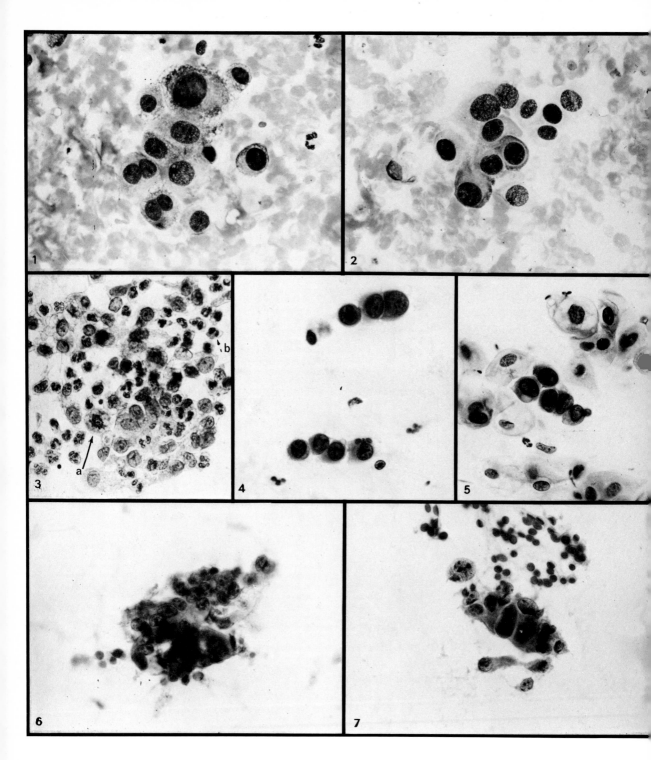

59

Metastatic Cancer and Invasive Cancer

1, 2. May–Grünwald–Giemsa (MGG)-stained cells in a vaginal smear from an invasive carcinoma of the bladder. In such cases we prefer this stain since it is then possible to differentiate these cells from epidermoid cancer cells. Malignant urothelial cells have a darker outer zone in cytoplasm dotted with small vacuoles; this gives the cytoplasm a 'lace collar' appearance. This pattern is easier to see with the MGG stain than with the Papanicolaou stain. The nuclei are large and the chromatin is granular. (x 500)

3. Localisation of histiocytosis X in the vagina. Note the slightly abnormal histiocytes and the mitotic figure. Many eosinophils are present. In this patient the disease had developed in several sites over a period of 10 years [B]. (x 500)

4, 5. Vaginal smear. Metastasis of breast cancer with the characteristic 'Indian file' arrangement of the tumour cells [A]. These cells are relatively small but both the nucleocytoplasmic and the Nc/N ratios are unfavourable. Nuclear moulding can be seen. Note the clean background [A]. (x 500)

6, 7. Vaginal smear. Invasive carcinoma of the rectum. The cancer cells in both figures are well-differentiated mucus-producing columnar cells [A]. (x 500)

[A] Koss, L.G. (1968). *Diagnostic Cytology and its Histopathologic Bases*. 2nd edn, Lippincott, Philadelphia, p. 274

[B] Dupree, E.L. and Lee, R.A. (1973). Histiocytosis X in the female genital tract. *Acta Cytol.*, **42**, 201–204

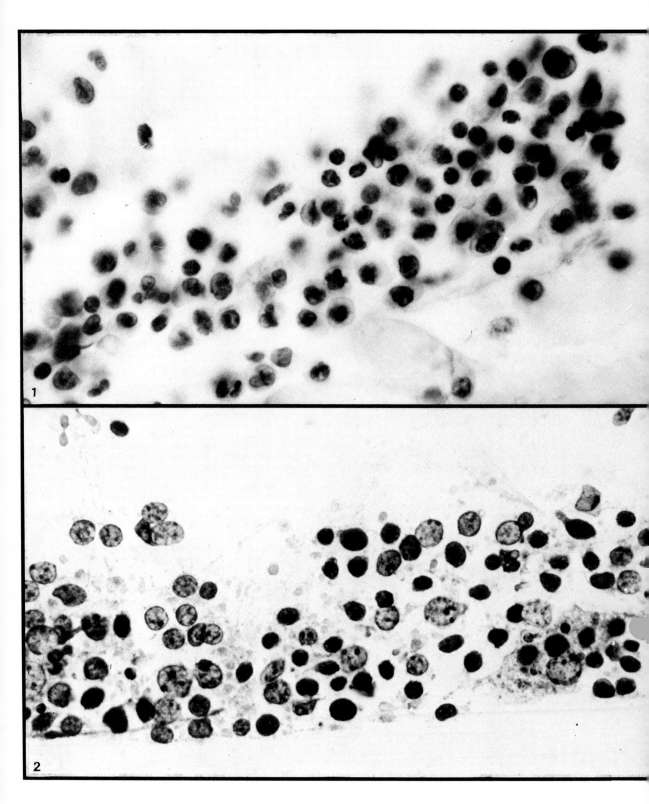

60

Differential Diagnosis - Leukaemia or Follicular Cervicitis

1. Leukaemia cells in a cervical smear. This patient visited the gynaecologist with complaints of marked menstrual bleeding. The diagnosis of leukaemia was established on the basis of this smear. The pattern is fairly monomorphic. The nuclei are sometimes lobulated, contain nucleoli and are approximately equal in size [A]. (x 500)

2. Chronic lymphocytic (follicular) cervicitis. Multi-form pattern with lymphocytes, lymphoblasts and reticulum cells. The nuclei vary markedly in size. There may also be cells with phagocytic material in the cytoplasm (histiocytes). Only the large nuclei contain a nucleolus. (x 500)

In figures 1 and 2, the cells lie separately and not as part of a tissue fragment.

[A] Koss, L.G. (1968). *Diagnostic Cytology and its Histopathologic Bases*. 2nd edn, Lippincott, Philadelphia, p. 274

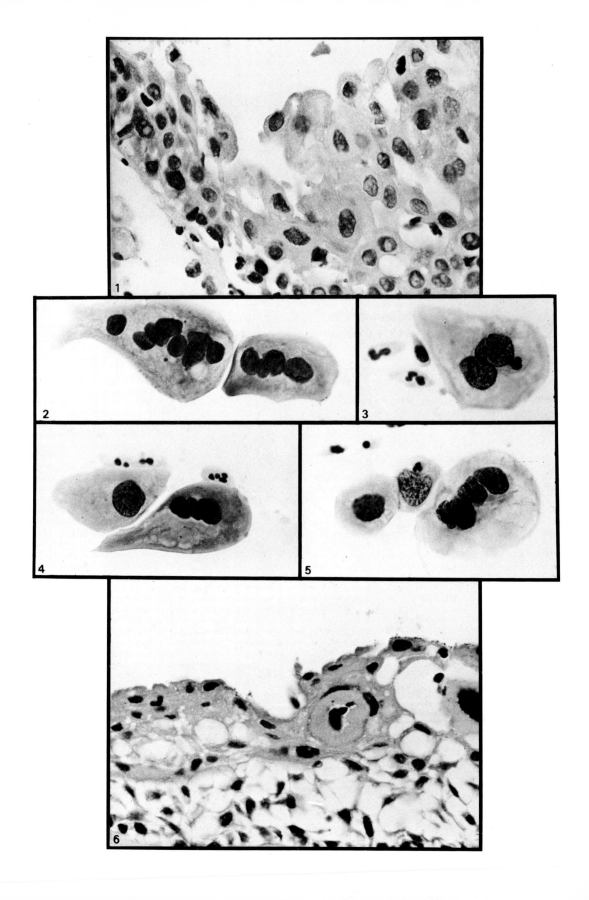

61

Irradiation Effect and Folic Acid Deficiency

1, 6.   Epithelial changes due to ionising radiation in tissue sections (see section 14.5). The nuclei are enlarged and contain macronucleoli. Note also nuclear hyperchromasia in figure 6. (x 500)

2, 3, 4, 5.   Folic acid deficiency. The squamous cells display multinucleation as well as cellular and nuclear enlargement (see section 14.5. The chromatin is granular. The cell changes disappeared after treatment. (x 500)

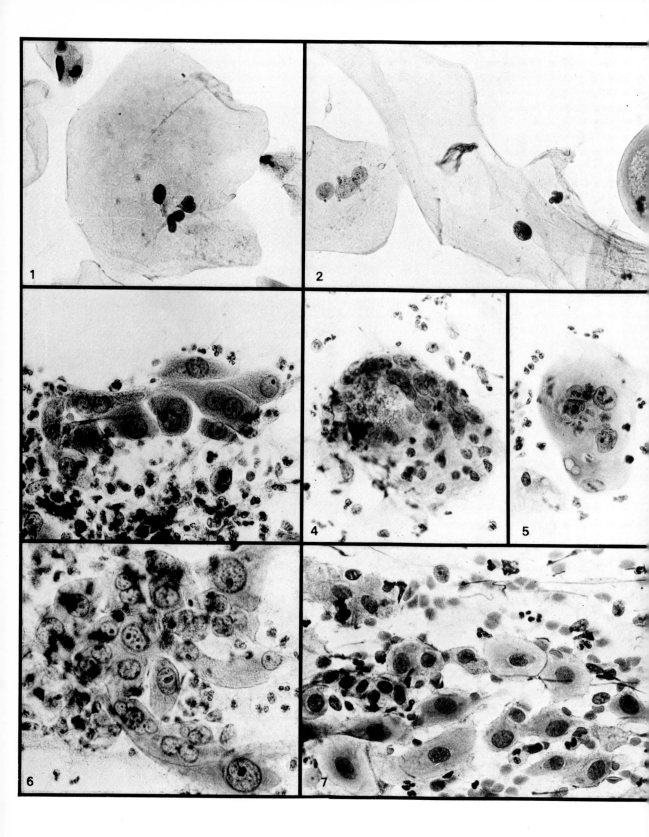

62

Cell Changes due to Irradiation

1, 2. Late radiation effect [A]. The cells are enormous. Many binuclear cells are present. These cell changes were found 18 years after radiation therapy. (x 500)

3. Changes in endocervical epithelial cells due to irradiation. Note the numerous binuclear cells. (x 500)

4. Histiocytic giant cell in a smear after irradiation. (x 500)

5. Changes in squamous epithelial cells due to irradiation: fairly abundant cytoplasm, multinucleation and prominent nucleoli. The chromatin pattern is fine. (x 500)

6. Changes in endocervical epithelial cells due to irradiation: macronucleoli, many binuclear cells and anisokaryosis. The chromatin structure is fine. (x 500)

7. Atrophy of squamous epithelium as a result of irradiation. Patient was 35 years old. (x 500)

[A] Koss, L.G. (1968). *Diagnostic Cytology and Histopathologic Bases*. 2nd edn, Lippincott, Philadelphia, pp. 277–281

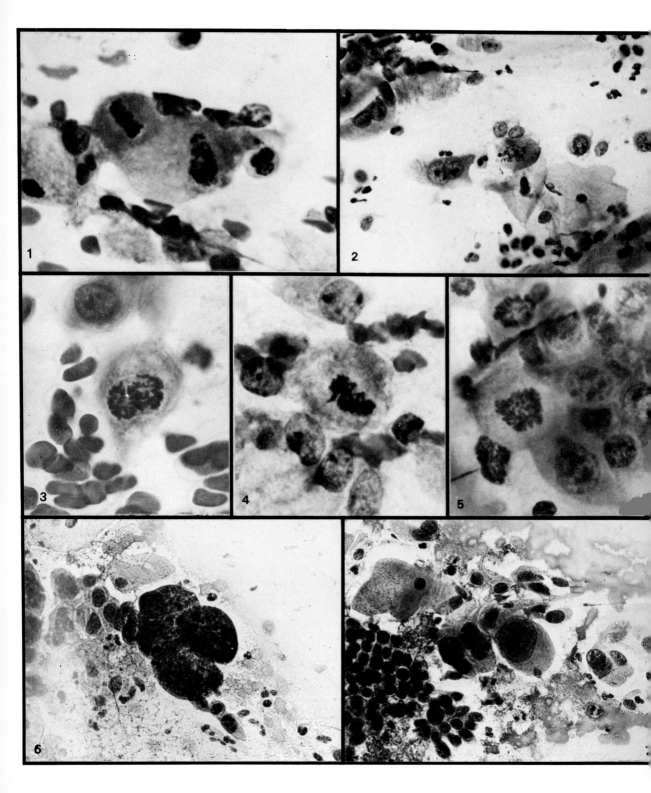

63

Iatrogenic Effects

1, 2, 3, 4, 5. Mitotic figures in a smear from a patient with an intrauterine device. *These endocervical epithelial cells have large multiple nucleoli. The nuclei, however, never lie in stacks as in malignancy and the chromatin structure remains fine (compare figure 5 of plate 18). The abnormal cells disappeared after the intrauterine device was removed. We have found that mitosis is likely to be frequent when an intrauterine device is present.* (1, 3,4, 5: x 1250; 2: x 500)

6. Enormous naked nuclei with nuclear moulding and hyperchromasia; the chromatin structure has become coarse but the chromatin is still evenly distributed over the nucleus. (x 500)

7. Columnar endocervical cells in the same smear as figure 6. (x 500) *This patient used Depoprovera to prevent conception. Six months after cessation of the hormonal contraceptive abnormal cells were still present in the smear, although they had decreased in number. In the biopsies, atypia of the endocervical epithelium was seen but an infiltrating carcinoma was not found. One year later there were no abnormal cells in the smear and the endocervical epithelium in the hysterectomy specimen was completely normal.*

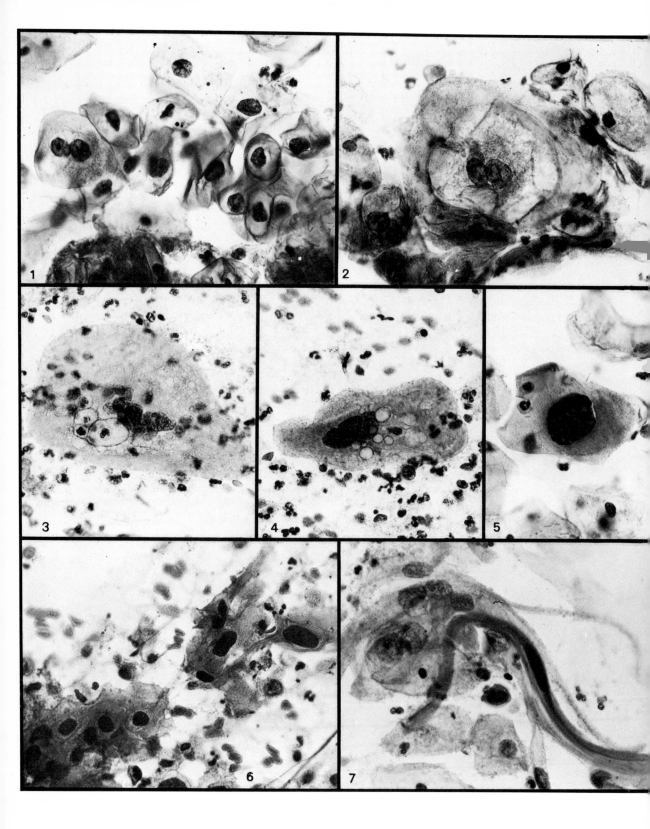

64

Special Types of Dysplasia

1. Dysplastic cells with koilocytosis and binucleation. Pattern can be compatible with viral infection (flat condyloma; section 10.2.2.2) [A]. (x 500)

2. Koilocytosis in an enormous binuclear cell. Same case as figure 1. (x 500)

3, 4. Multinucleated cell with abundant cytoplasm which appears granular and contains several vacuoles. These giant cells are often found in combination with koilocytotic atypia. (x 500)

5. Dysplastic cell with a large highly abnormal hyperchromatic nucleus. This patient was treated with a cytostatic drug for leukaemia [B]. (x 500)

6, 7. Two smears from different patients who received high doses of Azathioprine (an immunosuppressive drug). Both smears show dysplastic cells, sometimes with an abnormal shape [C]. (x 500)

[A] Meisels, A. and Fortin, R. (1976). Condylomatous lesions of the cervix and vagina. 1. Cytologic patterns. *Acta Cytol.*, **20**, 505–509

[B] Koss, L.G. (1968). *Diagnostic Cytology and its Histopathologic Bases.* 2nd edn, Lippincott, Philadelphia, p. 285

[C] Gupta, P.K., Pinn, V.M. and Taft, P.D. (1969). Cervical dysplasia associated with Azathioprine (Imuran) therapy. *Acta Cytol.*, **13**, 373–376

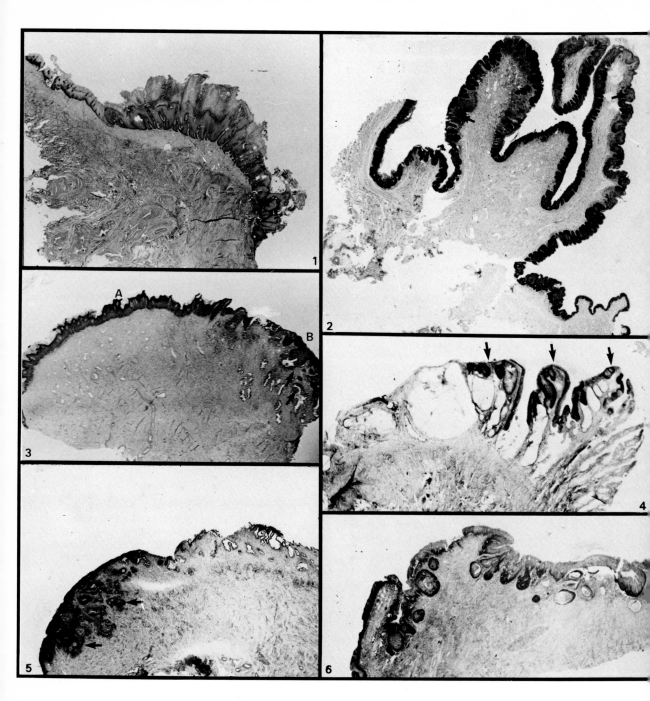

65

Location of Different Lesions

1. Condylomata acuminata located on the ectocervix, originating in the native squamous epithelium (see section 7.3.5.2). Note the elongated rete pegs and the severe hyperkeratosis.

2. Papillomata located on the ectocervix, with carcinoma *in situ*. In this case the layer of anucleated squames is thinner in comparison with case 1, and macroscopically not visible. The epithelium consists of cancer cells. In three places (see arrows) there is early stromal invasion, surrounded by dense lymphocytic infiltrates.

3. Condylomata acuminata located on the ectocervix, originating from the native squamous epithelium (A), in combination with flat condylomatous epithelium originating in the zone of the original columnar endocervical epithelium (B), with extensions in the endocervical glands (arrows).

4. Carcinoma *in situ* (arrows) originating in the zone of original endocervical epithelium. Patient used oral contraceptives resulting in characteristic glandular changes, for example, glandular hypersecretion and microglandular hyperplasia (see section 14.2.1.2).

5. Microinvasive carcinoma, originating in the zone of original endocervical epithelium. Note dense lymphocytic infiltrate around invasive foci (arrows).

6. Dysplasia, originating in the zone of original endocervical epithelium.

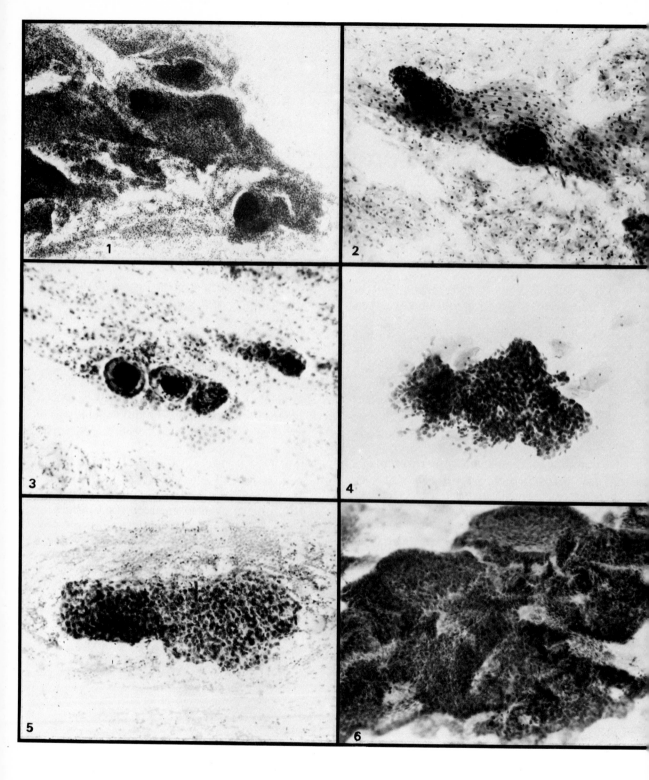

66

'Histological' Cytology

The smears can contain large fragments of tissue. Most cytotechnicians tend to consider these 'microbiopsies' uninteresting because they have been trained to study single cells or cells in loose aggregates.

We will try to illustrate here that it is also important to study large groups. In a low power field (x 125), the following aspects of the cell group should be noted: shape (flat, three-dimensional, papillary, ragged or sharp edges, etc.), arrangement and crowding of the nuclei. The distribution of the nuclei over the entire fragment is also important: are most of the nuclei crowded into one area or are they spread out evenly throughout the fragment? The high power field (x 500) will reveal the chromatin structure necessary for the correct cytological diagnosis.

1. Atrophic smear pattern at a low magnification (x 50). Large flat sheets with dark areas (nuclear crowding) interspersed with lighter areas (less crowding).

2. Higher magnification (x 125) reveals that dark regions originate from the epithelium at the rete (left: seen from the side; centre: seen from above). The lighter areas come from the superficial part of the epithelium.

3. Endometrial fragments in the menstrual phase of the cycle. Note the dense inner area and the loosely arranged outer zone of the groups. This 'two density' aspect of the tissue fragment is characteristic for endometrium. (x 125)

4. Microbiopsy from carcinoma *in situ*. One side of the tissue fragment is flat; the rete pegs (or the extension of carcinoma *in situ* into endocervical glands) give the other side an undulating appearance. There is crowding of the nuclei throughout the whole tissue fragment. (x 125)

5. Microbiopsy from carcinoma *in situ* (left) adjacent to an area of atypical reserve cell hyperplasia (right). The nuclear density in the former is pronounced; in the latter the nuclei are further apart. (x 125)

6. Microbiopsy from a well-differentiated papillary adenocarcinoma of the endocervix. Such large tissue fragments containing predominantly endocervical epithelial cells (note the honeycomb appearance) are seldom seen. Even at this magnification many mitotic figures can be observed. (x 125)

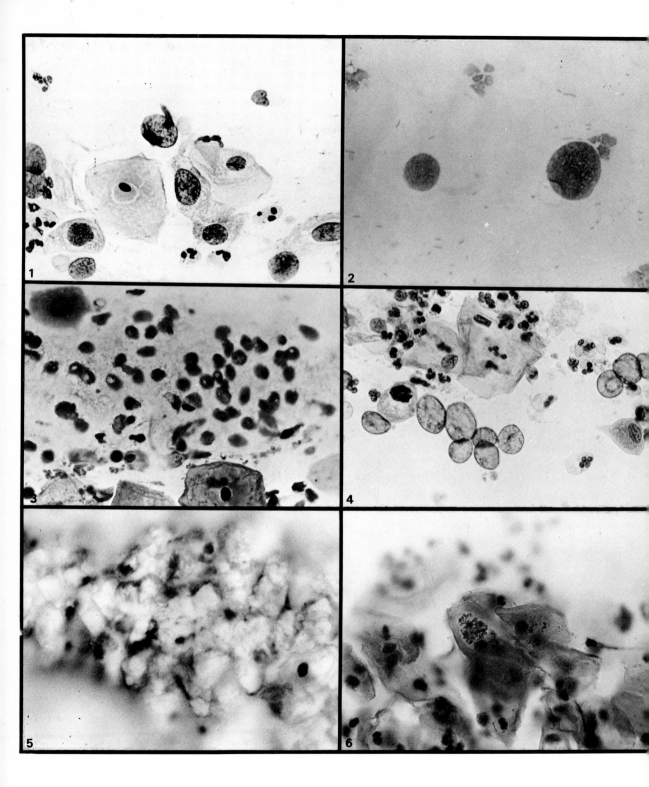

67

Fixation and Mounting

1, 2, 4. The smears were taken from a patient with an atypical reserve cell hyperplasia (borderline type).

1. Fixation with spray fixative (see section 15.4). The chromatin is spread evenly over the entire nucleus. (x 500)

2. Air-dried smear. The chromatin is evenly distributed, but the chromatin pattern is not crisp (see section 15.4). (x 500)

3. Air-dried columnar endocervical cells in mucus. The nuclei resemble those in figure 2; the outlines of the cytoplasm cannot be discerned. (x 500)

4. 95 per cent ethyl alcohol fixation, resulting in 'empty' nuclei. The chromatin has condensed beneath the nuclear envelope. (x 500)

5. Air-dried part of a smear taken on the day of ovulation. Fern formation. (x 500)

6. 'Granulae' are seen in the thick parts of the cytoplasm (mounting artefact) (see sections 15.5.1.9 and 15.7). (x 500)

EAST GLAMORGAN GENERAL HOSPITAL
CHURCH VILLAGE, near PONTYPRIDD

Acknowledgement

We are grateful to R.M.L. Heruer and K.G. van der Ham who skilfully developed and printed the photomicrographs, and to C.C. Padding for her helpful cooperations. P.W. Arentz, M.J.A. Voorn-den Hollander and C.F.H.M. Knepfle contributed some of the cytology photomicrographs. Some of the plates in the atlas were previously published in *Photographic Review of Gynaecological Cytology*.